Speech and Language Evaluation in Neurology: Childhood Disorders

Principal Scientific Consultant

Ronald Netsell, Ph.D.
Staff Scientist
The Boys Town National Institute for
    Communication Disorders in Children
Omaha, Nebraska

Scientific Consultants

Kurt P. Kitselman, Ph.D.
Associate Professor
Department of Speech Communication
California State University
Fullerton, California

Rachel E. Stark, Ph.D.
Director
Division of Hearing and Speech
Associate Professor
Department of Neurology
Johns Hopkins University School of Medicine
Baltimore, Maryland

Linda Swisher, Ph.D.
Director
Early Childhood Language Research Laboratory
Department of Speech and Hearing Sciences
The University of Arizona
Tucson, Arizona

Speech and Language Evaluation in Neurology: Childhood Disorders

Edited by

John K. Darby, M.D.

Postdoctoral Scholar
Departments of Genetics and Neurobiology
Stanford University School of Medicine
Stanford, California

Grune & Stratton, Inc.
(Harcourt Brace Jovanovich, Publishers)
Orlando   San Diego   New York
London   Toronto   Montreal   Sydney   Tokyo

Library of Congress Cataloging in Publication Data
Main entry under title:

Speech and language evaluation in neurology: childhood
  disorders.

  Companion v. to: Speech and language evaluation in
neurology: adult disorders.
  Bibliography
  1. Speech disorders in children. 2. Language disorders
in children. 3. Stuttering in children. 4. Brain—
Wounds and injuries—Complications and sequelae.
5. Brain damage—Patients—Language—Evaluation.
6. Pediatric neurology. 7. Children—Language—
Evaluation. I. Darby, John K. II. Speech and language
evaluation in neurology: adult disorders. [DNLM:
1. Language Disorders—in infancy & childhood.
2. Nervous System Diseases—complications. 3. Nervous
System Diseases—in infancy & childhood. 4. Speech
Disorders—in infancy & childhood. WL 340 S742]
RJ496.S7S627   1985   618.92'855   85-5548
ISBN 0-8089-1719-6

Grune & Stratton, Inc.
Orlando, FL 32887

Distributed in the United Kindgom by
Grune & Stratton, Ltd.
24/28 Oval Road, London NW 1

Library of Congress Catalog Number 85-5548
International Standard Book Number 0-8089-1719-6

Printed in the United States of America
85 86 87 88   10 9 8 7 6 5 4 3 2 1

Contents

Preface

This book and its companion volume, *Speech and Language Evaluation in Neurology: Adult Disorders,* complete a cycle begun with the original two *Speech Evaluation* volumes, in psychiatry and medicine. The four-volume compendium is a testimonial to my belief that the study of speech and language behavior is important to the practice of medicine in general, and to the study of central nervous system diseases in particular.

Our knowledge of communication disturbances and neurologic disease is accelerating due to broad interdisciplinary efforts involving neurology, neuroscience, genetics, nuclear medicine, speech pathology, speech science, rehabilitation medicine, psychology, computer science, and engineering. Neuroimaging techniques have recently contributed much to our understanding of speech and language function in the central nervous system. The current use of computers and instrumentation is rapidly assuming import in the field at the level of documentation of treatment progress, as an aid to treatment and diagnosis, and in basic research.

Speech and Language Evaluation in Neurology: Childhood Disorders is divided into three sections. The first section provides an overview of language acquisition and identification of related disorders, an extensive review of the principal language disorders in children, an analysis of language problems after pediatric head injury, and an update review of apraxia of speech in children.

The second section covers dysarthria in children. Chapters in this section provide a neurologic analysis of the dysarthric syndromes, a speech pathology perspective of the classification, theory, and treatment of dysarthria, and a review of speech problems in the multihandicapped child.

The third section is concerned with a new dimension of speech and language disorders; namely, genetic tramsmission. This section presents recent data on the genetics of selected developmental disorders, and new information on the application of molecular genetics in neurogenetic disorders of communication.

I am indebted to many people for their counsel and assistance in developing this volume. Ronald Netsell, the principal scientific consultant, provided valuable review, support, and assistance in planning the project. The other scientific consultants provided beneficial commentary and aided in the selection of authors and topics.

Many experts helped review content and specific chapters: Ray Kent, Jon Miller, Jon Eisenson, Dick Flower, Paula Square, Nina Simmons, Robert Wertz, John Bosma, Christy Ludlow, Else Cabos, and many others.

I am grateful to Diana Van Lancker for the continued use of her figure of the spectrogram, which has become the hallmark on the covers of the *Speech Evaluation* volumes.

Finally, the staff of Grune & Stratton deserves special appreciation for their work in preparing for publication the 1600 pages of material that comprise these four volumes.

Contributors X

Sarah W. Blackstone, Ph.D.
Chief, Speech and Language
  Pathology
The John F. Kennedy Institute;
Instructor, Rehabilitation Medi-
  cine
Johns Hopkins Medical Institu-
  tions
Baltimore, Maryland

**John Keith Brown, M.B.,
  Ch.B., F.R.C.P., D.C.H.**
Consultant, Pediatric Neurolo-
  gist
Royal Hospital for Sick Chil-
  dren;
Senior Lecturer, Department of
  Child Life and Health
University of Edinburgh
Edinburgh, Scotland

**Luigi Luca Cavalli-Sforza,
  M.D.**
Professor, Department of Genet-
  ics
Stanford University School of
  Medicine
Stanford, California

Judith A. Cooper, Ph.D.
Communicative Disorders Program
National Institute of Neurological and Communicative Disorders and Stroke
Bethesda, Maryland

John K. Darby, M.D.
Postdoctoral Scholar
Departments of Genetics and
  Neurobiology
Stanford University School of
  Medicine
Stanford, California

Barbara Davis, M.A.
Research Associate
Program in Communication Dis-
  orders
Department of Speech Communi-
  cation
University of Texas
Austin, Texas

Carla Dunn, Ph.D.
Assistant Professor
Program in Communication Dis-
  orders

Department of Speech Communi-
cation
University of Texas
Austin, Texas

Linda Ewing-Cobbs, Ph.D.
Department of Psychiatry and
Behavioral Sciences
University of Texas Medical
School
Houston, Texas

Jack M. Fletcher, Ph.D.
Chief, Developmental Neuropsy-
chology Section
Texas Research Institute of Men-
tal Sciences
Houston, Texas

Kenneth K. Kidd, M.D.
Associate Professor
Department of Human Genetics
Yale University School of Medi-
cine
New Haven, Connecticut

Susan H. Landry, Ph.D.
Developmental Neuropsychology
Section
Texas Research Institute of Men-
tal Sciences
Houston, Texas

Harvey S. Levin, Ph.D.
Professor, Division of Neurosur-
gery
University of Texas Medical
Branch
Galveston, Texas

Christy L. Ludlow, Ph.D.
Chief, Speech Pathology Unit
Communicative Disorders Pro-
gram

National Institute of Neurological and Communicative Disorders and Stroke
Bethesda, Maryland

Thomas P. Marquardt, Ph.D.
Associate Professor and Director
Program in Communication Dis-
orders
Department of Speech Communi-
cation
Austin, Texas

Michael J. Painter, M.D.
Chief, Department of Neurology
Children's Hospital of Pitts-
burgh;
Associate Professor
University of Pittsburgh Medical
School
Pittsburgh, Pennsylvania

Rachel E. Stark, Ph.D.
Director, Department of Communication Sciences and Disorders
The Kennedy Institute of Handicapped Children
Baltimore, Maryland

Linda Swisher, Ph.D.
Director, Early Childhood Lan-
guage Research Laboratory
Department of Speech and Hear-
ing Sciences
University of Arizona
Tucson, Arizona

Amy M. Wetherby, Ph.D.
Assistant Professor
Department of Audiology and
Speech Pathology
Florida State University
Tallahassee, Florida

Speech and Language Evaluation in Neurology: Childhood Disorders

I. LANGUAGE DISORDERS

Amy Miller Wetherby

1
Speech and Language Disorders in Children— An Overview

Language is a conventional system of arbitrary symbols that are combined and used in a rule-governed manner for communication (Bloom & Lahey, 1978). Speech is one medium for the expression of language that utilizes auditory input and vocal output. A deviation confined to the peripheral speech and/or hearing mechanism (e.g., cleft palate, hearing loss) may not impair the child's capacity for language development, but an alternative language system such as sign language may be necessary. Because of the developmental and neurologic relationship between speech and language, a language disorder may be accompanied by speech problems. Similarly, an impairment in cognitive and/or social development may disrupt language acquisition because of the interrelationships vis-à-vis linguistic, cognitive, and social knowledge (Bates, Benigni, Bretherton, Camaioni, & Volterra, 1979; Prutting, 1982).

Children with language disorders represent a heterogeneous population sharing the common feature of a delay or disorder in the acquisition of language. Children's language disorders may be classified as primary or secondary, based on contributory factors (Ludlow, 1980). A primary language disorder is present when the language impairment cannot be

Speech and Language Evaluation in Neurology:
Childhood Disorders
ISBN 0-8089-1719-6

accounted for by a peripheral sensory or motor deficit, a cognitive impairment, or adverse environmental conditions, and is often presumed to be due to dysfunction of the CNS. Secondary language disorders include language impairments of hearing-impaired and mentally retarded children. Children's language disorders may be further classified as developmental or acquired, based on time of onset (Ludlow, 1980). Developmental language disorders include those with an onset time before the emergence of language (birth to 1 year old), although the symptoms may not be detected until later. Acquired language disorders in children have an onset time after the emergence of language (3–12 years old). Childhood language disorders with an onset time between 1 and 3 years of age share some characteristics of both developmental and acquired language disorders in children.

Children with developmental language disorders display difficulties in the comprehension, production, and use of language, to varying degrees, and in any or all areas of phonology, semantics, syntax, and pragmatics (Bashir, Kuban, Kleinman, & Scavuzzo, 1983; Leonard, 1979; Ludlow, 1980). Developmental language disorders are relatively common. Between 3 and 8 percent of preschoolers in the United States and England are at least 1 year delayed in language development (Ludlow, 1980). Preschool language disorders may have a significant effect on subsequent academic achievement. Sixty percent of children who displayed language disorders at a preschool level were found to be placed in special education classes during late childhood (Aram & Nation, 1980). Fifty percent of children who displayed language disorders at age 6 continued to have language problems in adulthood (Hall & Tomblin, 1978). Thus, children with developmental language disorders are at a high risk for academic failure.

Primary developmental language disorders are usually presumed to be caused by CNS dysfunction but are often idiopathic. The neurologic bases of developmental language disorders are poorly understood. Explanations of postnatal damage to the left hemisphere, based on adult models of aphasia, are inadequate to account for the severity and sequelae of developmental language disorders in view of the potential for reorganization of language functions in the infant brain (Ludlow, 1979).

This chapter will provide an overview of speech and language disorders in children and introduce current issues relevant to this subject. The role of cerebral maturation in language acquisition and reorganization of language functions following early cerebral damage will be examined first. Diagnostic classifications, etiologic factors, and sequelae of developmental language disorders also will be discussed. And finally, clinical issues in the early identification of language disorders and language intervention with children will be examined.

CRITICAL PERIOD FOR LANGUAGE ACQUISITION

Lenneberg's Critical Period Hypothesis

In his biological theory of language development, Lenneberg (1967) hypothesized that the capacity for language learning is regulated by the unique maturational history of the human brain as well as environmental influences. At birth the human brain is relatively immature, weighing only about 24 percent of adult values. During the first 2 years of postnatal life, there is approximately a 350 percent weight increase, followed by a 35 percent increase during the next 10 years. By age 14 the brain has reached adult weight. The maturational history of the human brain is unique among primates. Brain–body weight ratios in humans approach adult proportions at a much slower rate than all "lower" species. Lenneberg (1966, 1967) hypothesized that the capacity for language acquisition is facilitated by the immature status and plasticity of the human brain at birth and the rapid maturation rate during the first 2 years of postnatal life.

Lenneberg (1967, 1969) proposed that a critical period for primary language acquisition exists based on evidence of a disproportionate capacity for language learning from infancy to senescence. According to Lenneberg, the critical period for language learning begins at about age 2 and declines with cerebral maturity at puberty, corresponding with the emergence and establishment of cerebral lateralization. Furthermore, he suggested that the cerebral hemispheres are equipotential for language lateralization during the first 2 years of life, and that with progressive decrease in involvement of the right hemisphere, language functions become firmly lateralized to the left hemisphere by puberty. Before the age of puberty, interhemispheric reorganization of language functions is still possible.

A Critical Look at Lenneberg's Theory

While Lenneberg's (1967) treatise was a monumental contribution to the literature, it stimulated much research challenging his theories. Lenneberg provided support for the critical period and equipotentiality hypothesis from evidence of the effects of early cerebral damage on language acquisition. He derived most of this evidence from a study reported by Basser (1962), who examined the effects of unilateral cerebral damage and hemispherectomy from case studies reported in the literature and cases attained in his clinical practice.

Unilateral Cerebral Damage

Basser (1962) reported that unilateral cerebral damage has a differential effect on language learning in children who acquire lesions before and after the onset of language (i.e., about age 2 years, according to Lenneberg). In approximately half of the children who sustained unilateral cerebral damage in either the left or right hemisphere before the age of 2 years, the emergence of language was found to be delayed, while in the other half of this population language acquisition began at the normal time. However, Basser assessed only the age of acquisition of single-word utterances and did not document the acquisition of word combinations. In unilateral lesions acquired between the ages of 2 and 10, 86 percent of the cases with left-sided lesions and 46 percent of the cases with right-sided lesions resulted in transitory language impairments as measured by deficits in verbal intelligence quotient (IQ) scores. These findings support Lenneberg's hypothesis that the two hemispheres are equipotential for language lateralization until about age 2 years.

Aphasia in childhood occurs with greater relative frequency following right hemisphere lesions than does aphasia in adulthood. Recent studies, however, have shown that the incidence is much lower than reported by Basser (1962). In a sample of 102 right and left hemiplegic children, Annett (1973) reported an increasing incidence of recorded speech problems with right hemiplegia (i.e., left hemisphere damage) and a decreasing incidence of speech problems with left hemiplegia (i.e., right hemisphere damage) as age of hemiplegia onset increased. Speech problems as a consequence of brain damage sustained before 13 months of age (including prenatal and perinatal damage) occurred in 32 percent of right hemiplegics and in 14 percent of left hemiplegics. Speech problems were recorded for 86 percent of the right hemiplegics who acquired cerebral damage after 13 months but before 4 years, and for 100% of the right hemiplegics who acquired brain damage after the age of 5 years. In contrast, no speech problems were recorded for left hemiplegics who acquired brain damage after 13 months of age.

With the exception of the study reported by Basser (1962), the proportion of childhood aphasia resulting from early right hemisphere lesions reported in other recent studies has ranged from 0–13 percent (Hecaen, 1976; Kinsbourne & Hiscock, 1977; Woods & Teuber, 1978). If the number of known left-handed children is excluded, the proportion is decreased to 7 percent or less. The discrepancy between the findings reported by Basser (1962) and other recent investigators may be partly due to Basser's inclusion of cases with systemic infections resulting in bilateral cerebral damage (Woods & Teuber, 1978). The incidence of diffuse encephalopathies from bacterial infections has decreased since the 1930s with the advent of antibiotics.

The language deficits following unilateral cerebral damage in childhood range from articulatory impairments to mutism (Hacaen, 1976). Dennis and Whitaker (1977) concluded that articulatory impairments may occur following early damage to either the left or right hemisphere, but that delays in the acquisition of word combinations occur only following early left hemisphere damage. Studies that have characterized the nature of the language deficits following early cerebral damage support this conclusion. For example, Woods and Carey (1978) examined the language functions of patients who sustained damage to the left hemisphere before and after the onset of language acquisition. They found that the children with perinatal injury to the left hemisphere showed mild cognitive impairment and not specific aphasic deficits. The children who acquired damage to the left hemisphere after the age of 1 year showed persisting aphasic deficits during the second decade of life. The discrepancy between the findings reported by Basser (1962) and those of Woods and Carey (1978) appears to be due to the measures selected for the assessment of language functioning. While Basser (1962) considered only the acquisition of single-word utterances and verbal IQ scores, Woods and Carey (1978) employed comprehensive language assessments of semantic and syntactic skills.

Aphasia following early cerebral damage has generally been considered to be relatively transitory, with rapid and complete recovery even after left hemisphere lesions (Hacaen, 1976; Woods & Teuber, 1978). This is presumed to be due to the capacity for intrahemispheric and interhemispheric reorganization of language functions during childhood. Hacaen (1976) reported that although recovery from childhood aphasia is more striking than in adulthood, mild verbal deficits, particularly in writing, may persist. Woods and Teuber (1978) found that before the age of 8 years, recovery from aphasia ranged from less than 1 week to 2.5 years. However, they did not find a direct relationship between age of onset and duration of recovery. The subjects who acquired aphasia after the age of 8 years were still considered aphasic at the time of the study, which was after an interval of more than 4 years. These studies indicate that recovery from childhood aphasia is less complete than has generally been presumed.

Hemidecortication

Hemispherectomy patients provide a rare opportunity to study the language capacity of an isolated (i.e., remaining after hemispherectomy) left or right hemisphere. These patients have sustained cerebral damage, however, and removal of the damaged hemisphere is often performed many years after the onset of lateralized cerebral damage and seizures. These patients, therefore, are not ideal subjects on whom to test the theory of the equipotentiality of the hemispheres, and generalizations to normal hemispheric specialization should be guarded.

According to Basser's (1962) report, the effects of a hemispherectomy on language functions were found to be related to the age at which the primary damage was sustained. In cases with lesions acquired before age 10 years, removal of the damaged hemisphere generally did not result in aphasia, regardless of laterality of damage and surgery. Verbal intelligence as measured by IQ tests was found to be equivalent in left and right hemispherectomy cases. In cases with lesions acquired in adulthood, left hemispherectomy resulted in permanent aphasia while right hemispherectomy did not produce any aphasic symptoms. These findings support Lenneberg's critical period and equipotentiality hypothesis.

Recent investigations of the linguistic capacities of right and left hemidecorticates have demonstrated that language development is superior in an isolated left hemisphere compared with an isolated right hemisphere. Although language functions measured by verbal IQ scores have been shown to be equally developed in either isolated hemisphere, the comprehension of complex syntactic forms (e.g., passive constructions) was found to be impaired in left hemidecorticates as compared with right hemidecorticates matched for verbal IQ (Dennis & Kohn, 1975; Dennis, 1980). The age at hemidecortication for these subjects ranged between 1 month and 20 years. The demonstrated syntactic deficits in some subjects thus may be related to intrahemispheric reorganization within the damaged hemisphere that may have occurred preoperatively.

Dennis and Whitaker (1976) examined the acquisition of a variety of language functions in one right and two left hemidecorticates who had undergone surgery before 5 months of age. All 3 subjects, ranging in age from 9 to 10 years, had been seizure free since the onset of language acquisition and had achieved normal verbal and performance IQ scores. The results of comprehensive language testing indicated that the left and right isolated hemispheres have different capacities for linguistic functions. Phonemic and semantic abilities were found to be equally developed in either hemisphere; in relation to the left, however, the isolated right hemisphere was impaired in the comprehension, production, and metalinguistic awareness of syntactic information. Thus by the end of the first decade, the two isolated hemispheres are not equal substrata for linguistic functions, even when surgical removal of one hemisphere precedes the onset of language acquisition.

Lenneberg's Theories Revised

Lenneberg's critical period and equipotentiality hypotheses need to be examined and revised in light of recent research findings. In defining the lower limit of the critical period for language acquisition, Lenneberg

(1967) referred to the onset of language acquisition as the time when the child produced two-word utterances (about age 2 years). The recent focus of child language research on the prelinguistic and one-word stage has shown that the emergence of language is a gradual unfolding rooted in early communicative, cognitive, and social development (Bates et al., 1979). In a discussion of a critical period for language learning, it is therefore more accurate to consider language acquisition as an active process commencing at birth, or to deal specifically with a critical period for the development of syntax beginning at about age 2 years.

Lenneberg's (1967) theory of the equipotentiality of the hemispheres has not been supported by recent research. Evidence from anatomical, behavioral, and electrophysiologic studies of presumably normal infants has revealed that the two hemispheres differ in structure (Chi, Dooling, & Gilles, 1977a; Wada, Clarke, & Hamm, 1975; Witelson & Pallie, 1973) and function (Entus, 1977; Gardiner and Walter, 1977; Molfese, Freeman, & Palermo, 1975; Segalowitz, 1983; Segalowitz & Chapman, 1980) very early in development, if not at birth. The recent investigations of the effects of early unilateral cerebral damage and hemidecortication reviewed previously provide further evidence that the two hemispheres are not equal substrata for language representation. The right hemisphere apparently cannot achieve the level of proficiency attained by the left hemisphere, particularly in syntactic development. The plasticity of the infant brain is due to the immature status at birth; however, this does not necessarily imply equal potential for language representation in the two hemispheres. Interhemispheric and intrahemispheric reorganization of function following early cerebral damage is facilitated by the neural plasticity of uncommitted cortical areas rather than by hemispheric equipotentiality. The prepotency of the left hemisphere is evident from the outset, and the potential of the right hemisphere to assume language functions declines as cortical areas become committed to other functions (Woods & Carey, 1978). In opposition to Lenneberg's equipotentiality hypothesis, Dennis and Whitaker (1977) concluded that at birth the two hemispheres "are not equally at risk for language delay or disorder and that they are not equivalent substrates for language acquisition" (p. 103).

Lenneberg proposed that the critical period for language acquisition closes with the establishment of cerebral lateralization at puberty and, hence, that the right hemisphere can assume language functions until puberty. If an age threshold for recovery from early cerebral damage reflects the ontogeny of cerebral lateralization, then lateralization may be considered to be established as late as age 8 years (Woods & Teuber, 1978) and as early as the onset of language acquisition (Woods & Carey, 1978). Perhaps a more conservative estimate is age 5 years, since there is consistent evidence that after the age of 5 the occurrence of childhood aphasia is similar to that in adulthood, and the right hemisphere can no longer completely assume language functions (Annett, 1973; Krashen, 1975).

The concept of a critical period for language acquisition implies that the capacity for language learning is triggered by "mere exposure" to language only during a critical time period of "limited duration" (Lenneberg, 1967). The effects of environmental deprivation on learning have provided evidence in support of critical periods in nonhumans; however, such experiments obviously cannot be applied to human subjects. The case of Genie (Curtiss, 1977), a girl who was confined to isolation by her parents from the age of 20 months to 13.5 years, provides an unusual test case for the critical period hypothesis. When Genie was discovered at 13.5 years of age, she could not talk or understand language. Genie has shown subsequent language development in both comprehension and production from mere exposure; her use of syntactic constructions, however, is severely impaired in relation to vocabulary and semantic development. Behavioral and electrophysiologic testing indicated that Genie uses her right hemisphere for language as well as for certain nonlinguistic functions. Her language development shows some similarities to left hemidecorticates. Curtiss concluded that Genie's acquisition of language after puberty supports a weak version of Lenneberg's critical period hypothesis; i.e., language acquisition from exposure cannot develop "normally" after puberty.

Although Lenneberg's (1967) hypotheses have been criticized, the underlying principle of his biological theory of language acquisition has been supported by recent research. According to Lenneberg, the sequential regularity of the emergence of certain developmental milestones in language acquisition is governed by maturational processes of the brain. Lenneberg (1967) correlated language development with indicators of brain maturation such as gross weight and neurodensity. Recent studies of myelogenesis, synaptogenesis, and gyral development indicate that the regularity of onset of certain language milestones corresponds with the regional maturation of fiber systems presumed to mediate speech and language functions (Chi, Dooling, & Gilles, 1977b; Lecours, 1975; Milner, 1976; Yakovlev & Lecours, 1967).

NEURODEVELOPMENTAL LANGUAGE DISORDERS

Neurodevelopmental disorders in childhood are characterized by learning and behavior problems with known or presumed etiology in the CNS (Flower, 1981). In this chapter *neurodevelopmental language disorders* will be used to refer to a subset of neurodevelopmental disorders in which the primary symptom is a disorder of language. That is, children with neurodevelopmental language disorders show language skills lagging behind other areas of development, and etiology is known or presumed to involve the CNS whether from delayed development, a lack of development, or abnormal development of the brain.

Diagnostic Classification of Speech and Language Disorders in Children

It is necessary to consider neurodevelopmental language disorders in relation to the full spectrum of childhood speech and language disorders in the differential diagnosis. Current classification systems of such disorders are inadequate and represent a major area of deficiency in the literature (Ingram, 1975; Ludlow, 1980). The literature contains a plethora of diagnostic labels for these children that has resulted in confusions over the definitions of boundaries between and relationships among subclassifications of this population. Because of the lack of adequate classification systems, the major flaws in research studies of language-disordered children have been insufficient subject descriptions and poor control over subject selection (Ludlow, 1980).

One of the most comprehensive classifications and detailed descriptions of childhood speech–language disorders was proposed by Ingram (1959) and later revised (Ingram, 1969; 1975). His classification system was defined in terms of the primary language function or process that is impaired and associated clinical features. An adaptation of Ingram's classification system is presented in Table 1-1 using terminology and subclassifications currently popular in the United States. Such a system is based on a medical diagnostic model in which speech and language impairments are classified into mutually exclusive categories based on etiologic factors (Aram & Nation, 1982).

Primary developmental language disorders should be differentiated from developmental speech disorders and acquired speech–language disorders in childhood. Developmental speech disorders include impairments in the quality, rhythm, and production of speech sounds and may be associated with structural abnormalities such as cleft palate or with neuromuscular disorders such as cerebral palsy (see Table 1-1). These will be discussed in chapters 4, 5, 6, and 7 respectively. Children with developmental speech disorders without accompanying mental retardation may have the potential for normal language skills; however, a nonspeech language system may be necessary (Shane, 1980). Children with acquired speech–language disorders (see Table 1-1) are characterized by an onset following a period of normal language acquisition and would include acquired aphasia in childhood. Such children display a clinical profile that is different from both the developmental and adult disorders (see chaps. 2 and 3). And finally, the differential diagnosis of a primary developmental language disorder implies that the existence of a language disorder cannot be attributed to a general cognitive impairment

Table 1-1
Diagnostic Classification of Speech and Language Disorders in Children

Voice disorders (dysphonia)

Fluency disorders (dysrhythmias)

Speech sound production disorders secondary to structural abnormalities

Motor speech disorders (dysarthrias)

Speech–language disorders secondary to cognitive impairment

Speech–language disorders secondary to hearing impairment

Speech–language disorders secondary to adverse environmental factors

Primary developmental language disorders

Acquired speech–language disorders in childhood

Mixed speech–language disorders with two or more of the above categories

(i.e., mental retardation), a hearing impairment, or adverse environmental conditions (see Table 1-1).

Neurodevelopmental language disorders are comprised of the various primary developmental language disorders (see Table 1-1). These may be subclassified into specific and pervasive developmental disorders as presented in Table 1-2. Detailed information about the various neurodevelopmental language disorders syndromes will be presented in chapters 2 and 4.

Table 1-2
Subclassifications of the Primary Developmental Language Disorders

Specific
  Developmental phonologic disorders
  Developmental apraxia of speech
  Specific developmental language disorders (developmental aphasia)
  Developmental reading disorders (dyslexia)
Pervasive
  Infantile autism

The specific developmental language disorders are characterized by normal measured nonverbal intelligence and an impairment in one or more domains of linguistic development (American Psychiatric Association, 1980). Four subgroups of the specific developmental language disorders have been identified in the literature and are listed in Table 1-2. These subgroups may not be mutually exclusive, and a particular child may change from one diagnosis to another with maturation. It is not yet known, however, whether these disorders fall on a continuum, and the relationships among these disorders remains to be elucidated.

Developmental phonologic disorders have recently been considered as linguistic disorders rather than functional articulation disorders and have been described as systematic deviations in knowledge and use of phonologic rules (Ingram, 1976; Shriberg & Kwiatkowski, 1982). Developmental apraxia, or dyspraxia of speech, has been characterized by a deficit in programming the position and sequence of volitional speech movements, which is not due to muscular weakness (Rosenbek & Wertz, 1972). There is continued controversy in the literature over the specific symptoms of developmental apraxia of speech and whether or not developmental apraxia of speech can be differentiated from developmental phonologic disorders (Guyette & Diedrich, 1983; Williams, Ingham, & Rosenthal, 1981). Children with developmental apraxia of speech or developmental phonologic disorders are likely to be impaired in expressive language development, while receptive language is relatively normal (Shriner, Halloway, & Daniloff, 1969; Rosenbek & Wertz, 1972). Specific developmental language disorders (sometimes referred to as developmental or childhood aphasia or dysphasia) are characterized by varying degrees of receptive and expressive impairments of spoken language, while developmental reading disorders (often referred to as dyslexia) involve impairments of written language (Carrow-Woolfolk & Lynch, 1982).

Pervasive developmental disorders involve impairments of multiple psychologic functions, as differentiated from disorders affecting a single specific function (American Psychiatric Association, 1980). Infantile autism is currently classified by the American Psychiatric Association (1980) as a pervasive developmental disorder rather than as a childhood psychosis, as was done previously. Infantile autism is categorized in Table 1-2 as a primary developmental language disorder because current definitions of autism describe impairments of speech, language, and communication as a primary diagnostic feature (Baltaxe & Simmons, 1981; Ritvo & Freeman, 1978; Rutter, 1978). In contrast to the specific developmental disorders, between 60 and 80 percent of autistic children have measured intelligence in the moderate to severely mentally retarded range (DeMyer, Hingtgen, & Jackson, 1981; Ritvo & Freeman, 1978).

Thus autism and mental retardation coexist in the majority of autistic cases; however, autistic children display a distinct profile of language functions (Ritvo & Freeman, 1978). Pervasive developmental disorders, other than autism, with language impairments as a primary symptom have not yet been identified in the literature.

The terminology used in the classifications presented in Tables 1-1 and 1-2 has its roots in the medical literature from the 1800s. There is continued controversy over the appropriateness of applying such terms as aphasia and apraxia to childhood disorders (Aram & Nation, 1982). Diagnostic categories based on verifiable etiology are useful with adult-onset disorders. However, the medical diagnostic model has several limitations with childhood disorders, including unidentifiable or multiple etiologies, a lack of homogeneity in language abilities within diagnostic categories, difficulty in classifying childhood disorders into mutually exclusive categories based on etiologic factors, and failure to account for the interaction of behavioral and neurologic influences on language development (Aram & Nation, 1982; Beadle, 1981). In spite of these limitations, such diagnostic classifications commonly form the bases for decisions about treatment approaches, classroom placement, and professionals responsible for remediation.

An alternative to the medical diagnostic model came in the 1960s and 1970s with the explosion of research in linguistic and psycholinguistic descriptions of normal child language (Aram & Nation, 1982). New approaches to the description, analysis, and treatment of child language disorders evolved in phonology, syntax, semantics, and pragmatics based on the normal developmental model. While behavioral descriptions of childhood speech and language disorders provide a useful framework for assessment and intervention, they do not offer explanations about neurologic, perceptual, cognitive, or linguistic processing breakdowns that may contribute to the disorder.

A unidimensional classification system, whether based on etiology or linguistic descriptions, appears to be inadequate to accomodate the complex behavioral and neurologic interactions of childhood disorders. Multiple factors, including behavioral descriptions and etiologic components, need to be considered in developing any taxonomy of speech and language disorders in children. Shriberg and Kwiatkowski (1982) presented a multilevel diagnostic classification system for developmental phonologic processes, severity ratings, and etiologic correlates coding the speech and hearing mechanism, cognitive–linguistic functioning, and psychosocial factors. A multidimensional diagnostic taxonomy for speech and language disorders in children, similar to the one described by Shriberg and Kwiatkowski, is needed as both a clinical and a research tool and will take the concerted efforts of many clinicians and researchers.

Neurologic Bases of Language Disorders in Children

There has been little research directed at identifying the cause of developmental language disorders (Ludlow, 1980). This may reflect technologic limitations of existing diagnostic tools for detecting and measuring brain dysfunction in children. Many etiologic factors have been implicated as contributory to brain dysfunction in children, including the following: (1) prenatal, perinatal, and postnatal trauma; (2) prenatal, perinatal, and postnatal infections; (3) anoxia; (4) vascular diseases; (5) toxic and metabolic diseases; (6) chromosomal anomalies; and (7) congenital neoplasms (Bashir et al., 1983; Dreifuss, 1975; Lemire, Loeser, Leech, & Alvord, 1975). It is not clear, however, how these etiologic agents affect brain function to produce language disorders in children.

Neurologic models of adult-onset aphasias are insufficient to explain the developmental language disorders because of the neural plasticity of the infant brain; i.e., the theory of damage to the left hemisphere is inadequate to account for the severity and duration of developmental language disorders, particularly in view of the demonstrated recovery of language functions (albeit incomplete) following early circumscribed lesions of the left hemisphere (Hecaen, 1976; Woods & Carey, 1978; Woods & Teuber, 1978). Some researchers have concluded, therefore, that developmental language disorders are a consequence of bilateral cerebral damage or dysfunction (Bashir et al., 1983; Leonard, 1979). There has been little direct neurologic evidence to support this theory, with the exception of a postmortem neuropathologic study that revealed bilateral temporal lobe damage in a case that presented developmental aphasia (Landau, Goldstein, & Kleffner, 1960).

The National Institute of Neurological and Communicative Disorders and Stroke sponsored a symposium in 1978 and subsequently published a monograph devoted to better understanding the neurologic bases of language disorders in children. The participants at this symposium offered several intriguing theories and directions for future research in this area. Zaidel (1979) suggested that developmental language disorders reflects an abnormal interaction between the cerebral hemispheres and cited evidence of abnormal states of cerebral lateralization in developmental aphasia, dyslexia, and autism. Geschwind (1979) hypothesized that language and learning disabilities are a result of certain brain regions maintaining a smaller size and hence limiting functional potential. He suggested that such anatomical differences may reflect either normal genetic variations in endowment or delays in the structural development of these brain regions.

Ludlow (1979) suggested that developmental language disorders have their bases in deficient or disordered development of left hemisphere language areas rather than in a circumscribed lesion in these areas.

Language remains primarily lateralized to the left, albeit dysfunctional hemisphere. She hypothesized that the acquisition of language in these children begins in the right hemishere, within its limited linguistic capacities, and later the dysfunctional left hemisphere matures and develops some linguistic skills. The child may be left with persisting deficits in complex language functions, which lead to reading and writing difficulties.

The theory of dynamic localization of higher cortical functions, described by Luria (1966), states that the neural substrata of higher cortical functions do not remain constant in ontogeny but rather higher cortical functions are mediated by different constellations of cortical areas at different stages of development. This concept has been supported by the extensive work of Goldman (1979) and colleagues with nonhuman primates. This theory implies that the sequalae of cerebral dysfunction sustained at different stages of ontogeny will be manifested differentially. A lesion sustained in a particular cortical region during early childhood may have a systematic effect on higher cortical centers superposed above it in ontogeny. A theory of the neurologic bases of developmental language disorders must account for the dynamic nature of the neural representation of language and other higher cortical functions, such as that suggested by Ludlow (1979).

Part of the difficulty in unraveling the neurologic substrata of developmental language disorders lies in the time lag intervening between the onset of cerebral "dysfunction" and the time of examination of the effects of this dysfunction on brain organization and language functions. The effects of a circumscribed lesion, abnormal development, or even delayed development on a particular region of the immature brain may be cumulative (Goldman, 1979; Luria, 1966). It may be difficult or nearly impossible, therefore, to differentiate the primary etiologic agent from the secondary disruptive effect when the child is not examined until years after the fact. Furthermore, what may have initially been a secondary effect may subsequently become a causative factor in the disruption of brain regions that have not yet matured. Thus minor malfunction or adjustment in the precise orchestration of events that unfold during neural maturation may have major, and potentially deleterious, clinical manifestations.

Issues in Timing and Developmental Interaction

The study of normal child language acquisition has recently demonstrated individual variation in strategies or learning styles, e.g., analytic versus gestalt styles (Nelson, 1981; Peters, 1983). These have been explained by differences in the child's cognitive makeup based on the combined effects of heredity and experience. Bates (1979a) proposed that variations in the relative timing of the emergence of cognitive abilities may lead to differences in language-learning strategies. Taking this a step further, variations in the developmental timing of cerebral lateralization of higher cortical functions may partly account for the differential timing of acquisition of cognitive skills and hence the divergent language-learning strategies of normal children (Bates, 1979a; Peters, 1983).

Bates (1979b) hypothesized that the human capacity to use a symbol system was generated through the process of heterochrony, which refers to the construction of new capacities through changes in the relative timing of emergence and rate of development of pre-existing capacities (Gould, 1977). Bates (1979b) proposed that in phylogeny the relative proportions of available cognitive and social component skills reached a certain threshold level that resulted in new interactions among the components creating the new symbol-using capacity. Thus quantitative variations in developmental timing led to a qualitatively new capacity. Bates suggested that the heterochronous process that occurred in phylogeny is replicated in ontogeny.

While Bates (1979b) used the concept of heterochronism to explain the construction of the symbol-using capacity in phylogeny and ontogeny, the use of this concept may be extended to explain deviations from normal development. Slight variations in developmental timing of component skills in early stages may lead to pervasive differences in later stages based on the interaction of the components available at particular times in development. This concept suggests that the particular combination of available components may lead to a distinct interaction and contribute to the heterogeneity seen among children with developmental language disorders.

For example, the scattered profile characteristic of autistic children may be explained by the accelerated and protracted development of skills requisite for normal communication. Wetherby and Prutting (1984) examined aspects of communicative, cognitive, and social development in autistic children functioning in the prelinguistic and early stages of language development compared with normal children. The autistic subjects displayed a communicative profile that was distinct from the normal children and was characterized by (1) a proficiency in regulating another's behavior to achieve an environmental end and (2) deficiencies in attracting another's attention to oneself, directing another's attention to an object, and focusing one's own attention to a referent. These communicative functions emerge in synchrony between 9 and 12 months of age in normal development (Bates, 1979a). Wetherby and Prutting (1984) explained the heterochrony in communicative development demonstrated by the autistic subjects by the differential timing and rate of acquisition of specific cognitive and social skills. The cumulative effect of variations in the relative timing of cognitive and social skills results in a qualitatively distinct interaction among linguistic, cognitive, and social development in autistic children. The particular heterochronous process that occurs in the autistic child presumably reflects a disruption in the maturational timetable of neural regions whether from an anatomical lesion, physiologic dysfunction, and/or delayed development, which leads to qualitative variations in the neural representation of language (Wetherby, 1984).

The concept of heterochrony has recently been used to account for the heterogeneity in outcome of children with specific developmental language disorders (Bashir et al., 1983; Kirchner & Skarakis-Doyle, 1983). The presence of deviant linguistic rules or compensatory strategies may induce variations in the disordered child's subsequent acquisition of language. This principle is exemplified by the findings of Shriner and associates (1969) that children with developmental phonologic disorders showed deficits in syntax and used shorter sentences. Delayed or deviant phonologic development thus may be related to deficits in the acquisition of syntax due to developmental interaction. The child with a primary developmental language disorder that is specific in nature may be characterized by heterochronous development within the linguistic domain, while the autistic child demonstrates heterochrony across the linguistic, cognitive, and social domains.

The issue of timing is critical in understanding language disorders in children because of the developmental interplay among component skills within and across linguistic and nonlinguistic domains. The behavioral profile of the language-disordered child is a manifestation of that child's relative strengths and weaknesses as well as experiences. The particular combination of skills and experiences available to the language-disordered child are not seen at any point in normal development. Because of the developmental interaction of available skills, the profile of the language-disordered child is not merely a slower version of normal development (Kirchner & Skarakis-Doyle, 1983).

EARLY IDENTIFICATION OF SPEECH AND LANGUAGE DISORDERS IN CHILDREN

The concept of a critical period for language learning implies that the optimal period for intervention with language-disordered children is during early childhood. It has been assumed that the earlier language intervention begins, the better the outcome should be (Miller, 1983). While there have been several recent reports of the effectiveness of early language intervention with a variety of populations (Schiefelbusch & Bricker, 1981), there has been only one reported investigation directed at the question of the optimal timing of language intervention. Fowler (1981) reported the preliminary findings from a series of studies investigating the effectiveness of early language stimulation. It was found that 87 percent of the infants exposed to language stimulation for 12 months made substantial gains and showed accelerated rates of development compared with test norms. Additionally, the children receiving language stimulation between the ages of 15 to 27 months showed faster rates of development than infants receiving stimulation between the ages of 3 to 12 months. These preliminary results suggest that early language intervention may be more advantageous beginning at 15 months of age rather than earlier, and therefore clinical efforts should focus on the identification of children with communicative problems or the potential for such problems during the first year of life so that intervention may begin by 15 months of age.

The pediatrician is most likely to be the first professional to come in contact with and evaluate the infant and thus plays a critical role in the early identification of children with communication problems. The pediatrician needs a sensitive, efficient means of detecting communication problems or the potential for such problems in order to make the necessary referrals as early as possible. Strategies for the detection of developmental problems that are currently in practice involve two general approaches: the use of high-risk registers at birth, and the use of developmental scales checked during pediatric visits for routine examination and immunization.

The means for identifying children with speech and language problems lags behind that for identifying hearing impairments in infants. Recent advances in diagnostic techniques make it possible to detect a hearing impairment during the first few months of life (e.g., see Williston & Schimmel, 1981). The use of high-risk register for hearing was established in 1973 and revised in 1982 by the Joint Committee on Infant Hearing (1982) and has led to more accurate detection than has behavioral screening in the newborn nursery (Gerber, 1977; Meyer & Wolfe, 1975). The difficulty of establishing and using a high-risk register for speech and language is compounded by many factors including the age at which language normally emerges, multiple etiologies and unidentifiable etiologies of developmental language disorders, and the lack of sensitive diagnostic tools for detecting such problems in early infancy.

Certain etiologic agents are known to cause speech and language disorders and are manifested at birth or in early infancy such as Down's syndrome, maternal rubella, cleft lip or palate, and cerebral palsy. However, often the first evident symptom of an underlying neurologic dysfunction is a delay in or failure to develop language. The child's communicative status, therefore, may be a sensitive indicator in the diagnosis of neurodevelopmental disorders (Miller, 1983). Many etiologic factors have been identified as contributing to a high risk for speech and language disorders in children, including abnormal gestational age or birth weight, elevated bilirubin level, respiratory distress, blood incompatability, lowered Apgar scores, forceps delivery, maternal age, intrauterine virus or infection, congenital perinatal infections, family history, and poor prenatal care (Ehrlich, Shapiro, Kimball, & Huttner, 1973; Lassman, Vetter, & LaBenz, 1980). The predictive value of these high-risk factors in the early identification and subsequent outcome of developmental language disorders remains to be determined.

Ehrlich and associates (1973) evaluated the communication skills of 81 5-year-old children who were identified as "at risk" as newborns based on one or more of the following factors: (1) abnormal birth weight or gestational age, (2) blood incompatability, (3) respiratory distress, and (4) hyperbilirubinemia. They reported that only 16 percent of these children were functioning normally at age 5, 30 percent were to be monitored for slight deficiencies, and 54 percent showed substantially poor performance and were recommended for therapy. They found that significant deficits occurred primarily in those children with histories of abnormal birthweight or gestational age and respiratory distress, suggesting that these two conditions should be included on a high-risk register for speech and language. Further research is needed to establish and evaluate the success of high-risk register for speech and language.

Many developmental scales are available to assess the emergence of major milestones in cognitive, language, and motor development. Such scales, however, typically do not sample a sufficient diversity of language skills to detect mild or moderate problems. And yet, more comprehensive developmental scales require too much time for administration by the pediatrician. Miller (1983) discussed the limitations of the Denver Developmental Screening Test (Frankenburg, Dodds, & Fandal, 1973), which is one of the most widely used developmental screening tests by pediatricians, and noted that, for example, it may not identify a child with a severe language comprehension problem until well past the age of 2 years.

Developmental follow-ups of infants with identified congenital defects or neurologic dysfunction, those with a high risk for speech and language disorders, and any others with a potential problem necessitate a sensitive developmental scale for language acquisition, and yet such a scale needs to be short enough to administer quickly in the pediatric office. Miller (1983) devised a developmental and criterion-referenced scale based on developmental research for this purpose (see Table 1-3). Failure to develop any particular language behavior by the age specified would indicate the need to refer the child to a speech–language specialist for further evaluation.

Child language research has recently focused on communicative be-

Table 1-3

Developmental Scale for Identification of Communication Deficits in the First 2 Years of Life

Behaviors that should be present at 6 mo
  Comprehension
    Consistent orienting to sound
  Production
    Syllable repetition (*ba ba ba*)
    Duration of cooing, singing, and babbling, 203 sec
    Variable intonation, both during crying and cooing
    Voiced–voiceless contrast: /p/ vs /b/
    Discrete tongue movements: /d/, /n/
Behaviors that should be present at 12 mo
  Comprehension
    Understands own name or name of present familiar person
  Production
    Ma-ma or da-da, pet name referentially, low frequency and intelligibility
    Imitates speech sounds
  Language use
    Turn-taking vocalizations in communication games, peek-a-boo, pat-a-cake
Behaviors that should be present at 18 mo
  Comprehension
    Understands single words, names for objects within visual field
  Production
    Few intelligible words
    Words frequently note familiar people and objects
    Frequency of vocalization increasing
  Language use
    Requests, comments
    Rejects with motor and vocal or vocal behavior
    Hi and bye with gesture or vocal behavior
Behaviors that should be present at 24 mo
  Comprehension
    Understands at least two words in utterance, such as *throw ball* indicating action object relation
  Production
    Expresses single words, including action verbs and reference to absent objects
    Vocabulary increases to 20 words minimum
    Two-word utterances
    At least two intelligible utterances
  Language use
    Request names, locations: "What's that," "Where's that"
    Uses words for multiple function

From Miller, J. F. (1983). With permission.

havior emerging during the prelinguistic stages (e.g., Bates et al., 1979), which may have implications for the early identification of language disorders. The child's communicative behavior before the emergence of language may indicate the likelihood of subsequent difficulties in language acquisition. Behaviors that are deviant from normal prelinguistic development have been identified in several different populations. For example, some autistic children show deficiencies in gestural and vocal communication to attract and direct another's attention, compared with a proficient use of communication to request and protest (Wetherby & Prutting, in press). Down's syndrome children as well as autistic children have been found to show a reduced rate of vocalizations to request compared with normal children (Greenwald & Leonard, 1979; Wetherby & Prutting, in press). The study of prelinguistic development in children with specific developmental language disorders poses a particular dilemma in that this information may have direct implications for early identification and yet these children are typically not identified, and therefore not studied, until well past the prelinguistic stage. Future research should be directed at expanding a developmental language scale, such as that presented in Table 1-3, to include measures of prelinguistic communicative behavior that should be present by 12 months of age.

FROM ASSESSMENT TO INTERVENTION

Language assessment is an ongoing process that is integrally related to language intervention (Miller, 1981; Snyder, 1983). The initial decision in language assessment is to identify or rule out the existence of a communication problem. The issue of deciding what constitutes a speech and/or language disorder in children is not a straightforward process. Norm-referenced standardized tests serve as a clinical tool in determining whether speech and language differences are considered significant or fall within a normal range of variation for a child's chronologic age. While there is an abundance of published norm-referenced tests to assess speech and language skills of preschool and school-aged children, the majority of these tests fail to meet a number of psychometric criteria generally considered necessary for educational and psychologic testing (McCauley & Swisher, 1984; Muma, 1978). Given the state of the clinical art in available norm-referenced tests, McCauley and Swisher (1984) suggested that speech–language clinicians be attentive to the psychometric flaws of the tests they use in making clinical decisions, use norm-referenced test results in conjunction with other kinds of objective and subjective assessment information, and to be informed consumers to encourage publishers to include empirical evidence of test reliability and validity.

Once a child has been identified as having a language problem, it must be decided whether to recommend that child for speech–language pathology and other professional services. There is disagreement in the literature over the decision-making process of whether to provide language intervention. For example, Aram and Nation (1982) take the position that all language–disordered children can benefit to some degree from speech–language therapy. In contrast, Beadle (1981) argues that all patients do not improve from speech–language therapy. Empirical evidence is needed to identify variables that may have predictive value in determining which children will benefit from language intervention and which will evolve out of the language disorder without therapeutic intervention. Presently, the selection of children for language intervention is a clinical decision that should be based on many factors including the severity of the child's problem, the appropriateness of the child's language to other developmental milestones and to environmental factors, and the chances for improvement considering the motivation of the child and the child's family (Beadle, 1981; Carrow-Woolfolk & Lynch, 1982).

As the child is being considered for language intervention, the purpose of assessment shifts to establishing a developmental profile to be used in making a differential diagnosis and planning intervention strategies. A comprehensive developmental profile should include evaluation of the child's developmental level across domains (cognitive, social, linguistic), components within the linguistic domain (phonology, semantics, morphology, syntax, pragmatics), processes (comprehension, production), and modalities (auditory, visual, gestural, vocal, graphic). It should also include a determination of the integrity of the child's speech and hearing mechanisms and consideration of the child's motor abilities, attention skills, motivation, and environmental factors (Miller, 1981, 1983). As language intervention proceeds, assessment continues as a critical component of intervention to monitor the child's progress and evaluate the effectiveness of the individualized treatment plan.

Language intervention with children has evolved within the field of speech–language pathology over the past 3 decades. The nature and scope of language intervention with children has metamorphosed from focusing solely on vocabulary and syntactic structure to encompassing not only the structure and content of language but also the child's cognitive and social knowledge contributing to the use of communication for social interaction (Launer & Lahey, 1981; Prutting, 1982; Rees, 1983). The introduction of pragmatics to the child language literature in the mid-1970s has had far-reaching consequences on the conceptualization of language intervention. Pragmatics, i.e., the way a speaker "can code a message in a particular context for a particular effect" (Muma, 1978, p. 23), is the rule governing language use. This recent shift of focus to pragmatics has clinical implications not only for the content of language goals but also for making such decisions as who will be the intervention agent and what will be the context and nature of intervention (Craig, 1983; Prutting, 1982).

Content of Language Intervention With Children

The American Speech–Language–Hearing Association sponsored a conference of invited experts to discuss critical issues in language intervention with child and adult populations in 1982. Rees (1983) discussed the content of language intervention with children and proposed that the proper language goals with children be to

> provide them with the knowledge of language structures pertinent to their own language community and the conventional means and the ready inclinication to put this knowledge to use in interpersonal communication as well as in thinking, learning and problem-solving, insofar as the child's capacity and resources will allow (p. 311– 312).

She went on to state that for those children who cannot learn or use "conventional means," alternative means should be explored.

Ree's position statement highlights several new shifts in the conceptualization of language intervention with children that have emerged from the study of pragmatics. First of all, the primary and ultimate goal of language intervention is the effective use of communication (Craig, 1983). Speech is an efficient means of communicating; however, much attention is now being given to nonspeech communication either to facilitate the development of speech or as an alternative communication system for children in whom speech is not a viable option (see Schiefelbusch, 1980). Pragmatics has most obviously contributed new areas to assess and remediate in the use of communication, whether through speech or nonspeech means. Secondly, formulating goals for language structures should incorporate what is relevant to the child's environment. Thirdly, goals should be selected on the basis of the child's motivation. Generalization of language goals thus should not be considered a last step in therapy but rather a primary focus of language intervention from the outset (Seibert & Oller, 1981). A fourth point made by Rees is that language goals should embrace the many functions of language including use as a social tool for communicating and as a cognitive tool for thinking and problem solving.

Intervention Agents

Traditional language intervention programs utilize the speech–language clinician as the primary intervention agent and may involve the parent and/or teacher as a secondary agent to achieve consistency across settings and facilitate generalization. The study of pragmatics has stimulated the question of who is (are) the appropriate intervention agent(s). The pragmatics literature indicates that the child's language behavior will vary as a function of major characteristics of the listener such as familiarity and age (Craig, 1983). Furthermore, normal children appear to need experience in social interaction with peers in order to communicate competently with this age-group, in spite of experience and competence in communicating with adults (Mueller & Brenner, 1977). It should not be assumed, therefore, that language intervention with a speech–language clinician is sufficient to teach a language-disordered child how to be a competent communicator with any listener. Multiple intervention agents including parents, teachers, siblings, and peers should be utilized in language intervention, along with and under the direction of a speech–language clinician (Craig, 1983). The role of the speech–language clinician is changing to include not only direct therapy but also consultation with parents, teachers, and other professionals (Lyngaas, Nyberg, Koekenga, & Gruenwald, 1983).

The use of parents as primary intervention agents has recently gained attention in the literature. Koegel, Schriebman, Briten, Burke, and O'Neill (1982) taught behavior management skills to parents of autistic children and compared the effectiveness of parent training with direct clinic treatment. They found that the children whose parents received 25–30 hours of training improved at least as much as the children who received 255 hours of direct clinic treatment. Schumaker and Sherman (1978) presented guidelines for training parents to serve as language interventionists; there have been no reported studies, however, to compare the effectiveness of clinician- versus parent-directed language intervention. In addition to the obvious cost-effectiveness of parent-training, Spradlin and Siegel (1982) noted several potential advantages for parents carrying out language intervention in the home including more opportunity to use a variety of language structures and functions, increased maintenance and generalization of language skills, involvement in various communicative situations, and parental control of numerous reinforcers.

The developmental progression of communicative interactions of normal children may serve as guidelines for selecting intervention agents for language-disorderd children. The normal child proceeds from caregiver–child interactions, to caregiver-mediated child interactions with other adults and peers, to peer interactions (Corsaro, 1979; Craig,

1983). Thus language intervention may progress from adult–child inter-actions, where the adult may be the clinician, teacher, and/or parent, to familiar-adult–mediated child interactions with an unfamiliar adult, and ultimately to child–peer interactions. Advances in techniques for the early identification of language disorders will increase the urgency of utilizing parents as a primary intervention agent.

Context of Language Intervention With Children

The traditional context of language intervention has been to isolate the child with the speech–language clinician in a room that is barren of potentially interesting stimuli and to have the clinician direct the child's nonverbal and verbal behavior throughout the session. The recent litera-ture in pragmatics has questioned the appropriateness of this traditional context. Decisions about the setting of language intervention and the nature of the interactions should be based on the language goals. If the long-term goal of language intervention is for the child to communicate effectively using language with a variety of communicative partners, then the traditional context of language intervention is inadequate.

Several recent authors have indicated that "natural" communicative interactions should be preserved in the context of language intervention (Craig, 1983; Muma, 1978; Seibert & Oller, 1981). The setting of lan-guage intervention should be expanded to include environments that the child is exposed to regularly such as the home, classroom, playground, grocery store, etc. The nature of the interactions should be planned so that the child assumes not only the role of respondent but also that of initiator. Communicative interactions should center around an activity of mutual interest and shared attention, and natural reinforcers should be optimized. The recent pragmatic literature has raised many important questions about the optimal context of language intervention with chil-dren that need to be systematically studied.

SUMMARY

Primary developmental language disorders are characterized by (1) varying degrees of difficulty in the comprehension, production and use of language, and onset time before the emergence of language, and (2) pre-sumed underlying CNS dysfunction. Recent literature indicates that the left and right hemispheres do not have equal potential for language rep-resentation and that damage to the left hemisphere in infancy is much more likely to result in language deficits than early right hemisphere damage. There is some support for the existence of a critical period for language learning. Postnatal maturation of the brain serves to regulate the development of language.

Primary developmental language disorders include such classifications as developmental apraxia of speech, developmental phonologic disorders, specific developmental language disorders (developmental aphasia), developmental reading disorders (dyslexia), and infantile autism. While many etiologic factors have been implicated as contributory to CNS dysfunction in children, the dynamic processes involved in how these etiologic agents affect or disrupt brain function to produce language disorders in children are poorly understood. The issue of timing is critical in understanding childhood language disorders because of the cumulative effects of early brain dysfunction and developmental interaction of available skills.

The pediatrician plays a critical role in the early identification of children with communication and language problems. Strategies for the detection of developmental problems used by pediatricians include the use of high-risk registers at birth and developmental scales checked during routine pediatric visits. The child with a potential problem should be referred to the speech–language specialist as early as possible to enable early intervention.

The conceptualization of language intervention with children was dramatically changed with the introduction of pragmatics to the child language literature in the mid-1970s. The primary goal of language intervention is for the child to effectively communicate with different communicative partners in various situations. Decisons about the content, intervention agent(s), and context of language intervention need to be made in consideration of this primary goal.

REFERENCES

American Psychiatric Association. (1980) *Diagnostic and statistical manual of mental disorders* (3rd ed.). Washington, DC, Author.

Annett, M. (1973). Laterality of childhood hemiplegia and the growth of speech and intelligence. *Cortex, 9,* 4–33.

Aram, D. M., & Nation, J. E. (1980). Preschool language disorders and subsequent language and academic difficulties. *Journal of Communication Disorders, 13,* 159–170.

Aram, D. M., & Nation, J. E. (1982). *Child language disorders.* St. Louis: C. V. Mosby.

Baltaxe, C., & Simmons, J. (1981). Disorders of language in childhood psychosis: Current concepts and approaches. In J. K. Darby (Ed.), *Speech Evaluation in psychiatry.* New York: Grune & Stratton.

Bashir, A., Kuban, K., Kleinman, S., & Scavuzzo, A. (1983). Issues in language disorders: Considerations of cause, maintenance, and change. In J. Miller, D.

Yoder, & R. Schiefelbusch (Eds.), *Contemporary issues in language interven-tion* (American Speech–Language–Hearing Association, ASHA Reports 12, pp. 92–106). Rockville, MD: ASHA.

Basser, L. (1962). Hemiplegia of early onset and the faculty of speech with special reference to the effects of hemispherectomy. *Brain, 85,* 427–460.

Bates, E. (1979a). The biology of symbols: Some concluding thoughts. In E. Bates, T. Benigni, I. Bretherton, L. Camaioni, and V. Volterra (Eds.), *The emer-gence of symbols: Cognition and communication in infancy.* New York: Aca-demic Press.

Bates, E. (1979b). On the evolution and development of symbols. In E. Bates, T. Benigni, I. Bretherton, L. Camaioni, and V. Volterra (Eds.), *The emergence of symbols: Cognition and communication in infancy.* New York: Academic Press.

Bates, E., Benigni, T., Bretherton, I., Camaioni, L., & Volterra, V. (Eds.). (1979). *The emergence of symbols:* Cognition and communication in infancy. New York: Academic Press.

Beadle, K. (1981). Speech and language disturbances in childhood development. In J. K. Darby (Ed.), *Speech evaluation in medicine.* New York: Grune & Stratton.

Bloom, L., & Lahey, M. (1978). *Language development and language disorders.* New York: John Wiley.

Carrow-Woolfok, E., & Lynch, J. (1982). *An integrative approach to language disorders in children.* New York: Grune & Stratton.

Chi, J., Dooling, E., & Gilles, F. (1977a). Left–right asymmetries of the temporal speech areas of the human fetus. *Archives of Neurology, 34,* 346–348.

Chi, J., Dooling, E., & Gilles, F. (1977b). Gyral development of the human brain. *Annals of Neurology, 1,* 86–93.

Corsaro, W. (1979). Sociolinguistic patterns in adult–child interaction. In E. Ochs & B. Schieffelin (Eds.), *Developmental pragmatics.* New York: Academic Press.

Craig, H. K. (1983). Applications of pragmatic language models for intervention. In T. Gallagher & C. Prutting (Eds.), *Pragmatic assessment and intervention issues in language.* San Diego: College-Hill Press.

Curtiss, S. (1977). *Genie: A psycholinguistic study of a modern-day "wild child".* New York: Academic Press.

DeMeyer, M., Hingtgen, J., & Jackson, R. (1981). Infantile autism reviewed: A decade of research. *Schizophrenia Bulletin, 7,* 388–451.

Dennis, M. (1980). Capacity and strategy for syntactic comprehension after left or right hemidecortication. *Brain and Language, 10,* 287–317.

Dennis, M., & Kohn, B. (1975). Comprehension of syntax in infantile hemiplegics after cerebral hemidecortication: Left-hemisphere superiority. *Brain and Language, 2,* 472–482.

Dennis, M., & Whitaker, H. (1976). Language acquisition following hemidecorti-cation: Linguistic superiority of the left over the right hemisphere. *Brain and Language, 3,* 404–433.

Dennis, M., & Whitaker, H. (1977). Hemispheric equipotentiality and language acquisition. In S. Segalowitz & F. Gruber (Eds.), *Language development and neurological theory.* New York: Academic Press.

Dreifuss, F. E. (1975). The pathology of central communicative disorders in children. In D. B. Tower (Ed.), *The nervous system, Vol. 3: Human communication and its disorders.* New York: Raven Press.

Ehrlich, C., Shapiro, E., Kimball, B., & Huttner, M. (1973). Communication skills in five-year-old children with high-risk neonatal histories. *Journal of Speech and Hearing Research, 16,* 522–529.

Entus, A. (1977). Hemispheric asymmetry in processing of dichotically presented speech and nonspeech stimuli by infants. In S. Segalowitz & F. Gruber (Eds.), *Language development and neurological theory.* New York: Academic Press.

Flower, R. M. (1981). Neurodevelopmental disorders in childhood. In J. K. Darby (Ed.), *Speech evaluation in medicine.* New York: Grune & Stratton.

Fowler, W. (1981). A strategy for infant learning and developmental learning. In R. Schiefelbusch & D. Bricker (Eds.), *Early language intervention.* Baltimore: University Park Press.

Frankenburg, W., Dodds, J., & Fandal, A. (1973). *Denver developmental screening test.* Boulder: University of Colorado Medical Center.

Gardiner, M., & Walter, D. (1977). Evidence of hemispheric specialization from infant EEG. In S. Harnad (Ed.), *Lateralization in the nervous system.* New York: Academic Press.

Gerber, S. (1977). High-risk conditions. In S. Gerber (Ed.), *Audiometry in infancy.* New York: Grune & Stratton.

Geschwind, N. (1979). Anatomical foundations of language and dominance. In C. Ludlow & M. Doran-Quine (Eds.), *The neurological bases of language disorders in children: Methods and directions for research* (US Department of HEW NINCDS Monograph No. 2, pp. 145–153). Bethesda, MD: US Department of Health, Education, & Welfare.

Goldman, P. S. (1979). Developmental and plasticity of frontal association cortex in the infrahuman primate. In C. Ludlow & M. Doran-Quine (Eds.), *The neurological bases of language disorders in children: Methods and directions for research* (US Department of HEW NINCDS Monograph No. 2, pp. 1–16). Bethesda, MD: US Department of Health, Education, & Welfare.

Gould, S. J. (1977). *Ontogeny and phylogeny.* Cambridge, MA: Belknap Press, division of Harvard University Press.

Greenwald, C. A., & Leonard, L. B. (1979). Communicative and sensorimotor development of Down's syndrome children. *American Journal of Mental Deficiency, 84,* 296–303.

Guyette, T., & Diedrich, W. (1983). A review of the Screening Test for Developmental Apraxia of Speech. *Language, Speech, and Hearing Services in Schools, 14,* 202–209.

Hall, P. K., & Tomblin, J. B. (1978). A follow-up study of children with articulation and language disorders. *Journal of Speech and Hearing Disorders, 43,* 227–241.

Hecaen, H. (1976). Acquired aphasia in children and the ontogenesis of hemispheric functional specialization. *Brain and Language, 3,* 114–134.

Ingram, D. (1976). *Phonological disability in children.* London: Edward Arnold.

Ingram, T. T. S. (1959). Specific developmental disorders of speech in childhood. *Brain, 82,* 450–467.

Ingram, T. T. S. (1969). Developmental disorders of speech. In P. J. Vinken &

G. W. Bruyn (Eds.), *Handbook of clinical neurology, vol. 4*. Amsterdam: North-Holland.

Ingram, T. T. S. (1975). Speech disorders in childhood. In E. H. Lenneberg & E. Lenneberg (Eds.), *Foundations of language development, vol. 2*. New York: Academic Press.

Joint Committee on Infant Hearing. Position statement 1982. *Pediatrics, 70,* 496–497.

Kinsbourne, M., & Hiscock, M. (1977). Does cerebral dominance develop? In S. Segalowitz & F. Gruber (Eds.), *Language development and neurological theory*. New York: Academic Press.

Kirchner, D., & Skarakis-Doyle, E. (1983). Developmental language disorders: A theoretical perspective. In T. Gallagher & C. Prutting (Eds.), *Pragmatic assessment and intervention issues in language*. San Diego: College-Hill Press.

Koegel, R., Schreibman, L., Britten, K., Burke, J., & O'Neill, R. (1982). A comparison of parent training to direct child treatment. In R. Koegel, A. Rincover, & A. Egel (Eds.), *Educating and understanding autistic children*. San Diego: College-Hill Press.

Krashen, S. (1975). The critical period for language acquisition and its possible basis. *Annals of the New York Academy of Sciences, 263,* 211–224.

Landau, W., Goldstein, R., & Kleffner, F. (1960). Congenital aphasia: A clinico-pathologic study. *Neurology, 10,* 915–921.

Lassman, F., Fisch, R., Vetter, D., & LaBenz, E. (Eds.). (1980). *Early correlates of speech, language and hearing: The Collaborative Perinatal Project of the National Institute of Neurological and Communicative Disorders and Stroke*. Littleton, MA: PSG.

Launer, P. B., & Lahey, M. (1981). Passages: From the fifties to the eighties in language assessment. *Topics in Language Disorders, 1,* 11–30.

Lecours, A. (1975). Myelogentic correlates of the development of speech and language. In E. H. Lenneberg & E. Lenneberg (Eds.), *Foundations of language devlopment, vol. 1*. New York: Academic Press.

Lemire, R., Loeser, J., Leech, R., & Alvord, E. (1975). *Normal and abnormal development of the human nervous system*. New York: Harper & Row.

Lenneberg, E. H. (1966). Speech development: Its anatomical and physiological concomitants. In E. Carterette (Ed.), *Brain function, vol. 3*. Berkeley: University of California Press.

Lenneberg, E. H. (1967). *Biological foundations of language*. New York: John Wiley.

Lenneberg, E. H. (1979). On explaining language. *Science, 164,* 635–643.

Leonard, L. (1979). Language impairment in children. *Merrill-Palmer Quarterly, 25,* 205–232.

Ludlow, C. (1979). Research directions and needs concerning the neurological bases of language disorders in children. In C. Ludlow & M. Doran-Quine (Eds.), *The neurological bases of language disorders in children: Methods and directions for research* (US Department of HEW NINCDS Monograph No. 2, pp. 183–192). Bethesda, MD: US Department of Health, Education, & Welfare.

Ludlow, C. (1980). Children's language disorders: Recent research advances. *Annals of Neurology, 7,* 497–507.

Luria, A. (1966). *Higher cortical functions in man*. New York: Basic Books.

Lyngaas, K., Nyberg, B., Hoekenga, R., & Grunewald, L. (1983). Language intervention in the multiple contexts of the public school setting. In J. Miller, D. Yoder, & R. Schiefelbusch (Eds.), *Contemporary issues in language intervention* (American Speech–Language–Hearing Association, ASHA Reports 12, pp. 239–252). Rockville, MD: ASHA.

McCauley, R., & Swisher, L. (1984). Psychometric review of language and articulation tests for preschool children. *Journal of Speech and Hearing Disorders, 49,* 34–42.

Meyer, D., & Wolfe, V. (1975). Use of a high-risk register in newborn hearing screening. *Journal of Speech and Hearing Disorders, 40,* 493–498.

Miller, J. F. (1981). *Assessing language production in children: Experimental procedures.* Baltimore: University Park Press.

Miller, J. F. (1983). Identifying children with language disorders and describing their language performance. In J. Miller, D. Yoder, & R. Schiefelbusch (Eds.), *Contemporary issues in language intervention* (American Speech–Language–Hearing Association, ASHA Reports 12, pp. 61–74).

Milner, E. (1976). CNS maturation and language acquisition. In H. Whitaker & H. Whitaker (Eds.), *Studies in neurolinguistics, vol. 1.* New York: Academic Press.

Molfese, D., Freeman, R., & Palermo, D. (1975). The ontogeny of brain lateralization for speech and nonspeech stimuli. *Brain and Language, 2,* 356–368.

Mueller, E., & Brenner, J. (1977). The origins of social skills and interactions among playgroup toddlers. *Child Development, 48,* 854–861.

Muma, J. (1978). *Language handbook: Concepts, assessment, intervention.* Englewood Cliffs, NJ: Prentice-Hall.

Nelson, K. (1981). Individual differences in language development: Implications for development and language. *Developmental Psychology, 17,* 170–187.

Peters, A. M. (1983). *The units of language acquisition.* Cambridge, MA: Cambridge University Press.

Prutting, C. A. (1982). Pragmatics as social competence. *Journal of Speech and Hearing Disorders, 47,* 123–134.

Rees, N. S. (1983). Language intervention with children. In J. Miller, D. Yoder, & R. Schiefelbusch (Eds.), *Contemporary issues in language intervention* (American Speech–Language–Hearing Association, ASHA Reports 12, pp. 309–316).

Ritvo, E., & Freeman, B. (1978). N.S.A.C. definition of childhood autism. *Journal of Autism and Childhood Schizophrenia, 8,* 162–167.

Rosenbek, J., & Wertz, R. (1972). A review of 50 cases of developmental apraxia of speech. *Language, Speech and Hearing Services in Schools, 3,* 23–33.

Rutter, M. (1978). Diagnosis and definition of childhood autism. *Journal of Autism and Childhood Schizophrenia, 8,* 139–161.

Schiefelbusch, R. L. (Ed.). (1980). *Nonspeech language and communication.* Baltimore: University Park Press.

Schiefelbusch, R., & Bricker, D. (Eds.). (1981). *Early language intervention.* Baltimore: University Park Press.

Schumaker, J. B., & Sherman, J. A. (1978). Parent as intervention agent: From birth onward. In R. Schiefelbusch (Ed.), *Language intervention strategies.* Baltimore: University Park Press.

Segalowitz, S. (1983). Cerebral asymmetries of speech in infancy. In S. Segalowitz (Ed.), *Language functions and brain organization.* New York: Academic Press.

Segalowitz, S., & Chapman, J. (1980). Cerebral asymmetry for speech in neonates: A behavioral measure. *Brain and Language, 9,* 281–288.

Seibert, J. M., & Oller, D. K. (1981). Linguistic pragmatics and language intervention strategies. *Journal of Autism and Developmental Disorders, 11,* 75–88.

Shane, H. (1980). Approaches to assessing the communication of non-oral persons. In R. Schiefelbusch (Ed.), *Nonspeech language and communication.* Baltimore: University Park Press.

Shriberg, L., & Kwiatkowski, J. (1982). Phonological disorders I: A diagnostic classification system. *Journal of Speech and Hearing Disorders, 47,* 226–241.

Shriner, T., Halloway, M., & Daniloff, R. (1969). The relationship between articulatory deficits and syntax in speech defective children. *Journal of Speech and Hearing Research, 12,* 319–325.

Snyder, L. (1983). From assessment to intervention: Problems and solutions. In J. Miller, D. Yoder, & R. Schiefelbusch (Eds.), *Contemporary issues in language intervention* (American Speech–Language–Hearing Association, ASHA Reports 12, pp. 147–164).

Spradlin, J. E., & Siegel, G. M. (1982). Language training in natural and clinical environments. *Journal of Speech and Hearing Disorders, 47,* 2–6.

Wada, J., Clarke, R., & Hamm, A. (1975). Cerebral hemispheric asymmetry in humans. *Archives of Neurology, 32,* 239–246.

Wetherby, A. M., & Prutting, C. A. (1984). Profiles of communicative and cognitive–social abilities in autistic children. *Journal of Speech and Hearing Research. 27,* 364–377.

Wetherby, A. M. (1984). Possible neurolinguistic breakdown in autistic children. *Topics in Language Disorders. 4,* 19–33.

Williams, R., Ingham, R., & Rosenthal, J. (1981). A further analysis for developmental apraxia of speech in children with defective articulation. *Journal of Speech and Hearing Research, 24,* 496–505.

Williston, J., & Schimmel, R. (1981). Auditory evoked responses. In J. K. Darby (Ed.), *Speech evaluation in medicine.* New York: Grune & Stratton.

Witelson, S., & Pallie, W. (1973). Left hemisphere specialization for language in the newborn. *Brain, 96,* 641–646.

Woods, B., & Carey, S. (1978). Language deficits after apparent clinical recovery from childhood aphasia. *Annals of Neurology, 6,* 405–409.

Woods, B., & Teuber, H. (1978). Changing patterns of childhood aphasia. *Annals of Neurology, 3,* 273–280.

Yakovlev, P., & Lecours, A. (1967). The myelogentic cycles of regional maturation of the brain. In A. Minakowski (Ed.), *Regional development of the brain in early life.* Philadelphia: F. A. Davis.

Zaidel, E. (1979). The split and half brains as models of congenital language disability. In C. Ludlow & M. Doran-Quine (Eds.), *The neurological bases of language disorders in children:* Methods and directions for research (US Department of HEW NINCDS Monograph No. 2, pp. 55–86). Bethesda, MD: US Department of Health, Education, & Welfare.

Linda Swisher

2

Language Disorders in Children

Language disorders are attributable to several factors, which operate singly or in combination (see Table 2-1). Brain dysfunction is the most commonly assumed etiology. Although a standard neurologic examination including computerized tomography scan and electroencephalogram (EEG) usually does not result in positive findings, Rapin (1977) reported that most of the children with a language disorder seen in her neurological practice have other symptoms of brain dysfunction. She considers this an expected finding if one assumes that brain dysfunction in a child would need to be quite extensive to preclude normal language acquisition.

In addition to brain dysfunction, hearing loss and deafness can clearly underlie a language disorder. Atypical input from caregivers must also be considered as a possible contributing factor. Evidence clearly links the impoverished language stimulation characteristic of some institutions to depressed language acquisition in some children

B. Rende assisted with the section on aphasia, M. Tindell with the section on mental retardation, N. Matkin and I. Rapin with the section on auditory disorders, and L. Jaffee and S. Kirk commented on the section on dyslexia. The following provided constructive suggestions concerning the entire chapter: M. Barnett, N. Gibb, and G. Wallace. S. Strinka typed, she and B. Bardram retyped the chapter, smiling most of the time. C. Lowe and W. Swisher kept me smiling. I thank them all.

Preparation of this paper was supported by Grant No. G008301459 from the U. S. Department of Education.

Speech and Language Evaluation in Neurology:
Childhood Disorders
ISBN 0-8089-1719-6

Table 2-1
Possible Etiology by Diagnostic Category

	Brain	Ear	Caregiver
Specific language impairment	X		/
Deafness		X	/
Hearing loss		X	/
Dyslexia	X		/
Mental retardation	X		/
Autism	X		/
Hyperverbal, hydrocephalic	X		/
Aphasia	X		/
Auditory agnosia	X		/

X = "Major" problem; / = contributing or maintaining problem.

(e.g., Lyle, 1959). In addition, as pointed out by Swisher, Wooten, and Thompson (1977), the children who are not provided with adequate nutrition are at risk not only for a generalized delay but also for an even poorer level of language acquisition. In a more normal setting, however, a caregiver very seldom would appear to be the primary problem. The possibility that language facilitation has been adversely altered by the child's disorder is more likely. The child's language levels lead the caregiver one way, while the child's physical development leads the caregiver another. Not all caregivers respond well to these conflicting cues.

PREVALENCE AND INCIDENCE

Figures for the prevalence of different syndromes that include a language disorder are "guesstimates." Only recently, for example, have language disorders been considered separately from speech disorders. The American Speech and Hearing Committee of the Midcentury White House Conference (Johnson et al., 1952) estimated that 5 percent of children and youth in the United States have "speech disorders" and 0.5 percent have "impaired hearing" with speech defects. No category dealt with language disorders. Prevalence estimates vary from 5.3 percent (Morley, 1965) to 8.4 percent (Silva, 1980), depending on the age of the children studied and the severity and type of the disorder. Leske (1979) points out that the magnitude of the problem is probably underestimated. It is, however, clear that many neurologic disorders that include a language disorder are far more common in boys than girls.

DELAYED OR DIFFERENT LANGUAGE DEVELOPMENT

The Handbook of Applied Psycholinguistics (Rosenberg, 1982) contains excellent, thorough reviews of the language characteristics of children with specific language impairment (Leonard, 1982), mental retardation (Rosenberg, 1982), autism (Fay & Mermelstein, 1982), and deafness (Quigley & King, 1982). Hearing impairment receives a similar, thorough review by Norlin and Van Tasell (1980).

In the 1960s the work of Chomsky (1957) resulted in a focus on the word order (syntax) of a child's language. Then Bloom (1970) touched off investigations concerning the meanings (semantics) of the words being expressed. In the late 1970s the use of language in everyday context (pragmatics) began to be described. Most of these studies, e.g., the study by Leonard, Bolders, and Miller (1976), focused on children with specific language impairments. These studies of one language domain with controls matched for the average length of their utterances, revealed mostly delays, that is, that children with specific language disorders appeared to have language features similar to those of younger, normal children.

The compelling evidence for differences, i.e., language features not characteristic of normal children of any age, comes from comparing development across the major domains of expressive language. For example, most children with autistic behaviors are appropriately described as having (1) expressive language that is different from normal children because of superficial form, i.e., form at a higher level than the meaning being represented, and (2) a form–context mismatch, i.e., well-developed form inappropriately used.

Table 2-2 summarizes by diagnostic category the type of disorder for the major domains of expressive language. Until recently most investigators have focused only on the form of a child's expressive utterances and have studied only one disability group, so different procedures have been used with different groups. Therefore, the summary is necessarily guided by my clinical experience as well as published results. Although the history and physical findings are useful in differentiating disorders, this summary is included because the expressive language characteristics also serve as important clues to the diagnostic category. Table 2-2 will be referred to within the section for each category.

As indicated in Table 2-2, the meaning base of language that the form represents is available to children in most categories except those with mental retardation, autism, and hydrocephalus. This is consistent with a definition by exclusion. By definition, the children in the other groups must have normal, nonlanguage cognitive development; i.e., they

Table 2-2
Spoken Expressive Language Characteristics: A Summary
Simplification by Diagnostic Category

Diagnostic Category	Form	Meaning	Use
Specific language impairment	*Delayed**	Needs form to be expressed	Needs form to be expressed
Deafness	*Delayed*	Needs form to be expressed	Needs form to be expressed
Hearing Loss	*Delayed*	Needs form to be expressed	Needs form to be expressed
**Dyslexia, language based	*Delayed*	Needs form to be expressed	Needs form to be expressed
Mental retardation	Delayed	*Delayed*	Needs form and meaning to be expressed
Autism	Delayed	Different; poorer than form	*Different; poorer than form*
Hyperverbal, hydrocephalic	Delayed	Different; poorer than form	Different; poorer than form
Aphasia	*Different*	?	?
Auditory Agnosia	?	Needs form input	Needs form and meaning to be expressed

* What might be considered to be the "major" deficit is italicized for each category.
** No spoken language disorder is expected for "pure" dyslexic children.

must have ideas even though they do not have the words and sentence types to express them. Likewise, children in most of the groups listed use words and sentences appropriately if they are adequately mapped onto their meaning base. The exceptions include children in the autistic, hyperverbal–hydrocephalic, and aphasic categories. Autistic children, probably because of their disinclination to communicate, are especially noteworthy in their different use of words and sentences.

Congenital etiologies tend to affect expression of language form in a grossly similar fashion. When scored as either present or absent, delayed rather than different form characterizes the output. When scored in terms of frequency of occurrence, the least frequently occurring structures used by normal children are usually even less frequently used by developmentally disabled groups. This is one way in which their language is different.

SYNDROMES

Not only are there many different groups of children with a language disorder, but there are also intra-group differences. For example, although children with autistic behaviors are not easily confused with children who have a hearing loss, not all children with autistic behaviors are alike in language, behavior, or histories. Within categories there are individual differences which relate primarily to the level of severity of the disorder. Having acknowledged that noteworthy differences exist within syndromes, this chapter will proceed to highlight what is usual within nine syndrome categories. What will be described must be understood as probable rather than inevitable. Never expect, however, to find that what is summarized in this chapter applies to any one child. Assume that the descriptions apply to *group averages,* be sure to assess, evaluate the results, and intervene until you can judge for yourself whether what is summarized here is true of the individual child before you. This chapter only provides a framework for beginning the evaluation and management process. There are remarkable developmental surprises in children. Therefore, we must wait and document what develops over time for each child.

This chapter is addressed primarily to the neurologist and thus relies heavily on a medical orientation. The reader is advised to read it as a whole. To avoid redundancies, comments were placed where they would apply to the most children in a given diagnostic category. For example, comments about prognosis in relation to level of intellectual functioning, which occur in the section concerning autism, apply to all children with a developmental disability.

SPECIFIC LANGUAGE IMPAIRMENT

Language disorder occurs in relative isolation in the diagnostic categories of specific language impairment, dyslexia, and aphasia. Specific language impairment is a term applied to children who have the following characteristics: normal performance IQs, delayed language form, and no other obvious primary problems. In line with the definition by exclusion (Benton, 1964), should motor symptoms be present, they are noted as additional problems. Specific language impairment was noted in approximately 5.7 percent of approximately 200 three year olds assessed by Stevenson and Richman (1976).

Various authors have used different terms to describe this group of children, for example, infantile speech (Menyuk, 1964), developmental aphasia (Benton, 1964), deviant language (Leonard, 1972), and language disorder (Rees, 1973). The terms reflect the authors' theoretical orientations more than differences among groups of children.

The experience of Stark and Tallal (1981) suggests that the diagnosis of specific language impairment is most frequently misapplied to children with mental retardation. Of 132 children referred to their study of specific language impairment, 37 percent scored below an IQ of 85 on the revised Weschsler Intelligence Scale for Children or the Wechsler Pre-School and Primary Scale of Intelligence.

Etiology

Relatively few children with specific language impairment have chromosomal abnormalities, and it is not clear if or how particular gene combinations or types of gene transmissions are related to developmental speech and language problems (Cooper & Ludlow, Chapter 8; Darby, Kidd, and Cavalli-Sforza, Chapter 9). The consensus is that the primary deficit is a brain dysfunction. As mentioned earlier, Rapin (1977) has reported that most children with a language disorder seen in her neurological practice have other symptoms of brain dysfunction. In addition, there is some evidence that parents of children with specific language impairment show less accommodation to their needs. For example, Kriegsmann, Wulbert, Inglis, and Mills (1975) found that the mothers of language-disordered children were more restrictive and punitive, and less responsive, than those of normal children of the same age. It is not clear whether the differences are due to the adults, the children, or an interaction between the two. Possibly, for example, the mothers of the language-disordered children were attempting to increase the children's language performance levels by more prompting and directiveness than is necessary for controls matched for age.

Correlates

Articulation

Children with specific language impairment are necessarily similar only in that their performance IQs are within the normal range and exceed their verbal IQs, and that hearing loss or other major involvements are not present. They do not have an execution or motor impairment severe enough to qualify as apractic (see Marquardt, Dunn, & Davis, Chapter 4) or dysarthric. An articulation disorder, however, is not uncommon (Affolter, Brubaker, & Bischofberger, 1974; Aram & Nation, 1975; Demetras, Matkin, & Swisher, 1982; Stark & Tallal, 1981). Stark and Tallal excluded 9 of 132 subjects because the severity of the articulation disorder indicated a mixed problem.

Nonlanguage Cognitive Skills

Piaget (1962) postulated that language is only one part of a more global system of representation. Central to his position is the view that language is one of several symbolic skills and that the acquisition of language is correlated with the development of other representational skills. If representation skills turn out to be interdependent, then no child would be appropriately described as specific language impaired. Each would be expected to have a disorder in some other behaviors, e.g., pretend play. In fact, several studies of specific language impaired children (e.g., Inhelder, 1963; Kamhi, 1981) have indicated that they are less skilled than their normal, same-age peers in several other areas of mental representation. Kamhi (1981) reported that language-disordered children performed at a lower level than normal children matched for mental age on the Leiter International Performance Scale. This finding contrasts, for example, with Furth's (1966) findings that most deaf children have other areas of respresentational skills intact.

Thus the view that language is independent of all other cognitive skills is in need of some modification, such as has been suggested by Curtiss (1981). She reviews cases that illustrate that semantic skills appear to be deeply linked to broader conceptual development, but that morphologic and syntactic skills do not. She would therefore predict a high correlation between semantics and nonlanguage representational skills, but not necessarily between syntactic skills and nonlanguage representational skills. As Ludlow (1980) noted, most children with specific language impairment have a syntactic type of language disorder.

In summary, it is now clear that language-disordered children with a presumed brain dysfunction perform well on some but not all so-called nonverbal tasks. Undoubtedly, overall cognitive development is necessary, but not sufficient, for the development of meaningful language. The degree of correlation obtained will vary depending on the types of both language and nonlanguage tasks assessed. It is possible, however, to identify children who score within the normal range on nonverbal IQ measures (Stark & Tallal, 1981).

Motor Skills

There is some evidence that children with specific language impairment can be somewhat clumsy. Affolter, Brubaker, and Bischofberger (1974) studied fine and gross motor skills in their clinical population of language-disordered children. They observed hand–eye coordination on tasks such as climbing, inserting a key in a lock, building simple block constructions, and doing intricate close-fitting puzzles. The children appeared to lose hand–eye coordination whenever a problem or situation reached a certain level of complexity or involved more than one modality. In another study, King, Jones, and Lasky (1982) described the motor skills of 50 communicatively impaired children during the initial evaluation and again in a follow-up survey 15 years later. Initially, they noted possible motor coordination problems in 64 percent of the 18 subjects classified as language disordered, and 28 percent of the 7 subjects classified as language and articulation disordered. Of the 11 subjects reported to exhibit motor coordination problems, only 4 participated in athletics in school. Of these 11 subjects, 33 percent had been diagnosed as language disordered, and 14 percent as language and articulation disordered.

History of Recurrent Otitis Media

A history of severe recurrent otitis media has been linked recently to learning disability by many but not all investigators. As will be discussed in the section on auditory disorders, data from Tonini (1983) do not indicate that such a history accounts for children with specific language impairment. If, however, a child has a preexisting language problem, otitis media with specific language impairment may well complicate the child's progress.

Auditory Processing

The findings concerning auditory processing and language disorder have been equivocal (see Rees, 1973). More recently, Tallal and Piercy (1973, 1975) have claimed that language-disordered children have particular difficulty with tones and speech sounds presented at rapid rates. Leonard (1982), however, noted that the characteristics of language-disordered children's expressive language are not predicted by this hypothesis. Ludlow, Cudahy, Bassich, and Brown (1982) found no exclusive relationship between language disorder and auditory temporal processing deficits. They also found that temporal order perceptual capabilities were poorest for hyperactive boys with normal language and normal reading skills compared with language-disordered and reading-disabled boys. As they noted, this finding suggests that poor auditory temporal processing can exist in the presence of normal language function.

Socioemotional Development

It is unrealistic to expect a child who is experiencing difficulty communicating with others to have social behavior clearly within "normal" limits. King, Jones, and Lasky (1982) reported that families noted problems in social and interpersonal relationships for 4 of 18 children initially diagnosed as language-disordered. One was reported to experience difficulty in relationships with family, siblings, and peers, and to have received professional help. Another was reported to have problems in sibling relationships, and the remaining two had difficulty in peer relationships.

Language

Because language comprehension may be equal to or better than language expression, a composite score based on the averaging of comprehension and expressive skills may be misleading. The severity of disorder and degree of discrepancy between comprehension and expression also varies. The results of Stark, Tallal, and Mellits (1982) indicate that standardized, norm-referenced language tests will reveal deficits that are not obvious on a verbal IQ test, particularly in language-disordered children 8 years of age or older. As will be discussed later, the results of Demetras, Matkin, and Swisher (1982) indicated that mild cases may have a language disorder so specific that it is only obvious from analysis of a spontaneous language sample.

Investigators have described difficulties in the expression of form (Johnston & Schery, 1976), meaning (Freedman & Carpenter, 1976), and the use of language (Gallagher, 1977). Form appears to be the area of greatest deficit (see Table 2-2). The meaning substrate is expected to be better developed in line with the criterion that nonverbal IQ scores fall within the normal range. If a child does not have adequate form, then use of form would be expected to be impaired as well. Typically, the case studies (Morley, Court, Miller, & Garside, 1955) indicate that these children acquire their words at a later age and at a slower rate than normal children. Children's language form appears delayed except for their occasional use of a less mature form relative to their other language skills, and failure to use an expected mature form.

Brinton and Fujiki (1982) compared the discourse characteristics of language-disordered and normal children by examining interactive request–response sequences. Twelve children, 5½–6 years of age were grouped into three dyads of language-disordered children and three of normal language children. All the disordered subjects were delayed at least 1 year on the Carrow Elicited Language Inventory and exhibited a variety of syntactic problems in spontaneous language production. The authors suggested that the language-disordered children appeared to be less aware of the interactive nature of discourse than normal children; e.g., they often did not respond or inappropriately responded to requests.

Management

The nonlanguage representational deficits obvious from systematic testing of a child with specific language impairment would not be noticed during an informal, clinical observation. If cognitive skills other than language appear to be a problem, the neurologist is wise to consider referral to a clinical psychologist for assessment of the child's performance IQ level. The presence of emotional maladjustment would indicate that language intervention should begin as soon as possible. Depending on the type and severity of the maladjustment, traditional psychotherapy could be delayed and implemented only if gains in language are not accompanied by gains in social interactions.

The language needs of these children are straightforward: to develop more words and sentences to express their ideas. Priorities have been listed in order of importance by Swisher and Matkin (1984): communication, quantity, language comprehension, language expression, and finally, articulation. Because the first priority is communication, all language objectives are to serve the child's needs. The amount of speech observed in the clinic is to be as much as heard elsewhere by caregivers before language facilitation begins. Articulation is addressed when language gains are not improving the intelligibility of a child's speech or if articulation has stabilized and is drawing adverse attention. Because expressive language is observable and the comprehension of language is not, and because more is known concerning the sequences of language expression than comprehension, the language objectives are initially derived from an expressive language sample obtained during play with another child, the clinician, and a caregiver.

The two major approaches to intervention, specific abilities and developmental, are addressed in a book on current therapies edited by Perkins (1984). Tomblin (1984) reviews the data that indicate that the specific abilities approach is theoretically unsound. Current theory and data in cognitive psychology support the developmental approach (e.g., Snyder-McLean, 1984; Swisher & Matkin, 1984), which relies heavily on the recent data concerning normal language acquisition (e.g., Bloom & Lahey, 1978). The developmental approach is in line with Piagetian theory, which predicts that what a child is ready to learn is best determined by what the child already knows. The assumption is made that stages of language evolve in a relatively consistent fashion for all children. It is also assumed that the natural conditions found universally in native language acquisition appear to be the best to simulate when aiding a child with a language disorder. Leonard's (1981) review indicates that all treatment strategies that have been used with these children are better than none at all. Improvements in rate (Leonard, 1975) or level of attainment (Friedman & Friedman, 1980) have been reported for all strategies employed. The pertinent issue at present is to determine the most appropriate intervention for each child.

Be cautious of clinicians whose language lessons are derived from information from standardized tests. As pointed out by McCauley and Swisher (1984), norm-referenced tests do not adequately sample a range of language skills, and performance on individual test items represents only possible deficits and competencies in real life. They also point out that the use of norm-referenced tests to plan therapy objectives invalidates the tests as indices of ability.

Prognosis

In general, results demonstrate that children with a preschool language disorder constitute a high-risk group for subsequent academic difficulties. Most academic subjects are based on language concepts and the child with a preschool language disorder appears to be at risk for experiencing later language-learning problems. Thus, one major reason to identify and help children with specific language impairment early in childhood is to decrease the number who require special services in school.

Many reading specialists (e.g., De Hirsch, 1971) have suggested that language skills in the preschool child are the best predictors of later reading levels. Although the studies have been retrospective and have not been restricted to children with specific language impairment, the majority of studies indicate that this suggestion is well-founded.

Hall and Tomblin (1978) conducted a follow-up study of 18 language disordered and 18 articulation-impaired subjects 13–20 years following initial contact with a speech and hearing clinic. They obtained two types of data regarding academic achievement: parental report of the highest education level achieved by their child and results from the Iowa Tests of Basic Skills and the Iowa Test of Educational Development. Parent reports indicated that all subjects were currently completing or had completed high school. Fewer of the language-disordered subjects obtained a higher education (44.4%) than articulation-disordered subjects (77.8%). Results from standardized educational testing showed that the language-disordered subjects consistently scored at lower levels than the articulation-disordered subjects, particularly in reading. A quote from this paper, however, must not go unnoticed. Remember the study was conducted in children initially seen from 1955 to 1962 when language therapy was in its neonatal stage. They state " . . . that most of the reported services given during that time were for articulation disorders, and thus the language deficits were not treated" (p. 238).

As will be discussed further in the section on mental retardation and autism, it is to the preschool child's benefit to consider an IQ test to have *no* predictive value. It is not uncommon to find that the estimate improves over time. Aram, Ekelman, and Nation (1984) provided follow-up data for 20 adolescents described 10 years earlier (Aram & Nation, 1975). They had originally excluded children with neurologic abnormalities, hearing problems, and craniofacial defects; and no IQ criterion was set. The prediction of stable, more generalized retardation was accurate for only 3 of 7 children who received a Leiter performance IQ score below 85 during their preschool years. Five of the remaining 16 children (31%) had been educated in regular classes with no special services. The remaining 11 (69%) had required repeating one or more grades, special tutoring, or placement in a learning disability class. They continued to have poor language skills and low academic achievement, and were rated by their parents as being less socially competent and having more behavioral disorders than their peers.

APHASIA

Aphasia refers to a language disorder acquired as a result of a cerebral insult after a period of normal development. More about these children is summarized by Ewing-Cobbs, Fletcher, Landry, and Levin (Chapter 3). This term also is applied to the language disorder that accompanies a rare syndrome involving a convulsive disorder. These language disorders will be discussed in this section. Postictal, transient aphasia, and the aphasia associated with a hemiplegia present at birth will not be discussed.

Premorbid and postmorbid assessments of language and nonlanguage skills in aphasic children with well-defined brain lesions are lacking. Most of the reports have discussed a small number of children, and nonstandardized tests or clinical impressions have formed the data base. Age of onset in relation to pattern of impairment and prognosis seldom has been addressed.

Cerebral Insult

Children with an aphasia secondary to a cerebral insult, in most instances a trauma, are initially nonfluent. Although exceptions occur, many then become telegraphic and agrammatic. Severity of receptive involvement varies from severe to nonexistent. Degree of recovery ranges from poor to possibly complete over a period of a few days to several years. As indicated in Table 2-2, it is possible but not clear that their language form is better described as different rather than delayed. More information is needed to describe the extent to which the meaning and use of words is impaired.

Aphasias due to cerebral insult in children between roughly 3 and 15 years of age differ from those observed in adults in at least the following ways. The younger the child at the time of onset, the more likely that a right hemisphere or bilateral insult rather than a left hemisphere insult has occurred (e.g., Guttmann, 1942). Fluent aphasias do not appear to occur in children (e.g., Rapin, 1977). Recovery tends to be more rapid and to a higher level (e.g., Riese & Collison, 1964). As with adults, trauma cases tend to improve more than stroke cases. The academic deficiencies that can remain have been attributed to general brain damage (Alajouanine & Lhermitte, 1965; Guttmann, 1942) and to residual language problems (Woods & Carey, 1979).

Guttmann (1942) described 16 aphasic children who were 14 years old or younger. Fourteen of these children had a left hemisphere lesion, one had a right hemisphere lesion, and one had bilateral lesions. Receptive and expressive abilities were assessed through observation and nonstandardized tests. There was an absence of spontaneous speech immediately after the insult and varying degrees of receptive impairment. The absence of spontaneous speech was without regard to the site of lesion. Only one child presented auditory comprehension as the primary problem. Guttman also studied recovery from one month to 10 years after hospital discharge in 10 of these children. He considered half to have recovered completely. A telegraphic style, hesitations, and dysarthria were characteristic of the speech of the three with long standing extensive speech and language disorders.

Basser's (1962) observations are in line with those of Guttmann (1942). He studied 19 children with an aphasia associated with hemiplegia. Receptive abilities were reported to be intact but no formal test results were presented in support of this observation. All the children had reportedly lost their speech and then improved over a period of several days to 2 years. The extent of improvement was not described.

Riese and Collison (1964) described four children between 4 and 10 years of age who acquired aphasia secondary to trauma. One was considered to have recovered completely after 2 months; another had regained most of the speech and language skills 4 years after sustaining brain damage at 6 years of age. Two (ages 8 and 9 years) never fully recovered.

Alajouanine and Lhermitte (1965) studied 32 children between the ages of 6 and 15 years who acquired aphasia due to a traumatic injury. Within an average of 3 months after their insult, 22 of the children were dysarthric and 20 of these had hemiplegia. Spontaneous speech was almost nonexistent in many of the children, and written language was impaired. Receptive impairment was reported to be rare but no test results were reported in support of this conclusion. If some degree of expressive language was present, it was considered to be syntactically simplified rather than grammatically incorrect. The 32 children were divided into two groups (nine children, ages 5–9 years; and 23 children, ages 10–15 years) to analyze the effect of age of onset on the aphasic symptoms. Six from the entire group were considered to have completely recovered their spontaneous speech. There was no significant difference in the rate of recovery between the younger and older groups. There was a difference in the onset of recovery, however, the younger children appeared delayed in beginning to recover. None of the children followed a normal academic progression. The authors cited Guttman's (1942) findings concerning generalized brain damage to account for the impaired intellectual development observed in the majority of the children.

Woods and Carey (1979) compared 11 children who acquired brain damage from a single, unilateral, nonprogressive cerebral lesion before their first birthday with 16 who sustained the same types of brain damage at a later age (mean age 5.7 years). The average age at time of testing for the group with early lesions was 17.8 years (range 10.2–25.5 years) and the mean age at testing for the group with later lesions was 15.3 years (range 8.6–24.5 years). Eight speech–language tasks were administered: picture naming, spelling, completing rhymes, sentence completion, relations task, syntactical judgments, ask–tell task, and the Token test. Children in the group that suffered lesions later in life scored significantly lower than the controls on all tasks except for rhyme completion. The earlier lesion group was significantly different from the controls only on the performance of the spelling task and the Token test. The authors interpreted their results as refuting the widely-held view that children who recover from acquired aphasia do so completely.

Convulsive Disorder

Children with a convulsive disorder and an associated aphasia which appears roughly between 3 and 15 years of age initially develop a marked receptive language impairment after a period of normal speech and language development. A gradual deterioration of speech and expressive language abilities follows. The residual expressive language presents in many ways, from none at all to telegraphic to jargon. Their language skills improve gradually over a period of several months or years and there is a wide range of recovery patterns, from almost complete to very little progress. The form of language appears to be different from that of a normally developing child of any age (see Table 2-2).

Most of these children have normal hearing, but some may have mild losses. A history of seizure activity usually but not always precedes the onset of the language disorder. The abnormal EEGs, primarily in the temporal lobe and the temporoparietal region, tend to become less abnormal as the language skills improve. Nonverbal IQ tests reveal that most of these children have normal intelligence. Their language skills improve gradually over a period of several months or years and there is a wide range of recovery patterns, from almost complete to very little progress. As indicated in Table 2-2, the form of language may appear to be different from that of a normally developing child of any age.

Landau and Kleffner (1957) were the first to identify this syndrome. They presented case histories of six children (ages 6–15 years). Normal speech and language development occurred until parents observed a decline in the amount of understanding of language by the children. The children were described as appearing to become "deaf." Two were given formal audiometric testing and were considered to have hearing within a normal range. Receptive language abilities were not formally tested. Expressive language abilities gradually declined after the receptive impairment was observed. Expressive language problems (i.e. jargon, anomia, imitation impairment, stutter-like dysfluencies) varied widely and increased over time until no speech was present in some cases. Formal nonverbal intelligence scores indicated that five children were within normal limits with the sixth being slightly below normal. Neurological examinations for all the children were normal; however, a history of seizure activity and abnormal EEG pattern was present in all the children. The severity of language disorder tended to positively correlate with EEG abnormalities and to improve as the EEG patterns normalized. One child spontaneously recovered both receptive and expressive language skills a few weeks after onset. The others improved after several months or years of special instruction.

Subsequent reports corroborated the findings of Landau and Kleffner (1957). Worster-Drought (1971) presented 14 case histories of children who had acquired aphasia between the ages of 3 and 7 years. A marked receptive language deficit was the salient feature. Comprehension skills ranged from none to adequate for simple language. Formal receptive tests used included the Terman-Merrill test of simple commands and the Peabody Picture Vocabulary Test. Expressive language abilities were tested informally. All had some articulation errors ranging from slight to severe. Abnormal EEGs were present in all the children but became more normal as the speech and language skills improved. Audiometric testing indicated that eight children had normal hearing while six presented mild hearing losses. Nonverbal IQ tests indicated normal levels of functioning in each child. Gradual recovery was reported; however, the means of measuring improvement was not described. Nevertheless, language abilities were considered to have improved to a normal or near-normal level for six children, while eight were considered to have improved only a little. Visual inspection of the data did not reveal a clear relationship between the age of onset or degree of expressive or receptive impairment and the amount of recovery.

Mantovani and Landau (1980) provided a fairly thorough description of language skills in nine children examined 10–28 years after the onset of aphasia and noted both poverty of expression and jargon. The Porch Index of Communicative Ability and the Modified Token Test were administered. Results were normal for three of the children and indicated mild or moderate impairment for four. Intelligence testing included the Wechsler Intelligence Scale (eight children), Slossen Intelligence Test (one child), and Revised Benton Visual Retention Test (eight children). All were found to have average or above-average nonverbal intelligence. Improvement varied: 10–28 years after onset, four were normal, one had mild language difficulties, and four were moderately language disordered. Seven had normal neurologic examinations except for the language dysfunction. Five of the nine had clinical seizures, four of whom had seizures prior to the onset of language difficulty. The continuation of seizure activity with age varied. The authors point out that children with this syndrome do not necessarily have clinical seizures but that a paroxymsal EEG is characteristic.

Management

Intervention should be focused immediately on the child and the family in relation to the major change that has occurred in their lives. The family may need to be (1) assured that the child has not "lost his mind," (2) prepared to wait and see how improvement proceeds, and (3) involved in the treatment process.

Tests of all language modalities that are age appropriate should be administered. Because tests of all four language modalities standardized on the same children are not available, implications concerning pattern of impairment across modalities must be severely limited (McCauley & Swisher, 1984b). In mild cases, the tests should be those considered sensitive to language disorder such as the Token Test (Needham & Swisher, 1972). A nonverbal intelligence test such as the Hiskey-Nebraska should be administered as one measure of generalized dysfunction. A hearing test is necessary for any child suspected of having a language disorder but especially for one with a convulsive disorder. In addition to the developmentally based language objectives recommended for all children with a language disorder, the clinician may need to help the child to become aware of his or her errors and to self-correct. All language modalities appropriate for the child's level must be addressed. If the child is improving rapidly, it may not be in his or her best interest to re-enter regular school while still obviously impaired. Tutoring at home or in a clinic may be more appropriate in order to lessen adverse attention from peers. If the child attends regular school, then academic areas as well as specific language skills also will need to be facilitated.

MENTAL RETARDATION

The most widely accepted definition of mental retardation is that adopted by the American Association on Mental Deficiency (Grossman, 1977), which requires that a person score at least 2 standard deviations below the average for his or her age group on a standardized intelligence test and show significant impairment in adaptive behavior to be considered mentally retarded. In addition, the deficits must occur during the developmental period. The definition makes no reference to the cause of the retardation or its permanence. This is the most common developmental disability that includes delayed language development.

The prevalence of mental retardation is currently estimated to be about 3 percent of the population. This figure has been broken down as follows (Schlanger, 1973):

- Mildly retarded = IQ from 50 to 70; makes up 2.6 percent of the total population and 85 percent of the mentally retarded population
- Moderately and severely retarded = IQ from 20 to 49; makes up 0.3 percent of the total population and 11.5 percent of the mentally retarded population
- Profoundly retarded = IQ below 20; makes up 0.1 percent of the total population and 3.5 percent of the mentally retarded population

Retarded children will start most areas of development later, progress more slowly, and reach a lower level than their age peers. The later a skill emerges in a nonretarded child, the more likely the skill is delayed or nonexistent. Mild retardation, therefore, may become obvious only as the child takes on the tasks presented in school. Misdiagnosis can occur if the population with which the test norms were developed is not similar (except for retardation) to the child being evaluated. A child must be tested with instruments appropriate for his or her background and must be compared with peers before a term such as retardation can be considered. As pointed out by Kinsbourne and Swisher (1977), among those who score below normal on a full-scale intelligence test, there will be those who have normal learning potential but whose language is different (often classified as a dialect) rather than deficient.

There are two groups of children who meet the criteria for retardation (Ingalls, 1978). One group has an organic impairment. Children in this group tend to have IQs below 50 and are found in approximately equal proportions in all levels of society. The second, much larger group, has no organic impairment. This group, referred to by Ingalls as "functionally retarded," is not equally represented at all levels of society. Racial minorities and individuals at lower socioeconomic levels are overrepresented. The "retardation" of the functionally retarded is almost always mild.

Ingalls (1978) discusses three theories to account for the observation that children from low-income families and racial minorities do poorly in school. The theory that people with lower intellectual abilities tend to be found in the lower-income groups and thus pass a lower intelligence on to their children has not received wide support. There is, instead, support for the theory that they only appear to be retarded because they are being measured with what Ingalls calls a "white, middle-class yardstick." Undoubtedly, children from racial minorities do not all speak the so-called Standard American English of most if not all standardized tests. There is also some support for the cultural deprivation theory, i.e., that certain aspects of parent–child interactions and the general environment of poverty predispose these children to failure. Their parents, for example, may not provide language models appropriate for success in school.

Correlates

The problems that can accompany mental retardation are as varied as the etiologies. Only a few will be highlighted here. The most creative diagnoses appear to be applied to those who test within the retarded range, have normal motor milestones, and have no physical stigmata. Although many retarded children have a history of gross motor delays, as Lenneberg (1964) observed, a noteworthy proportion of mentally retarded children have motor milestones within normal limits.

Mentally retarded children have a higher incidence of hearing problems than the nonretarded. Different etiologies can lead to the three basic hearing problems: conductive, sensorineural, and mixed. Children with Down's syndrome, for example, may have respiratory problems and small external auditory canals predisposing them to a conductive hearing loss (Lloyd & Fulton, 1972). Thus, hearing must be monitored not only to foster language acquisition but also to foster health care.

Ingalls (1978) lists many reasons for the widely accepted view that the retarded have a higher degree of emotional disturbances as well as a number of other character disorders. The list includes social isolation and rejection, family stress, lack of insight, and frustration and failure. One report is especially informative. Dentler and Mackler (1962) reviewed several studies and concluded that there is a positive correlation between IQs and peer acceptance. The higher a child's IQ, the more likely that he or she is widely accepted.

Language

After Rosenberg (1982) reviewed the language of the mentally re-tarded, he concluded that relative to normal, same-age peers, milestones occur at a later age, development is slower in all aspects of language skills, final achievements are lower, but that the "stages" as well as the order of the stages are similar. He also concluded that institutionalized, mentally retarded individuals may be at a disadvantage, particularly in the area of language skills. All retarded children learn language more slowly than their normal, same-age peers. All, to some extent, lack the language skills that permit easy integration into many work settings. Some are also language disordered, i.e., their language levels (verbal IQ) are lower than their nonlanguage levels (nonverbal or performance IQ). Others are relatively equally retarded in both areas of development. Dif-ferences in prevalence figures indicating how many mentally retarded children have verbal levels even lower than nonverbal levels are due to differences in criteria for a disorder, selection biases, severity of retarda-tion, tests administered, and so on. For example, Schlanger (1973) esti-mates that less than half of the mildly retarded have language difficulties in comparison with 90 % of those with more severe levels of retardation; Jordan (1967) estimates that 75–80 percent of children with IQs below 50 have at least severe language problems.

Intelligence tests developed by Wechsler have begun to replace the Stanford–Binet as the most popular tests of general intelligence. The three Wechsler tests currently in use are the Wechsler Preschool and Primary Scale (WPPSI) for children ages 4–6; the Wechsler Intelligence Scale for Children—revised (WISC-r) for children ages 6–16; and the Wechsler Adult Intelligence Scale (WAIS), appropriate for adults over age 15. One of the major differences between the Wechsler tests and the Stanford–Binet is that in addition to an overall intelligence score, the Wechsler tests separate the measures of verbal and nonverbal intelli-gence. The Stanford Binet has verbal and nonverbal items, not in equal proportion, at each level of development. A nonretarded, language-im-paired child thus would be expected to score within the abnormal range on the Stanford–Binet and on the verbal measure of the Wechsler tests but not on the nonverbal measure of the latter.

Miller (1981) compared cognitive level, as assessed by Piagetian tasks, with language performance in 42 retarded children referred for a speech and language evaluation. Nine patterns of cognitive and language performance were described. In the most common (36 percent), children exhibited similar cognitive, expressive, and receptive syntactic–semantic skills. Most frequently, language expression levels predicted language comprehension levels. Occasionally, vocabulary was a strength. As

Miller noted, the latter pattern could have resulted in response to certain teaching strategies.

Most findings indicate that the retarded are best described as having a delayed rather than a different pattern of language development. There are, however, some indications of different development. When we remember that a mentally retarded child is older than his or her control matched for either nonverbal IQ or language level and thus has a different and longer history, this is not surprising. Kamhi and Johnston's (1982) findings are examples of those suggesting that the pattern of language skills of the retarded is not a simple delay. They investigated the language performance of mildly retarded children matched for nonverbal IQ to a group of normal and a group of language-disordered children. (The normal and language-disordered groups were younger in chronological age than the retarded group in order for the match to occur.) The retarded children's language was consistent with their general cognitive level; that is, they were not also language disordered in addition to retarded. A significant difference in utterance lengths was found; the retarded children produced longer utterances than both the normal and language disordered. The syntactic maturity of the children's utterances was assessed by the Developmental Sentence Scoring procedure and nonstandardized measures of grammatical marker use. These analyses revealed three differences in the language of the retarded. Compared to the other groups, the retarded children asked significantly fewer questions and produced more sentences in the progressive tense. In addition, they tended to use less complex sentences. The differences were primarily in the frequency with which the retarded group produced different forms and, as pointed out by the author, would be unnoticed by a naive observer.

The studies of language use have focused on adults rather than children. For example, Bedrosian and Prutting (1978) undertook an analysis of the language use of moderately retarded adults with their peers, a speech–language pathologist, their parents, and a normal child. The analyses quantified the style of interaction with attention to the dominance and submission dimensions of the use of control within each speaking situation. Results indicated that only one of the four retarded adults held the dominant position in any of the conversational settings. The settings in which one was dominant involved the adult's peers and the normal child.

Rosenberg (1982) reviewed studies of mentally retarded children and their mothers and came to a different conclusion than applies to children with a specific language impairment and their mothers. It appears that mothers of the mentally retarded adjust their speech to their children as though the children were younger. Moreover, the complexity of the mother's speech appears to increase as a function of the language levels of their children. This is what would be recommended to caregivers—stay close to and sometimes a little above the child's level of language.

Management

Ingalls (1978) reviewed the biologic causes of retardation. In the majority of children the specific etiology is not identifiable. Despite these depressing odds, the child, parents, educators, and anyone else who is concerned with the child's development and well-being are entitled to the assurance that no condition that might benefit from medical treatment has been overlooked. Also, identification of a genetic etiology will facilitate counseling for parents and other family members regarding the risks associated with future pregnancies.

In addition to looking for the cause of mental retardation, the child's neurologist has a second important task: that of providing optimal health care, without which the mentally retarded child may not reach his or her maximum potential. Health and development are often closely intertwined, and the physician can help parents integrate the information they receive in these two areas. He or she generally has access to parents' thoughts and emotions. Talking to parents at frequent intervals to provide a resource for ongoing support is as important a role for the physician as it is for others who work with the child and family. Referral to a preschool that sets goals for both language and nonlanguage skills is warranted. In addition to referral to an audiologist, referral to a social worker should also be considered. The speech–language pathologist is needed as a direct interventionist for those children whose language skills are lower than nonlanguage skills and as a consultant to maximize the language skills of all mentally retarded children. The lower the level of the child, the more caregivers must be involved to maximize gains.

The pacesetter of meaningful language development is more the child's level of cognitive development than the child's chronologic age. Once language and cognitive levels are similar there are two necessary steps: (1) re-evaluate cognitive level because the levels may have improved, and (2) administer a standardized language test. The latter has been shown to reveal deficits not obvious in a test of verbal IQ (Stark et al., 1982). If no problem appears obvious by standardized testing, then proceed to an analysis of a spontaneous language sample. This has been shown to reveal deficits not obvious on standardized testing, presumably because more of the skills sampled are appropriate to the child's level of development (Demetras et al., 1982).

The overall goals for language intervention have been listed in the section on specific language impairment. They apply to all developmental disability groups as do the following. The lower the level of the child's nonverbal intelligence and language skills, the more functional commun-

ication skills are appropriately highlighted. The lower the level, the more
the framework provided by Bloom and Lahey (1978) is especially useful
for these children. It describes a developmental sequence with reference
to the meanings being expressed by the words. Mentally retarded children not only need to develop a greater variety of words and sentences,
but also to use them meaningfully. As pointed out by Kinsbourne and
Swisher (1977), effort should not be directed at memorization of words
and sentences. The clinician should also be prepared for slow progress. As
also pointed out by Kinsbourne and Swisher, "it is the essence of mental
retardation that its victim tends not to generalize from specific experience" (p. 12). Thus, the use of the same words in different, everyday
contexts should be part of the therapy program.

Prognosis

Before approximately 6 years of age, in addition to the significant
variability in the rates of development of individual normal children,
there are unpredicted gains in any developmental disability group. The
older the group of children, the less frequent the number of unexpected
"spontaneous" improvements. As will be discussed in the section on autism, level of IQ is a strong predictor of late functioning at age 6 years or
later. Variables that add to the likelihood of a poor prognosis for receptive
and expressive language development include the presence of a hearing
loss. A motor disability affecting speech complicates the development of
intelligible, expressive language.

AUTISM

Autism is a developmental disorder characterized by (1) social development that is inappropriate for the child's intellectual level; (2) language development that is delayed and/or deviant for the child's intellectual level; (3) an "insistence on sameness" as indicated by stereotyped
play patterns, abnormal preoccupations, or resistance to change; and (4)
an onset before the age of 30 months (Rutter, 1978). Other terms used to
describe children with these characteristics have included psychosis and
childhood schizophrenia.

The language disorder is one of the most striking and long-lasting of
the deficits observed in autistic children, who were first described in the
American literature by Kanner in 1943. None of the first 11 children
identified as autistic developed language normally (Kanner, 1971). Chur-

chill (1972) has gone so far as to indicate that the language disorder is "central" to the disability.

Wing (1976) reviewed several epidemiologic studies (e.g., Treffert, 1970) and concluded that the prevalence of autism is 4–5 in 1000 children. Of these, a small number function in the normal or mild to moderately mentally retarded range with a much larger number functioning in the severely retarded range. The group functioning within the normal range is more likely to show a high boy–girl ratio, and possibly, to have parents of a high socioeconomic level. Although seizures may develop, this group is also less likely to have overt neurologic symptoms.

As Rapin (1977) noted, *autism* is not a diagnosis; it is a description of a behavioral syndrome. Findings concerning the neurobiologic basis of autism (e.g., Swisher, Drzwicki, & Swisher, 1976), therefore, should not be expected to apply to all autistic children. Subgroups based on such variables as age of onset and degree of retardation clearly exist.

Correlates

Intelligence

As mentioned previously, autistic children are rarely of high intelligence as Kanner (1943) originally speculated. A study reported by Alpern (1967) was one of the first to illustrate that autistic children can be tested as validly and reliably as nonautistic children if the items are at suitable developmental levels. He administered a test that sampled primarily motor skills and then readministered the test after 3 days. The scores were found to be highly correlated with independent clinical judgments and parent reports of functioning. Lockyer and Rutter (1969) found objectively scored tests obtained in early childhood to be highly stable for autistic children and to be good predictors of intellectual functioning in adolescence and early adult life. This was true even in the small group of children who improved markedly in social and behavioral skills.

The IQ score obtained by an autistic child differs widely according to the type of task administered. The same child might have average performance on some tasks and yet have severely abnormal performance on others. Rutter and Lockyer (1967) found that most autistic children performed poorly on verbal tasks but did relatively well on nonlanguage tasks such as the block design and object assembly subtests of the Wechsler scale. They concluded that variability in intellectual functioning appeared to be due to problems with the child's use and understanding of language. As with all language-disordered children, therefore, estimates of intelligence are incomplete unless separate scores for both nonverbal and verbal items are obtained.

Motor Skills

No problems in motor development are obvious for most of these children. This confuses many beginning diagnosticians who assume that gross motor skills must be delayed if a child is retarded. However, as discussed earlier, cognitive and motor retardation can occur independently.

Socioemotional Development

As mentioned previously, having any type of a developmental disability is not conducive to one's emotional health. Autistic behaviors may appear to be characteristic of children with mental retardation whose caregivers have exceptionally unrealistic expectations for them. Autistic children, however, differ from the mentally retarded in many ways, the most obvious being in the severity of the language disorder relative to their nonlanguage skills. They are similar in being poorly equipped to deal with the frustrations of everyday living. As pointed out previously (Swisher & Butler, 1984), even autistic children have their good and bad days. Given their limited coping strategies, they probably are prone to have more of the latter than children with mental retardation.

Two typical courses of language development have been described for autistic children: early retardation (e.g., Pronovost, 1961; Swisher, Reichler, & Short, 1976) and an apparently normal development followed by a regression (e.g., Despert, 1947; Swisher, Reichler, & Short, 1976). In a retrospective study (Swisher, Reichler, & Short, 1976) of the clinical records of 20 autistic children, parents reported that a regression in development had occurred for 10 of the children. These children were initially considered by their parents to be normally developing, but on reflection the parents reported that around 18–24 months, as an average, a regression occurred. One child, who spoke no words at age 8 years, had said, e.g., *ball, my bottle,* and *I want to be like my daddy* before he regressed to vowel-like sounds around 26 months. At age 7 years, he spoke infrequently, primarily in simple, active declarative sentences. No history of regression was reported for the other 10, all of whom reportedly had always had delayed development.

No one point in time, appears to describe the onset of the regression. It most likely is gradual rather than abrupt. For one child studied by Swisher, Reichler, & Short (1976), a series of home movies had been taken several months prior to the age at which onset of behavioral regression was noted by his parents. The films were shown to a pediatric neurologist (C. Swisher, personal communication, 1973) who was not provided with any history and did not know that the child was currently considered autistic. He noted stereotyped motor activity, which he considered atypical of normally developing children of any age.

By 6 years of age, three groups can be identified in terms of both the quality and quantity of expressive language development (Doherty & Swisher, 1977; Rapin & Allen, 1983). The children referred to in the literature as mute have the lowest level of comprehension and expression of language and the poorest prognosis. They speak, but only once or twice a week, and sometimes only once or twice a year. They do not readily initiate speech or other activities, and they give few observable responses to sound.

Children described as intermittent language users by Doherty and Swisher (1977) speak at a higher developmental level than those referred to as *mute* but at a lower level than those they refer to as *fluent*. Intermittent language users have infrequent output with little or no echolalia, flat intonation, and articulation errors. Their utterances sometimes have a linguistic complexity that is above their usual level and is considered quite noteworthy by most who know the child well. The higher-level output usually occurs when the child is under stress or desires to fulfill a primary need such as getting food. For example, one child who typically used approximately 10 two-word phrases during the day, said, "I want *you* to stay!" to his mother when left at camp for the first time. Another sentence like this was not reported during the next 6 months. (This discrepancy between typical and occasional output presents the language clinician with a difficult task.) It is likely that parents of these children will report an early history of regression in language development. The utterances of many of the fluent speakers include jargon and elaborate intonation patterns (Doherty & Swisher, 1977). Their parents usually report that language development was always delayed with no history of regression.

Language intervention is the most successful with the fluent group. In 1966 Lovaas reported that he did not know why echolalic children proceeded faster than the previously mute children. Now it is clear that most echolalic children are initially at a higher overall level than either mute or intermittent speakers.

Ruttenburg and Wolf (1967) emphasized that one of the major problems in dealing with children labeled as autistic is their extreme inability or disinclination to communicate effectively, especially through verbal language. O'Connor (1975) believes that the mentally retarded suffer from an "inertia" in relation to language. Rosenberg (1982) refers to "passivity." These statements appear to refer primarily to the mute and intermittent language user but not to the fluent.

Recent reviews of the language of autistic children have been completed by Fay and Mermelstein (1982) and by Swisher and Demetras (1985). Both indicate that autistic children have different language development (see Table 2-2); i.e., they display language behaviors that are not characteristic of normally developing children of any age. Swisher and Demetras suggest that the data concerning expressive language can be summarized as indicating that there is a "superficial form" and a "form–context mismatch." Some of the utterances appear to have weak cognitive underpinnings, i.e., a superficial form. These utterances are syntactically correct but appear to be word "chunks" that do not show up separately in other utterances; that is, there is little recombination of the words in the chunk into other phrases. An example would be "Don't throw the dog off of the balcony," spoken several times when the child was tempted to throw an object (Kanner, 1946, p. 111) Wing (1976, p. 111) is apparently referring to this same characteristic when she refers to the "store of phrases" used by many autistic children.

Some utterances spoken by autistic children are often perceived by the listener to be inappropriate for a given context. This is what Swisher and Demetras (1985) refer to as a form-context mismatch. The utterances do not appear to communicate to the listener what other children of the same developmental level usually mean when speaking similar words in similar contexts. Because of the correct syntax, a failure to analyze the match between the form of what the child says and the context in which it is spoken may lead clinicians to conclude that the child's expressive language is more advanced than it actually is.

These two interdependent features differentiate the expressive language of autistic children from that of normal children and also from that of children with mental retardation or specific language impairment. Neither feature alone is unique to children with autistic behaviors. Superficial form is seen, for example, in children with hydrocephalus who are considered hyperverbal (Schwartz, 1974; Swisher & Pinsker, 1971). Each feature will vary in level of severity between and within the subgroups of autistic children that have been described (cf. Rapin & Allen, 1983; Swisher, et al., 1976).

Studies (e.g., Meyers & Goldfarb, 1961) that indicate parents of autistic children use abnormal language when speaking to their children have been criticized for the impressionistic rating categories, poor diagnoses of the children studied, small samples of speech, and unnatural contexts in which the speech was recorded (Baker, Cantwell, Rutter, & Bartak, 1976; Klein & Pollack, 1966). Fay and Mermelstein (1982) add that the most important problem affecting an interpretation of the results is the lack of an appropriate control group. Children must be matched at least according to the level of their expressive language, as it is well established that caregivers vary their language in relation to the child's level of output.

As mentioned earlier, it is possible that caregiver language will be not so much the cause of the child's disability as an effect of it. An approach that addresses this possibility compares the language of caregivers of autistic children with caregivers of another language disordered group. Such a comparison has been carried out by Cantwell, Baker, and Rutter (1978). They analyzed the speech of mothers of autistic and specific language impaired children matched for age and performance IQ. All of the children were part of a follow-up study which 2 years previously had matched them on utterance length and Reynell expression scores. The analyses included categories that may be significant for language acquisition such as imitations, expansions, corrections, and prompts; grammatical complexity and correctness; and tone of voice. Few differences in the speech of the two types of mothers were found.

Management

Therapeutic intervention for autistic children has included custodial care, electroconvulsive shock treatment, residential treatment, psychoanalytic therapy, megadoses of vitamins, and more recently, a developmental approach. The latter appears to be useful for all the children, as is attention to the family. The caregivers of autistic children are greatly in need of support in the treatment of their child.

An autistic child is at risk for being started and maintained at too difficult a developmental level. This occurs for several reasons including the lack of physical stigmata, better nonverbal than verbal skills, prior history in some of having appeared to have been normal, and severity and type of the language disorder. Both the examiner and language facilitator, therefore, must be well versed in developmental sequences of language and cognition. They must understand the stages of form, meaning, and use through which normal children move in the process of becoming increasingly efficient in communicating with others through words. Clinicians with this knowledge can more easily and accurately find the growing edge of the child's meaningful and appropriately used utterances, and therefore, they can more easily and accurately determine which language-learning task is likely to be most easily facilitated. Rather than starting at the level of the form of the language, the clinician will find, in most cases, that it is necessary to start at a lower level— where the form, meaning, and use components fit together appropriately.

The most productive approaches to language development for autistic children are used by clinicians who de-emphasize the possible theoretical implications of the label *autistic* and deal directly with the pattern and level of language disorder they observe. It is important to remember that autistic children enjoy tasks that are simple enough. If the child does not give any indication of enjoying the task, the difficulty of the task should be decreased and the degree to which the child is performing correctly should be increased.

Schopler and Reichler (1971) summarized their experiences as indicating that not only is the use of parents as co-therapists expedient, but that they also are often the most important developmental agents for their children. Kanner (1973) noted that autistic children placed in a custodial-type institution quickly regressed to an essentially non-functioning state. Rutter and Bartak (1973) found that autistic children who made progress in a residential environment did not improve at home. These reports of little or no gains outside of the teaching situation probably occur because of the retarded, autistic child's poor generalization skills and need for repeated trials to learn. In the home, remediation can be an on-going process of guiding the child to successfully manage the activities and interactions that are encountered daily and thus have the most interest and usefulness to the child.

Many autistic children are motorically active. In approaching the child who does everything except the task put before him or her, it is useful to remove the distracting stimuli. It also helps if the child is given a period of physical activity during language lessons (Kern, Loegel, Dyer, Blew, & Fenton, 1982).

Schopler, Brehm, Kinsbourne, and Reichler (1971) studied the effects of a structured and an unstructured situation on autistic children. The higher the child's developmental level according to both clinical judgment and social age, the less he or she was disorganized by lack of structure. Conversely, the lower the developmental level, the more external structure appeared to improve responses. Guidelines for following the child's lead if a structured, clinician-oriented approach fails have been given by Swisher and Butler (1984). They suggest letting the child choose what to talk about and when to talk about it. The clinician then becomes a narrator, proving language for what the child has chosen to do.

It is usually appropriate to assume that a nonautistic child has an interest in verbal expression. As discussed previously, however, attempts at talking vary widely among autistic children. The less the child spontaneously attempts to talk, the more the usual approach to language development is modified. The modification is not in terms of the language chosen for facilitation but in terms of the choice of a reward to increase attempts at verbal communication. More frequently than with the nonautistic child, and less frequently than the literature suggests, primary rewards such as food are needed. This appears to be true more often at the lowest levels of development and is a poor prognostic sign.

Several authors report success with the use of Total Communication (oral language and manual signed English presented simultaneously) in the treatment of autistic children who do not readily imitate an oral model. One such approach developed by Creedan (1973) follows a developmental sequence. She reports that some of the children begin to speak after they have started signing. Reports frequently suggest that the success of signing may be due to a modality effect, i.e., an unimpaired visual modality in the presence of an impaired auditory modality. Another interpretation arises from observations of several teachers who were using Total Communication with autistic children. Usually the clinician is learning to sign or, if fluent in sign, is committed to matching each sign to a spoken word. The result is to have a reduced rate of word presentation, a reduced linguistic complexity, and an increase in functional words relative to when the clinician used only spoken language. Remember also that normal children "sign" (e.g., wave good-bye) before they speak. There are reasons to believe, therefore, that some of the lessons provided through Total Communication are easier (i.e., at a lower developmental level) than some of the lessons provided through oral communication.

Prognosis

Most follow-up studies are of children who received neither early special schooling nor state-of-the-art language facilitation. Because "successes" often are no longer available for study, the results of any follow-up study may slightly underestimate what can be expected of children receiving intervention today.

The literature supports at least four statements: (1) Lack of speech is a poor sign and increasingly becomes a matter of concern as age increases beyond age 6 years. (2) Full-scale IQ after age 6 years is the best single predictor of functioning in adulthood. (3) Level of language development influences social functioning in adulthood, especially when the full-scale IQ is over 40–60. (4) A reported history of regression with no known neurologic insult in several areas including language is a poor sign. The literature relating *speech development* to prognosis is useful but the reader must be alert to the meaning of this term as it is used by each author. Although the terminology used by specific authors will be quoted, it is assumed that what DeMeyer, Burton, DeMeyer, Norton, Allen, and Steele (1973) and other authors have referred to with a similar term was expressive language rather than articulation of speech.

Several investigators (e.g., Kanner, 1973) report that children without speech at 5 years have a poorer outcome than those with speech. The autistic child who is not speaking by the age of 5 years is also frequently the same child who had or has a profound lack of response to sounds. He or she may improve considerably in relation to his or her initial level of impairment, but it is unlikely that he or she will achieve a near-normal level of social adjustment or of language development.

There is little information to aid us in counseling parents as to the outcome of future development if their child is under 6 years of age. Several studies (e.g., Rutter & Lockyer, 1967, Swisher, Reichler, and Short, 1976), however, indicate that intelligence test results become highly predictive of later functioning if obtained when the child is at least 6 years old. DeMeyer et al. (1973) reported the following data for children

12 years of age at follow-up who were $5\frac{1}{2}$ years of age at initial evaluation: 1–2 percent normal, 5–15 percent borderline, 16–25 percent fair, and 60–75 percent poor. Rutter and Lockyer (1976) reported that only 2–3 percent of children with autistic behaviors who were over 16 years of age held paying jobs.

Rutter and Lockyer (1976) reported a hierarchy of predictive variables from highest to lowest values as follows: IQ, severity of speech disorder, and amount of schooling. A low full-scale IQ (below 60) on the WISC was a predictor of poor outcome. In children with an IQ over 60, level of speech development more effectively than IQ score distinguished between children with a good social adjustment at follow-up and those with a fair or poor outcome. This suggests that in the presence of a severe or profound degree of mental retardation, the question of language development in relation to IQ scores is not particularly relevant. If intelligence test scores place a child above an IQ of 60, however, the level and type of language development assumes a greater importance in terms of predicting social adjustment.

Although test results of children less than 6 years old have little predictive value, their language development histories are important. As mentioned earlier, Swisher, Reichler and Short (1976) found that behavioral regression, which was reported retrospectively to have occurred late in infancy, was related to more serious consequences than the absence of such a history. Overall intellectual development and especially expressive and receptive language skills were more severely impaired in children who reportedly had regressed in language development compared with children with no such history. This is in line with Colby's (1973) statement that therapy was a failure for a child who showed normal linguistic development until 16 or 22 months of age and then stopped talking.

AUDITORY DISORDERS

Peripheral

Auditory disorders are classified within a medical model as peripheral or central. The peripheral category is subclassified into conductive and sensorineural hearing losses. A conductive loss is due to interference with the transmission of sound from the external auditory canal to the inner ear which is capable of normal function. It is characterized by hearing loss for air-conducted sounds but not for those conducted by bone. When air conduction is blocked to a maximum degree by a conductive component, a maximal hearing loss of approximately 60 dB by air conduction occurs. This type of loss is treatable medically, surgically, or by amplification. Sensorineural loss is due to lesions of the cochlea, auditory nerve, or both, and usually is irreversible. Air- and bone-conduction thresholds are comparable. When both sensorineural and conductive hearing losses are present, mixed hearing loss is diagnosed. The bone-conduction thresholds are below normal but not as much as the air-conduction thresholds.

Hearing loss is far more prevalent than deafness and far more common than the syndrome of auditory verbal agnosia. Congenital hearing losses outnumber acquired. Some of the causes of an auditory disorder, such as anoxia, result in problems in addition to deafness. As many as 25 percent of the deaf population may have complicating factors such as visual problems, retardation, and cerebral palsy (Vernon, 1969).

Hearing loss may be unilateral or bilateral. Children with unilateral hearing impairment experience some difficulties, particularly in identifying the source of a sound (localization) and listening in a noisy environment. Bess (personal communication, 1983) found a higher incidence of school failure in children with a unilateral hearing loss compared with children with normal hearing bilaterally. These children are likely to be brought to the attention of a neurologist. While children with a unilateral loss may have fewer problems than children with a bilateral hearing loss, it is important that they be identified, treated and followed.

The most common cause of conductive hearing loss in children is otitis media. Other causes include congenital malformations of the middle ear or a closing off of the ear canal by foreign bodies or cerumen. Causes of sensorineural loss present at birth may include a genetic base, and a maternal infection. Causes of sensorineural loss acquired during the birth process itself include asphyxia and head trauma. Loss acquired months or years after birth may be caused by diseases such as meningitis or mumps, head trauma, exposure to ototoxic drugs, extremely loud noises, or from a genetically determined condition that has its onset later in life.

Although hearing loss can be considered a continuum on the decibel scale, at some point along that continuum the child ceases to develop language received as auditory input and relies primarily on visual input. In addition to having an average hearing loss of 60 to 90 dB (ANSI, 1973) or greater, children considered deaf for educational purposes consist mostly of those who have sensorineural impairment suffered prior to the age of 2 years. There are about 54,000 students in school programs who meet these criteria (Karchmer, Milon, & Wolk, 1979). About 4% of deaf children have deaf parents (Rawlings & Jensema, 1977).

There are three major language systems used with the deaf: American Sign Language (ASL), manual English that uses signed codes for spoken English, and oral English. ASL is a language in and of itself with its own special characteristics. In contrast, manual English systems basically translate spoken English into signs and present both the spoken and visual stimuli simultaneously. Six of the best known manual English systems have been described by Quigley and King (1982).

Silverman (1971) reported that in 1968 approximately 85% of deaf children enrolled in special schools were receiving an exclusively oral method of instruction at least in the early years of schooling. The situation has been changing. Jordon, Gustason, and Rosen (1967) reported that 64% of classes for hearing-impaired students in the United States were using "Total Communication" defined as the use of manual signs, finger spelling, speechreading, and amplification. Jensema and Trybus (1978) reported that a combination of methods, rather than single methods, was the rule in the classroom. In contrast, the use of speech alone was the single most common pattern at home. There was relatively little consistency, therefore, between systems of communication used at home and in school.

Correlates

As mentioned earlier, hearing loss in and of itself is not correlated with gross or fine motor impairment. In general, those with an endogenous congenital loss have fewer additional problems than those with an acquired loss. Rapin (1977) pointed out that those who acquire a hearing loss due to purulent meningitis may have difficulty walking and the speech and language disorder may be incorrectly diagnosed as solely due to brain damage. Deaf speech often has a dysarthric quality to it in the absence of a neurologic disorder. Hearing loss affects the development of not only oral–auditory language but also speech. Thus the speech–language pathologist who works with the deaf must have up-to-date training in both speech and language acquisition and considerable knowledge concerning amplification.

Language

Conductive hearing loss. This section focuses on the extent to which a prior history of recurrent otitis media with presumably some associated fluctuating, conductive hearing loss can be a precursor to a learning disability in an otherwise normal child. Recent emphasis has been given to this problem and it is possible that the neurologist will become involved because of suspected learning disability.

In each of the retrospective studies of two groups of children with different histories of otitis media, the group with the greater number of previous episodes of otitis media has had poorer performance on speech and language measures (e.g., Friel-Patti, Finitzo-Hieber, Conti, &

Brown, 1982; Holm & Kunze, 1969; Sak & Ruben, 1981). Many, but not all, of the differences reached statistical significance. In general, the poorer performance by the group with a history of multiple episodes of otitis media has been attributed to the assumed fluctuating hearing loss associated with episodes of otitis media (e.g., Holm & Kunze, 1969).

Most investigators have required that the children in the groups with multiple episodes of otitis media had the first episode prior to 2 years of age and had three or more episodes to be selected for study (e.g., Brandes & Ehinger, 1981; Holm & Kunze, 1969; Needleman, 1977; Zinkus, Gottlieb, & Shapiro, 1978). Only frequency of episodes of otitis media was considered, thus the prevalence of unilateral and bilateral episodes was not reported. As noted by Tonini (1983), the assumption that bilateral and unilateral episodes and the associated fluctuating hearing loss have a similar impact on development appears unwarranted.

Only a few investigators have included a measure of performance IQ in addition to speech and language measures. In two studies (Zinkus et al., 1978; Zinkus & Gottlieb, 1980), the differences on the performance measure, in addition to those on the speech and language measures, reached statistical significance with poorer scores obtained by the group with histories of multiple episodes of otitis media. In other studies, the children in the group with a history of multiple episodes did more poorly than the control group, but the differences were not statistically significant (Brandes & Ehinger, 1981; Sak & Ruben, 1981; Tonini, 1983). Thus, as suggested by Tonini (1983), there is a possibility that a general developmental delay rather than a specific learning disability is associated with a history of multiple episodes of otitis media. If so, past periods of illness must be considered in interpreting the results since hearing loss alone does not affect the development of performance skills.

The extent to which all but the Tonini (1983) study can be generalized to "middle-class" children is unknown because as Ventry (1980) and Paradise (1981) have noted, most investigators selected children who were not representative of this group. For example, children who were medically indigent (Holm & Kunze, 1969), academically underachieving (Zinkus & Gottlieb, 1980; Zinkus et al., 1978), from aboriginal populations (Lewis, 1976), from low- *and* middle-class homes (Needleman, 1977), from intensive care of low-birth-weight nurseries (Friel-Patti et al., 1982), or from undescribed populations (Sak & Ruben, 1981). Thus it is not known whether reduced speech and language skills are sequelae of multiple episodes of otitis media in a population of "middle-class" children. It is important to note that these studies report only group trends. The number of individual children with a history of multiple episodes of otitis media who have a developmental disability has not been reported.

The assumption that a language disorder and/or learning disability in children with histories of recurrent otitis media are sequelae of fluctu-

ating hearing loss must be approached with caution because of the findings of poorer performance IQs in all studies that included such a measure. It is possible that the associated illness is of at least equal
importance as suggested by Menyuk (1979) and that a generalized developmental delay rather than specific language disorder follows. It is possible, but also not yet proven, that having otitis media interacts adversely
with other developmental difficulties already present in a child.

At present, it appears that multidiscipline assessment should be considered for children referred for a learning problem who have a history of
multiple episodes of otitis media. In addition to hearing sensitivity,
speech and language skills and performance IQ levels should be assessed.
If the otitis media is still present, hearing levels and illnesses should be
closely monitored. Communication with the child's pediatrician or otolaryngologist should occur frequently. There is, however, no reason at
present to expect that a large percentage of otherwise normal children
with histories of recurrent episodes of otitis media are at risk for a specific
speech and language impairment.

Sensorineural.   Little is known concerning the relationship between
hearing loss and language acquisition. Many textbooks suggest that deaf
children stop normal babbling around 6 months of age. Maskarinec,
Cairns, Butterfield, and Weamer (1981) acoustically analyzed the tape-
recorded vocalizations of five infants during the first 30 weeks of life.
Differences in vocal activity, e.g., total vocalization time, were obvious
for the hearing-loss infant by 6 weeks of age, suggesting that hearing
impairment affects vocalizations earlier than has been believed.

The problems in evaluating the language of children with a hearing
loss have been summarized by Quigley and King (1982). For example,
spoken language is difficult to assess in the presence of poor speech intelligibility; comprehension of spoken language is difficult to assess because
of the hearing loss. Much of the available data, therefore, focuses on
reading and writing levels.

The studies summarized by Swisher (1976) and by Quigley and King
(1982) indicate that large numbers of deaf children, most of whom have
not learned ASL as a first language, who are still in the special educational system do not reach the fourth-grade level of reading or writing,
and most are not considered to speak intelligibly. Overall, form is the
greatest deficit in expressive language (see Table 2-2).

Deaf children in private oral schools tend to develop adequate language skills. These children are more select in terms of IQ and socioeconomic status than deaf children in general, but their success is noteworthy. Ogden (1979) identified approximately 1000 former students of three
major private oral schools in the United States. The subjects came from
academically and occupationally elite families. He obtained extensive

information on 637 of them by use of a questionnaire and rating scale. Ninety percent of the subjects were prelingually hearing impaired and would be considered deaf. They were found to be highly successful in terms of their academic and occupational accomplishments. A majority of the 441 subjects who were out of school were engaged in professional-level occupations. Thirty percent had completed at least an undergraduate college as compared with the national average of 19.6 percent and 11.6 percent for white men and women, respectively. Forty percent of the 196 subjects still in school at the time of the survey were in institutions of higher education. They attributed their academic and occupational success to their development of oral English. The majority reported that their speech was readily understood by others and that they could understand speech well through speech reading.

Approximately three fourths of deaf adults in the United States use ASL (Rainer, Altschuler, & Kallmann, 1969), but only a small percentage acquired it in early childhood. Most learn ASL through interacting with deaf peers who have deaf parents, or with deaf adults after entering the school system. The language used in the home by deaf children of deaf parents is not always ASL. Some deaf parents use a form of manual English or communicate orally with their children. Others alternate between ASL and oral English.

Most of the available studies of ASL in young deaf children learning ASL as a first language are longitudinal studies of small groups or individual children. The children observed have ranged in ages from 6 months to adolescence. The studies indicate that these children proceed normally in language acquisition through the visual mode. From research conducted thus far, it appears, according to Caccamise, Hatfield, and Brewer (1978), that "the acquisition of language in a visual–manual modality parallels the acquisition of language in an oral–aural modality" (p. 814). For example, hearing children usually speak their first word between the ages of 10 and 13 months; deaf children learning ASL also produce their first signs around this age (Caccamise et al., 1978; Schlesinger & Meadow, 1972).

Management

As Rapin (1977) noted, congenital hearing loss is the most frequent reason for a language disorder in the presence of normal intelligence, no evidence of a brain disorder, adequate caregiver–child interactions, and normal emotional development. She states that "hearing must be tested adequately in every child who has defective speech or who does not speak" (p. 230). One should add also test the hearing of everyone for whom there is any concern about the comprehension or expression of language.

All children with hearing impairment should have a medical evaluation to look for signs of underlying diseases, some of which are treatable, and to identify genetic factors for which counseling may be necessary. In many cases of conductive hearing loss, successful medical or surgical intervention will return hearing to normal at some point in time. A sensorineural hearing loss, on the other hand, is permanent. The primary management technique for sensorineural loss is amplification and special education. Because of recent advances in the detection of hearing loss in infants and in the manufacture and selection of hearing aids, more children, infants included, can successfully use a hearing aid.

At the preschool level, a neurologist is not needed for most deaf children of deaf parents—the group that is most likely to be using ASL—because this group has the least number of complicating problems. Deaf children who succeed at spoken language are among the highest overall intellectually among the deaf, and thus they also are not likely to be seen by a neurologist. Those not doing well in language acquisition by any mode of communication are most likely to be referred because deafness is not their only problem.

There is nothing about hearing loss that in and of itself lowers the potential of the brain for language acquisition. The brain must, however, receive input through some sensory system for language to develop. There are two primary reasons to administer an IQ test to a child with a developmental disability. One is to estimate the potential for success in a regular school. When this is the goal, full-scale IQ tests involving language are needed. The other reason is to estimate the extent to which they are capable of problem-solving tasks that do not rely on language skills. This sort of assessment gives information concerning how far language skills might progress with special help. A deaf child with normal performance IQ scores, for example, would be expected to be able to learn sign language normally if given adequate input.

The primary goal for all language-disordered children is verbal communication. Developing language is thus initially more important than developing speech. Starting a deaf child with a Total Communication system is also assuming a diagnostic stance. Some—usually those who are the brightest—will move into exclusively oral communication. Some will move to manual. Others will need both.

Beginning with a major emphasis on individual speech segments is putting the cart before the horse. Language has an acoustic and linguistic redundancy that is taken advantage of when more than one word is spoken or signed in context. After oral language is well developed, the "holes" may not even be noticed by the child. If they are, then lip reading and auditory training is useful as part of the oral approach. Overall, the longest unit of language that can be handled by the child is recommended as the unit of intervention. Not only does this permit the child to take advantage of redundancies in the signal but it also facilitates the development of normal intonation patterns that in turn help the listener. Whenever possible both those who listen to a deaf child and the deaf child himself or herself must develop a strategy of "best guesses," i.e., filling holes when possible. A listener who cannot understand what was said is advised to ask for a restatement rather than an exact repetition of what was just said.

Whereas in previous years there was a tendency in some circles to favor placing children in schools for the deaf, the current tendency is to keep them, whenever possible, within the normal hearing community. The controversy of oralism versus manualism is finally reaching its long-awaited death in favor of focusing on the method or combination of methods that will help language develop most effectively in this individual child. The mode of communication is no longer seen to be as important as the effectiveness of the system in developing language. The suggestion of Matkin (personal communication, 1983) that deaf children in primarily a hearing environment be approached through a Total Communication system and then be given the opportunity to learn ASL as a second language is recommended. The hearing parents of deaf children usually do not have the skills in ASL to adequately transmit language to their children, and it is more difficult for them to learn a new language than to code their well-developed spoken language into signs. An additional advantage to a Total Communication system is that of preparing the child for the syntax of reading, which is based on spoken language. Children of deaf parents who have ASL as their native language will usually first learn ASL, which will later be translated into spoken language. An advantage of this approach includes easy communication with others who are deaf who use the same ASL. Still another noteworthy advantage to any system that facilitates communication between people is that parent–child communication is facilitated. The laborious route of oral education includes a preschool period where it is difficult for the parents to discipline or counsel their child in the presence of inadequate language development.

A cautionary note is in order. Many times Total Communication becomes signing and mouthing of some words on the part of the clinician–teacher rather than both signing and speaking. This rightfully concerns those who wish the child to develop oral–auditory language.

Prognosis

As Norlin and Van Tasell (1980) noted, the speech information available for language learning to a child with a hearing loss will be dependent to some extent on the degree and frequency configuration of the hearing loss. It cannot, however, be assumed that audiometric configuration is the sole variable. One must think in terms of aided audiometric configuration. Selective amplification makes some additional speech information available for language learning (e.g., Pascoe, 1975). In addition, a child's skills in coping with an impaired input and ability to learn language in general must be considered (Norlin and Van Tasell, 1980). The age at onset of the loss also is important. Particularly with the deaf, the age at which the impairment occurred can have a profound influence on the level of the child's language acquisition. Other important variables include etiology and the hearing status of the parents. Hearing status of parents and siblings is of special interest because the form of language being acquired can be quite different for the deaf child of deaf parents than for the deaf child of hearing parents. This factor alone can profoundly affect the language, educational, and socioemotional development of the child. Given the complexity of the interactions between these variables, it is not possible to predict the language level of a child from a description of the hearing loss that is present.

As mentioned previously, deaf children of deaf parents whose native language is ASL often acquire signed language as easily as hearing children of hearing parents acquire spoken language. Several factors are operating. Early identification is typical, and parental acceptance of the loss is seldom a problem so early, high-level language interactions occur. The majority of deaf children, however, have hearing parents who do not use ASL.

Central

The most severe expressive oral language and academic problems develop in the presence of a severe auditory comprehension difficulty. This occurs most frequently in children with deafness, autism, or auditory agnosia. Deafness and auditory agnosia are similar in that other, nonlanguage skills are intact and it is assumed that language expression would proceed normally if the comprehension deficit could be overcome. The disorders differ in that deafness prevents what is said to the child from reaching the brain. Auditory agnosia is a term applied when the auditory stimuli that presumably reach the brain are poorly processed but stimuli from other modalities are normally processed. This infrequently occurring disorder typically involves a greater deficit for verbal than nonverbal auditory stimuli.

As Rapin and Allen (1983) reported, some of the children with verbal auditory agnosia have little or no comprehension of speech and are mute or speak very few, poorly articulated words. Such children can be readily distinguished from mute autistic children because such symptoms as eye avoidance, resistance to change, and repetitive behavior are lacking. The child with agnosia can communicate by *ad hoc* gestures and some make sophisticated drawings as a means of communication.

Clinicians need to be aware of the existence of this syndrome since it mandates a very specific intervention - supplementation of the acoustic channel by the visual channel, i.e., the Total Communication approach. With time and training, many learn to produce and understand some speech, although they may continue to require signs for clarification. For some, speech usually remains poor and syntax primitive. Others do reasonably well (Mantovani & Landau, 1980). Some never achieve conversational use of speech.

Because the children can process language provided it is presented to a modality other than hearing, Rapin and Allen (1983) have suggested that the bilateral temporal lobe pathology that is the usual basis for this syndrome evidently spares the posterior temporoparietal and frontal regions. In the child described by Landau et al. (1960), both superior temporal gyri had undergone degeneration. In some children the cause of the syndrome may be a self-limiting process. The EEG often returns to normal.

Although the problem was first described as an acquired disorder it can also appear to be congenital or in any case to have developed before the start of expressive language. A number of children with auditory verbal agnosia have histories of regression of verbal skills after reportedly normal early milestones (Rapin & Allen, 1983). In this respect, histories of children with auditory verbal agnosia are similar to those obtained from the caregivers of some autistic children who say that their child regressed in language (Swisher, Reichler, and Short, 1976). Rapin (personal communication, 1985), in fact, speculates that mute autistic children have verbal auditory agnosia and autism.

Adults who acquire an auditory agnosia are reasonably self-sufficient people with a major handicap in relating to the hearing world. Reading and writing and performance skills are spared. Speech may or may not quickly degenerate. This, of course, does not happen if the problem is congenital. To the extent that nonverbal intelligence levels are low, prognosis is guarded and auditory agnosia should not be the only descriptor.

Careful communication among those caring for a child with a developmental disorder is essential, especially for children with rare problems. The more unusual the problem, the more likely that socioemotional problems will develop. This is true primarily because specialists disagree, which in turn confuses the parents and slows the time at which the child starts receiving a consistent, appropriate intervention. Management of a child with auditory verbal agnosia thus should be carefully orchestrated.

Diagnosis would include assessing the child's success with three modes of intervention: (1) spoken, (2) signed, and (3) spoken and signed. The condition in which words are only spoken should show the poorest gains to support the diagnosis.

Reading has been used effectively in special education (Rapin, personal communication, 1985) and a signed English could be tried.

Overall little is known about the specific form characteristic of the expressive language of these children (see Table 2-2). The assumption is that the meaning and use components are not attached well to the form because the latter is adequately processed on the input side.

DYSLEXIA

As Velluntino (1979, p. 321) points out, the term dyslexia is applied to children with a reading problem who also have the following characteristics: At least average nonverbal IQ, no sensory acuity problems, no "gross" brain damage, no "pronounced" emotional or social disorder, and a history of adequate academic instruction. As Kirk, (1981) points out, the Committee on Dylexia and World Illiteracy of the World Federation of Neurology defined dyslexia as "as disorder manifested by difficulty in learning to read despite conventional instruction, adequate intelligence and sociocultural opportunity. It is dependent upon fundamental cognitive disabilities which are fundamentally cognitive disabilities which are fundamentally of constitutional origin." Kirk (1981) and Velluntino (1981) stress that the term has little educational relevance and too often substitutes for an adequate assessment.

Mattis, French, and Rapin (1975) reported that 113 of 252 (45 percent) children referred to a neurologist's office for evaluation of learning and behavior disorders met these criteria. A small percentage of these children have only a reading problem ("pure" dyslexic); a large percentage also have difficulty with the auditory comprehension, oral expression, and writing of language (language-based dyslexic). In short, most but not all children with dyslexia also have trouble with language expression, language auditory comprehension, and the language of writing. Direct evidence of a neurological disorder is not essential for diagnostic purposes.

Denckla (1977) divided the neurologic findings for 52 children with dyslexia into developmental "soft signs," i.e.; they are abnormal only in reference to the child's, age and neurologic soft signs, that is; they are subtle but "classical" e.g., tremors and fixed strabismus. Very few the children were placed in the latter category. Many in both groups had a positive family history. She concluded that homogeneity of syndrome is not strongly associated with any one type of soft sign and rejected the notion of one syndrome, one etiology.

The vast majority of poor readers are so because of inappropriate or insufficient educational experiences. Most children who are not reading at age level are socioeconomically disadvantaged. It is difficult to succeed in school if one is poor, undernourished, or speaks a nonschool dialect. The criterion that there be a history of adequate academic instruction excludes these children from this category. Unfortunately many of the criteria are difficult to operationalize, e.g., example no gross brain damage, and therefore excluding such children is easier said than done.

A language-based dyslexia can easily go undetected during the first few years of school when the reading task does not require complex sentence-level language skills. Children who can speak in sentences certainly can be expected to understand the meanings conveyed by printed, simple sentences such as "Run, Spot, run." Even though, however, they appear to be expressing and understanding spoken language normally by the criterion of everyday usage, when they reach the level of reading tasks that require complex sentence-level language skills often a disorder is revealed. Subsequently, an assessment using standardized tests demonstrates that all is not well with oral expression and understanding.

For groups of children, Vellutino (1979) concluded that the evidence favors the more recent of four theories concerning dyslexia: the verbal processing theory. He points out that poor readers consistently perform more poorly on tasks influenced by verbal ability than controls with a similar past experience. He rejects the visual perception and visual memory, the intersensory integration, and the serial order recall theories as having only identified a secondary effect of a language disorder. The implication is that readers rely heavily upon language to store and retrieve information critical to the reading process and that dyslexics have difficulty on both short- and long-term memory tasks because of deficient language skills. A study from his own laboratory demonstrated that dyslexics had no basic difficulties in visually discriminating letters and words but were unable to remember their names. No differences were found between the ability of a dyslexic and normal group to graphically reproduce spatially confusing letters and words (b/d, was/saw, calm/clam) from memory after only a brief visual exposure to these stimuli. The dyslexic children, however, misnamed many of these same items when asked to read rather than copy them.

Additional group studies supporting the theory that many dyslexics are language disordered across modalities include one by Wiig, Semel, and Crouse (1973), which demonstrated that dyslexics had less facility than normal children in orally adding correct grammatical inflections to nonsense words, and one by Goldman (1976), which demonstrated that dyslexics had poorer auditory comprehension of complex grammatical constructions than normal readers. There are, however, clearly some children whose only problem appears to be with the printed word.

Correlates

Failing in school is not pleasant. Not meeting your own, your parents', or your teachers' expectations is also difficult. Everyone knows you are "intelligent." They may have thought you did not listen or express yourself as well as you should have during the early childhood years, but now the specificity of the reading task shows a difficulty that cannot be ignored. Much attention is now focused on you. Are you lazy? Are you in fact, dumb, or did you have inadequate teaching that went unnoticed? It's difficult suddenly being the center of such attention, but it is even more difficult not to be keeping up with your peers. Thus, emotional maladjustment in a dyslexic child is not unexpected. Herein lies a difficult task. Because of the definition by exclusion, emotional maladjustment cannot come before the dyslexia. Which comes first—school failure or emotional maladjustment—is usually impossible to describe in retrospect. A working assumption, however, is that emotional maladjustment is more likely to follow than precede a reading disability.

Norm-referenced tests standardized on the same children across all four language modalities are not yet available. Thus, one must rely on a clinical impression of the test results—a very unsatisfactory state of affairs. All tests are not equal in their ability to identify a language disorder. For example, one test of auditory comprehension, the Test of Auditory Comprehension of Language, has been shown to place normal children above age level in at least three separate studies (Allen, Bliss, & Timmons, 1981; Demetras et al., 1982; Stark & Tallal, 1981).

Language

The relationship between language acquisition levels and academic achievement is one that is widely accepted yet inadequately investigated. Lerner (1981) points out that "language plays a vital role in learning—consequently an intimate relationship exists between learning disabilities and deficits in language development" (p. 249). Research regarding this relationship, however, is limited as well as diverse in nature. Standardized tests are rarely used. The age of the children, time between initial diagnosis and follow-up, criteria for identifying language disorder, academic areas investigated, and method of follow-up vary greatly from study to study.

Table 2-3 summarizes what has been assessed in five randomly selected group studies of the relationship between preschool language disorders and subsequent academic achievement. As seen in this table, most studies have not assessed all four language modalities. Auditory comprehension of language is the area most neglected, with only one of the five studies assessing this area. Two studies included subjective measures.

Table 2-3

Language Areas Investigated in Five Studies of Children Identified as
Language Disordered as Preschoolers

Study	Listening	Language Spoken	Language Reading	Writing
King et al. (1982)		0	0	0
Aram et al. (1984)			X	
Hall & Tomblin (1978)			X	X
Garvey & Gordon (1973)	X	X	0	0
Griffiths (1969)		X	X	

0 = subjective judgment; X = standardized test results.

Group data show that deficits were found in all areas assessed. Two tentative conclusions follow. As discussed earlier, many of the children who have a language disorder at preschool age subsequently do poorly in school. More importantly, many children who do poorly in reading also do poorly on other tests of language.

As indicated in Table 2-2, the pattern of expressive language for many dyslexic children is similar to that of children with specific language impairment. In fact, many were in the latter category as preschoolers.

Management

Nonverbal IQ levels, hearing status, and oral language skills should be described for any child who is doing poorly in school. The neurologist would then proceed to distinguish those children with developmental soft signs from those with subtle neurologic soft signs, (Denckla, 1977) remembering that the latter are not common. Those with a positive family history also need to be identified.

Until recently, most authors were advocating the specific abilities or "basic" process approach to improve "readiness" for reading (e.g., Johnson & Myklebust, 1967; Kephart, 1960; Kirk & Kirk, 1971). Such an approach attempts to foster neurologic readiness for reading by remediating the basic process that is presumed to be impaired. As Hammill, Goodman, and Wiederholt (1974) noted, the assumptions underlying the perceptual–motor training programs include that visual–motor skills are important in cognitive development and that "visual-motor processes" are in fact trainable. Similar assumptions apply to other basic processes. Thus far, it appears to most reviewers that the effectiveness of this approach remains unvalidated (e.g., Bloom & Lahey, 1978; Rees, 1973; Tomblin, 1984; Vellutino, 1979). An example of such a study is reported by Hammill et al. (1974) in which pupils who were trained in visual perception scored no higher than their controls on academic or readiness tests. (Those who improved on visual perception were the perceptually adequate students rather than those who were perceptually handicapped.)

Currently, most of those who offer intervention suggestions for any group with a language disorder favor focusing directly on what the child needs to learn (e.g., Snyder-McLean, 1984; Tomblin, 1984). The assumptions underlying this approach include that auditory language is the keystone to reading with comprehension, and that the best model of successful language learning available at present is provided by the normally developing child. Such developmental sequences are seen as providing the essential foundation upon which the next skill may be built. This approach also remains unvalidated.

A word of caution in interpreting the results of any study that reports group data is in order. An individual's data are lost when averaged with those of others. It is thus possible that the specific abilities approach succeeds with carefully selected dyslexics, probably those who do not have a multimodality deficit. No one should ever expect one approach to work with all children.

Prognosis

At present little is published with a data base concerning what to expect for a child with dyslexia. (In my own experience, the more specific the problem, the rarer its existence, the more likely there is to be a positive family history, and the poorer the rate of progress and eventual outcome.) The group with deficits across all language modalities responds well to intervention unless the child also has a low performance IQ.

HYPERVERBAL-HYDROCEPHALUS

Some children with hydrocephalus have been referred to as having a "cocktail party" syndrome (Hadenius, Hagberg, Hyttnas-Bensch, and Sjogren, 1962). This apt term was coined to refer to children who were "mentally retarded but educable, with peculiar contrast between a good ability to learn words and talk, and not knowing what they are talking about. They love to chatter, but think illogically" (p. 118). Children with similar expressive language characteristics and a history of hydrocephalus have been referred to as "chatterboxes" or "bletherers," (Ingram & McNaughton, 1962, p. 288), dysverbal (Diller, Paddock, Badell-Ribera, & Swineyard, 1966), and hyperverbal (Swisher & Pinsker, 1971).

Hagberg and Sjorgen (1966) found the cocktail party syndrome in 25 percent of 63 children ages 6–24 years with spontaneously arrested hydrocephalus. It has been noted in both shunted (Parsons, 1968) and non-shunted (Hagberg & Sjorgen, 1966; Spain, 1974) hydrocephalic children. Intellectual impairment has ranged from minimal (Fleming, 1968) to severe (Hagberg, 1962). Some of the children had associated problems such as spina bifida cystica (Badell-Ribera, Shulman, & Paddock, 1966) or cerebral palsy (Ingram & Naughton, 1962). The cocktail party syndrome children had high spinal lesions (T6 to L2) compared with spina bifida cases without the syndrome in Tew's (1979) series.

Tew (1979) noted that children with this syndrome are most likely to be severely physically disabled girls who have valve-controlled hydrocephalus. He further noted that the insertion of a valve to control the increasing pressure of cerebrospinal fluid is probably less important than the severity of the hydrocephalus that led to neurosurgery. In Tew's series and those of others referred to earlier, a small number of children without valves but with mild hydrocephalus showed evidence of this syndrome.

Taylor (1961) suggested that the child's verbal fluency may be due to selective reinforcement by caregivers. The type of family who is likely to encourage the cocktail-party syndrome is described by Schaffer (1964) as "too cohesive." An abnormal degree of attention from all members of the family is focused on the child. It is certainly encouraging to hear a physically disabled child who was slow to start talking begin to speak in full, well-formed sentences. Rewarding these utterances would seem to follow naturally for many caregivers not sophisticated enough to realize that the form of language needs to be matched meaningfully to context for the child to benefit from his verbal fluency. Others have provided neurobiologic explanations for this behavior. Undoubtedly, such an explanation is pertinent to the core of the syndrome. Emery and Svitok (1968) speculated that ventricular dilation occurring as a result of hydrocephalus has an effect upon some of the association fibers that develop after birth. Laurence (1969) attributed the cocktail party syndrome as well as other neurologic abnormalities to thinning of the cerebral mantle. Autopsy evidence, however, is lacking.

Language

Structured test situations (Diller et al., 1966; Fleming, 1968) have not elicited the hyperverbal behavior noted during informal conversations with the children. It was, however, quantified as such during a pseudoinformal conversation on an individual basis (Swisher & Pinsker, 1971). Relative to controls born with one or more extremities absent, hydrocephalic children regarded as hyperverbal by their clinicians spoke

significantly more words and sentences and initiated more verbal interactions. This tendency to use a greater number of words appeared to
increase with the age of the hydrocephalic child. Type–token ratios indicated that the more talkative hydrocephalic children were more redun-
dant in word usage than the less talkative children. There was no significant difference between groups in the average number of words within
the sentences. The findings therefore suggest that the greater output of
the hyperverbal children included many of the same words used repeatedly in sentences similar in length to those of the controls. Overall, their
form is not as impaired as their meaning base and their use of form (see
Table 2-2).

Several findings in the study by Swisher and Pinsker (1971) indicate
why some hydrocephalic children fall below expected levels of achievement in school (e.g., Ingram & Naughton, 1962; Tew, 1979) and in rehabilitation training activities (Badell-Ribera et al., 1966). First, the total
number of words spoken did not relate to their full-scale IQs; secondly,
their production of the syntactical aspects of language as assessed by the
Illinois Test of Psycholinguistic Abilities was better than their comprehension and expression of the meaning of the words. Thirdly, as referred
to earlier, greater quantity of output was not accompanied by a greater
variety of words. A clinician or parent who relied primarily on the
amount and form of verbal output thus could have overestimated the
intellectual potential of these children.

Three types of verbal output have been noted in hyperverbal, hydrocephalic children. Swisher and Pinsker (1971) reported that the output of
the youngest children was primarily characterized by bizarre, hostile,
and inappropriate responses. The language of the children in the next
higher age-range showed a decrease in bizarreness and hostility but remained inappropriate. In agreement with reports (Diller et al., 1966;
Fleming, 1968) that the inappropriate quality of the output decreased
with age, the oldest children exhibited appropriate language behavior.
Overall, these findings are in line with the observations (Fleming, 1968;
Taylor, 1961) that most hydrocephalic children are friendly and chatty,
whereas some show signs of irritability, social aggressiveness, and irrelevant language behavior.

In agreement with the observations of Ingram and Naughton (1962),
a review of the case histories of the hyperverbal, hydrocephalic children
studied by Swisher and Pinsker (1971) indicated that many of them were
considered by parents or speech–language pathologists to have had delayed language development up to the age of $2\frac{1}{2}$ years. After that age their
output increased quite rapidly, so that generally by their third birthday
they were no longer considered by parents or physicians to be delayed in
language development. In retrospect, it seems that this view was incorrect and based primarily on the correct syntax (form) of the utterances.

The poor tie to the meaning base and, in some cases, inappropriate use apparently were not detected.

Sensory-motor

The sensory–motor correlates of hydrocephalus are well known to neurologists as is the possible accompanying mental retardation and will not be reviewed here.

Management

First the hydrocephalus must be arrested. Then a multidisciplinary approach including neurologists, physical therapists, speech–language pathologists, and special educators is recommended. Often physical therapy, language therapy, and special education must be started. Psychometric testing appears necessary in many cases. Parents, however, may have difficulty accepting the results.

As mentioned earlier, the emergence of a quantity of language in a hydrocephalic child may be a source of pleasure and comfort to the parents. When the child's body is physically impaired, they can believe that intelligence is not because of the emerging expressive language. Tew (1979) stated that the parents often went out of their way to demonstrate their child's achievements. An 8-year-old girl (IQ 40) could "sing" the whole of two pop songs, and a boy of 5 years of age (IQ 59) could name many of the players and their positions in the Welsh Rugby team. the latter could not, however, give an adequate definition of an apple or a book. When asked to estimate their child's IQ, the parents of children with the cocktail party syndrome estimated that their child scored on average 18 points higher than the actual result, with some parents giving IQ estimates up to 30 to 40 points above the child's actual score. Additionally, they were more likely to be critical of the results of the cognitive assessment.

Attention to the child's socioemotional development requires helping him or her adjust to physical limitations, and preventing adjustment problems by helping the child and the parents determine realistic expectations regarding the degree of academic success to be expected. Improving the quality of the child's language skills for communication purposes and as a basis for success in school fosters achievement of both of these goals.

The suggestions to improve the superficial form–context mismatch characteristic of the expressive language of autistic children given by Swisher and Demetras (1985) and summarized earlier apply not only to autistic children but also to hyperverbal, hydrocephalic children. The words and sentences already being spoken by the child must be given meaning and tied appropriately to the context in which they are spoken. The parents must be helped to understand that rewarding the child for inappropriate or bizzare utterances of a noteworthy syntactic complexity is to be avoided. The child must be helped to pause, self-correct, and speak words and sentences that are meaningful and appropriate to the context. A naturalistic rather than drill-like language-learning setting is recommended. Gains in the use of meaningful language would be expected to aid the child in school and in social contexts.

Prognosis

Tew (1979) demonstrated that 5-year-old children with the cocktail-party syndrome were distinguishable from other children with hydro-cephalus and spina bifida and normal controls in terms of lower IQ scores on both the verbal and performance scales of the Weschler Preschool Scales and lower Vineland Social Maturity Scale scores. The poor scores seemed to be due to the combined effects of low IQ and severe physical handicap, and possibly for some children, to oversolicitous caregivers. At 7 years of age, they also had poorer reading, spelling, and arithmetic scores. Their teachers also reported that they had shorter concentration spans and more behavior disorders than other cases of spina bifida. The children who had "grown out" of the syndrome by 10 years of age were of comparatively higher intelligence with a mean full-scale IQ of 71.3, while the children with aberrant language were mostly in the severely sub-normal range. The highest individual IQ in the children with this syndrome at age 10 years was 61, and the mean full-scale IQ was 44.9 (verbal IQ 57.3, performance IQ 42.3). Thus the presence of the syndrome at the age of 10 years was diagnostically significant of a subnormal level of intelligence.

By what means and to what extent the expressive language of these children is modifiable has not yet been determined. The limit to their development of meaningful, appropriate expressive language will include the level of their cognitive development as discussed previously.

PSYCHIATRIC DISORDERS

Look for a language disorder in every child considered to have a psychiatric problem because the distinction between a psychiatric and a neurologic disorder is ill defined. The one cause, one condition assumption is never appropriate. Neurologic signs may be present at one age but not at another because of maturational changes, yet the underlying condition remains the same. There is considerable controversy concerning the conclusions to be drawn from so-called soft neurologic signs such as EEG abnormalities. The effects of such problems were shown in the Maudsley follow-up study of children with infantile psychoses conducted by Rutter, Greenfeld, and Lockyer (1967). Many children who showed no evidence of neurologic abnormality when first seen developed epileptic seizures during adolescence. One is then left with determining whether their disorders should be classified as neurologic or psychiatric. I will leave undiscussed the futility of attempting to determine how much of a child's problem can be labeled as "organic" and how much can be labeled as due to environmental factors.

EVALUATION OF A CHILD WITH A SUSPECTED LANGUAGE DISORDER

Because most language disorders appear in the early developmental years, it is irresponsible to adopt a "wait and see" approach. In the presence of a suspected problem, a child's language, motor, performance, and hearing skills should be assessed and his or her emotional development described. A speech assessment may also be required. The results form a baseline that then permits the degree of progress over time to be evaluated. "Wait and see" without this baseline is waiting without the necessary prerequisite for seeing.

A brief overview describing how a speech–language pathologist evaluates a child with a suspected language disorder follows. Physicians (e.g., Ferry, 1981; Rapin, 1977) have provided detailed accounts with more emphasis on the medical and neurologic components of the evaluation. The framework for the evaluation will vary depending on the purpose. Five questions should be addressed before the evaluation is completed: (1) Is there a language disorder? (2) What is the etiology? (3) What are the areas of the deficit? (4) What are the goals of intervention? (5) What is the prognosis? Arriving at answers to all the questions for a child whose developmental age is at least $2\frac{1}{2}$ years will involve evaluating information obtained from norm-referenced test instruments, standardized and nonstandardized observational procedures, expressive language analyses, criterion-referenced language measures, and questionnaires.

The steps taken by the speech–language pathologist are similar to those performed during a neurologic evaluation. They include (1) taking a history, (2) observing the child, (3) assessing skills, (4) referring to additional professionals, (5) establishing a tentative diagnosis, and (6) developing a program of treatment or continued observation. These six steps allow for input from the caregivers, the child, and cooperating professionals in related areas of specialty. Conceptually, the first step (case history) encourages input from the caregiver, and the second step (observation) encourages input from the child. Information gathered from steps three and four represents primary input from referral sources. The combined information from these four steps serves as a basis for the final two steps: establishing a tentative diagnosis and developing a program of treatment or continued observation.

Step 1: Case History

Two types of information are needed: (1) specific information regarding developmental milestones, history of illnesses, language spoken by the caregivers, etc.; and (2) general information pertaining to the caregivers' perception of the nature of their child's problem and the evaluation to follow. The same interview technique cannot be used to obtain both types of information effectively. Detailed information is best obtained prior to the evaluation in a questionnaire form so caregivers can refer to their child's baby records. From a review of the questionnaire, the clinician develops a hypothesis about the nature of the child's problem and an outline for the interview to come. Then a face-to-face interview is conducted for general questions and to discuss the information submitted on the questionnaire.

While the specific genetic patterns of most childhood language disorders are not fully known, the family history of speech, language, or reading problems is explored in the questionnaire. Selected cases will require pedigree analysis and genetic counseling. In addition, any threat to the developing brain or ear is given special attention.

In order to obtain the maximum amount of unbiased information from the caregiver, it is important to start the interview with broad, general questions and then focus to finer detail. The interview can be structured with reference to the child's development in four areas: intellectual, speech–language, socioemotional, and motor. The onset and duration of milestones in all four areas should be explored. The interview is best conducted in private and with sufficient time allowed for elaboration of pertinent facts. The clinician who conducts the initial interview is optimally the one to summarize all information at the end of the evaluation process. During the interview, the caregivers are encouraged to voice opinions about the nature and degree of their child's problem and to state their expectations about the evaluation procedures to follow. In addition, the clinician gains information regarding the child's use of language in different situations. Does the child communicate predominantly with words or gestures? Is his or her speech intelligible to strangers? What are specific examples of the child's communication skills; e.g., how does he or she ask to go out and play?

Step 2: Observations

Observations can begin when the child arrives for the evaluation and continue throughout the session. They are not limited to a 10-minute session during which the clinician stands behind a two-way mirror and observes the child play. The observations can be grouped into the same four areas suggested above: intellectual, speech–language, socioemotional, and motor.

A clinician can learn a lot by observing the child alone and in interaction with the caregiver. A language disorder most likely results from dysfunction of the ear or brain of the child. A mismatch between child and caregiver styles of communication, however, can contribute to a developmental delay. One of the most productive sources of information about a child with delayed speech or language development is the observation of behavior in structured and unstructured situations. Disregarding infants, the lower the level of the child, the more there will be a discrepancy between behaviors in these two settings (e.g., Schopler et al., 1971). Typically most children seem less impaired in a structured situation.

Step 3: Assessment of Speech–Language Skills

The assessment of speech and language skills addresses two questions: Is there a problem? If so, what are the levels of expressive language skills? Tests are not yet adequately designed to address still another question: Is comprehension of language better than expression of language? (McCauley & Swisher, 1984b)

The two questions must be kept separate in the mind of the examiner because the answers come from different sources of information. The first question requires the use of norm-referenced test instruments for children at a developmental level of approximately $2\frac{1}{2}$ years or higher. Below that level, parent interviews and observations of the child must be substituted. The second question requires the use of criterion-referenced measures including standardized language sampling analysis procedures and usually nonstandardized probes of specific language structures and uses.

The speech–language pathologist must be aware of any special considerations that would influence the validity of the assessment results such as hearing or visual deficits. The norms for a test also must have been obtained from children of the same socioeconomic status and dialect as the child being tested. The objective documentation of a language disorder is currently primarily limited to middle-class, so-called standard English speakers because children with these characteristics were used to form the normative base. Furthermore, a majority of the tests used to determine the presence of a speech or language disorder meet only a minimum number of psychometric criteria (McCauley & Swisher, 1984a). Without carefully developed test instruments, the validity and reliability of the test scores and the resulting diagnoses are in jeopardy.

In mild cases or those who are close to recovery from a more severe disorder, the currently available tests of expression generally reveal deficits not detected by most comprehension tests. This is not necessarily surprising when we acknowledge that spontaneous expression is a recall task and a test of comprehension is a recognition task. Chance helps improve one's score primarily in the latter case.

In line with the results of other studies, Demetras, et al. (1982) found that the comprehension tests they administered, which did not include the Token Test, were not as useful as the expressive tests for identifying specific language impairment. The Test of Auditory Comprehension of Language, as mentioned earlier, identified none of the 10 children judged independently by three speech–language pathologists to be language disordered. One child would have been overlooked if a receptive vocabulary test had not been included in the battery. These results will not apply to all groups of language-disordered children. They do, however, serve to illustrate that considerable thought must go into one's choice of a test battery for each child. Thought must also go into the interpretation of the results (McCauley & Swisher, 1984b). Age levels, for example, are inappropriate as the sole criterion of impairment. If the report only defends the label of language disordered in terms of age levels, further documentation should be requested. Different tests are also more useful than others for different ages.

Step 4: Referral

If the child appears below normal in any of the four areas assessed, a referral is made to the appropriate professional. A child suspected of a language disorder should always be referred to an audiologist. If indications point to a possible deficit in intellectual functioning, the child should be referred to a psychologist for testing with both verbal and nonverbal measures. (Remember that many IQ tests are heavily language based, even so-called performance tests such as the Kaufman Assessment Battery for Children Nonverbal Scale and the Leiter International Performance Scale.)

Remember also that an IQ is the summary score derived from items that sample a broad range of behaviors. It enables one to compare a particular individual with the norms established by testing a population of presumably normal children of the same age and background. A full-scale IQ can be useful for making distinctions among normal children and for predicting academic performance. It is much less meaningful when tests are administrated to handicapped children whose performance across tests is uneven. Language-disordered children by definition are expected to do poorly on a full-scale measure because language skills are assessed. A summary score represents neither their areas of real deficit nor their strengths.

Step 5: Establishment of a Tentative Diagnosis

Essentially, the establishment of a diagnostic label is a one-line summary of all the information that has been gathered. This label, with or without supporting information, will probably accompany the child throughout his or her school years and possibly throughout life. For this reason, it is critical that the label be tentative and reviewed as often as is appropriate for the child's chronologic age and rate of progress.

Essentially, the establishment of a diagnostic label guides professionals in determining both medical and educational short- and long-term plans of action for the child. All plans should be reconsidered frequently. The diagnostic category may provide information relative to how intervention will be structured; e.g., children in the hearing loss category will need to be considered for a hearing aid. The focus of intervention for improving language, however, always will be language behaviors. It is an error to assume that similar language levels and expressive language patterns imply that the children fit into the same diagnostic category (see Table 2-2), or that they will respond equally to the same intervention procedures. Level of development within each language area directly reflects what a child is ready to learn.

It is the responsibility of the neurologist to in-service other professionals regarding childhood syndromes, their etiologies, and usual course of development so that a child will be placed in the most appropriate setting possible. In this manner, the teachers and administrators for the child's school can become more effective members of the team. Likewise, they must do the same for the neurologist regarding expected educational progress and related problems.

Step 6: Development of Intervention Program or Continued Observation

Two factors influence this decision: the severity of the problem and the age of the child. The former reflects both the level of the language disorder and the family's reaction to it. A mild delay in language development that is perceived by the family to be a major obstacle to family communication or academic success leads to a different management plan than a mild disorder to which there is no reaction.

In the absence of hearing, the rate of progress depends primarily on an interaction between the child's age and level of cognitive development.

The younger the child with a presumed brain dysfunction, the more likely there will be spontaneous improvements without direct intervention. For some children less than 3 years of age, therefore, some speech–language pathologists give parents advice as to how to provide better or more frequent language lessons for their child, and then they re-evaluate in approximately 3 months. For all children, the greater the severity of the disorder, the closer school approaches, the more bad habits observed, and the poorer the family interactions, the sooner therapy is started. Progress is then assessed over time with vacations from therapy or alternate treatment interventions.

Norm-referenced tests are designed to examine gross, relatively stable behavioral patterns. In measuring progress, however, comparisons need to be made of specific language behaviors within an individual over time. For this purpose, criterion-referenced tests are more appropriate. Norm-referenced tests merely show whether the child is impaired at a given point in time relative to normal children of the same age. Progress noted from test scores may be the result of imperfect test reliability and may not reflect clinically significant improvement in language abilities.

CONCLUSIONS

Syndromes

- The major task before the neurologist is to identify and treat whenever possible the "cause" of a language disorder. For most children, no specific cause will be identified. For most of those for whom the etiology can be identified, the condition is irreversible.
- Another task before the neurologist is to identify the syndrome into which the child fits. Such a diagnosis has implications for (1) referrals, (2) intervention with family and child, and (3) prognosis. The diagnostic category should be re-evaluated no less than every 6 months for a developing child.

Correlates

The minimum team available to a language-disordered child should include the following:

- Clinical psychologist who can administer and interpret the results of verbal and performance scales of IQ tests
- Neurologist who understands that a language disorder is usually associated with either a brain or an ear problem or both

- Pediatrician or otolaryngologist who is knowledgeable about otitis media
- Pediatric audiologist who is skilled at fitting hearing aids and able to perform evoked response as well as behavioral audiometry
- Social worker who understands the far-reaching implications of a language disorder on the child's emotional and educational development
- Speech–language pathologist who is knowledgeable about normal sequences of language acquisition and normal caregiver–child language interactions

Language

- A description of a child's language skills will include all modalities appropriate for the child's level of development, the areas of vocabulary and syntax, and observations concerning functional use.
- Standardized, norm-referenced tests are needed to document the presence of a disorder; analysis of spontaneous expressive language is needed to determine therapy objectives.
- Information concerning the syndrome into which the language disorder fits can influence how intervention should proceed (e.g., the use of a hearing aid with a deaf child).
- Information concerning the level and pattern of language disorder will influence decisions concerning what the child is ready to learn.

Management

- A developmental model is best for guiding intervention.
- All but the very profoundly impaired child can learn at least a little more than he or she currently knows; some can learn a lot more if special help is provided.
- The older the child when assessment, evaluation, and intervention begin, the more bad habits there are to change and the more lost opportunities there are for learning.
- Assessment and intervention techniques are available even for infants. It is no longer appropriate to tell parents that the child will outgrow the disorder.
- Many language-disordered children require management by a team of professionals working closely with the children's caregivers.

Prognosis

- Level of cognitive development is the major determinant of expected rate and level of progress within each developmental disability group.
- Below 6 years of age, progress is not predictable for an individual; above age 6, trends become obvious for many individuals.
- The older the child, the less likely there will be spontaneous gains.

REFERENCES

Affolter, F., Brubaker, R., & Bischofberger, W. (1974). Comparative studies between normal and language disturbed children. *Acta Otolaryngol,* (Suppl. *323*), 1–32.

Alajouanine, T. & Lhermitte, F. (1965). Acquired aphasia in children. *Brain, 88,* 653–662.

Allen, D., Bliss, L., & Timmons, J. (1981). Language evaluation: Science or art? *Journal of Speech and Hearing Disorders, 46,* 66–68.

Alpern, G. (1967). Measurement of "untestable" autistic children. *Journal of Abnormal Psychology, 72,* 478–486.

Aram, D., Ekelman, B., & Nation, J. (1984). Preschoolers with language disorders: 10 years later. *Journal of Speech and Hearing Research, 27,* 232–244.

Aram, D., & Nation, J. (1975). Patterns of language behavior in children with developmental language disorders. *Journal of Speech and Hearing Research, 18,* 229–241.

Badell-Ribera, A., Shulman, K., & Paddock, N. (1966). The relationship of nonprogressive hydrocephalus to intellectual functioning in children with spina bifida cystica. *Pediatrics, 37,* 787–793.

Baker, L., Cantwell, D., Rutter, M., & Bartak, L. (1976). Language and autism. In E. Ritvo, B. Freeman, E. Ornitz, & P. Tanguay, (Eds.), *Autism: Diagnosis, current research and management.* New York: Spectrum.

Basser, L. (1962). Hemiplegia of early onset and the faculty of speech with special reference to the effects of hemispherectomy. *Brain, 85,* 427–460.

Bedrosian, J., & Prutting, C. (1978). Communicative performance of mentally retarded adults in four conversational settings. *Journal of Speech and Hearing Research, 21,* 79–95.

Benton, A. (1964). Developmental aphasia and brain damage. *Cortex, 1,* 40–52.

Bloom, L. (1970). *Language development: Form and function in emerging grammars.* Cambridge, MA: MIT Press.

Bloom, L., & Lahey, M. (1978). *Language development and language disorders.* New York: John Wiley.

Brandes, P., & Elhinger, D. (1981). The effects of early middle ear pathology on audiology perception and academic achievement. *Journal of Speech and Hearing Disorders, 46,* 301–307.

American National Standards, (1973). *Standard specifications for audiometers.* (ANSI S 3.20-1973) New York: American National Standards Institute.

Brinton, B., & Fujiki, M. (1982). A comparison of request–response sequences in the discourse of normal and language disordered children. *Journal of Speech and Hearing Disorders, 47,* 57–62.

Caccamise, F., Hatfield, N., Brewer, L. (1978). Manual/simultaneous communication research: Results and implications. *American Annals of the Deaf, 123,* 803–823.

Cantwell, D., Baker, L., & Rutter, M. (1978). A comprehensive study of infantile autism and specific developmental receptive language disorder. IV. Analysis of syntax and language function. *Journal of Child Psychology and Psychiatry, 19,* 351–362.

Chomsky, N. (1957). *Syntactic structres.* The Hague: Mouton.

Churchill, D. (1972). The relationship of infantile autism and early childhood schizophrenia to developmental language disorders of childhood. *Journal of Autism and Childhood Schizophrenia, 2,* 182–197.

Colby, K. (1973). The rationale for computor based treatment of language difficulties in nonspeaking autistic children. *Journal of Autism and Childhood Schizophrenia, 3,* 254–260.

Creedan, M. (1973, March). *Language development in nonverbal autistic children using a simultaneous communication system.* Paper presented at the Society for Research in Child Development Meeting, Philadelphia.

Curtiss, S. (1981). Dissociations between language and cognition: Cases and implications. *Journal of Autism and Developmental Disorders, 11,* 15–30.

De Hirsch, K. (1971). Prediction in reading disability: A review of the literature. In A. Hayes & A. Silver (Eds.), *Report of the Interdisciplinary Committee on Reading Disability.* Washington DC: Center for Applied Linguistics.

Demetras, M., Matkin, A., & Swisher, L. (1982, November). *Speech and language behaviors of preschool children: A clinical review of tests.* Paper presented at The Annual American Speech–Language–Hearing Association Conference, Toronto, Canada.

De Meyer, M., Burton, S., De Meyer, W., Norton, J., Allen, J., & Steele, R. (1973). Prognosis in autism: A follow-up study. *Journal of Autism and Childhood Schizophrenia, 3,* 199–246.

Denckla, M. (1977). Minimal brain dysfunction and dyslexia: Beyond diagnosis by exclusion. In M. Blaw, I. Rapin, & M. Kinsbourne (Eds.), *Topics in child neurology.* New York: Spectrum.

Dentler, R., & Mackler, B. (1962). Mental ability and sociometric status among normal and retarded children: A review of the literature. *Psychological Bulletin, 59,* 273–283.

Despert, J. (1947). Psychotheraphy in child schizophrenia. *American Journal of Psychiatry, 104,* 36–43.

Diller, L., Paddock, N., Badell-Ribera, A., & Swinyard, C. (1966). Verbal behavior in spina bifida children. In C. Swinyard (Ed.), *Comprehensive care of the child with spina bifida manifesta* (Rehabilitation Monograph No. 31). New York: Institute of Rehabilitation Medicine.

Doherty, L., & Swisher, L. (1977). Children with autistic behavior. In F. E. Minifie & L. L. Lloyd (Eds.), *Communicative and cognitive abilities—Early behavioral assessment.* Baltimore: University Park Press.

Emery, J., & Svitok, I. (1968). Intra-hemispherical distances in congenital hydrocephalus associated with meningomyelocele. *Developmental Medicine and Child Neurology, 15,* 21–29.

Fay, W., & Mermelstein, R. (1982). Language in infantile autism. In S. Rosenberg (Ed.), *Handbook of psycholinguistics: Major thrusts in research and theory,* Hillsdale, NJ: L. Erlbaum.

Ferry, P. (1981). Clinical appraisal of language functions in the preschool child. In *Developmental disabilities in preschool children.* New York: Spectrum.

Ferry, P., Culbertson, J., Fitzgibbons, M., & Netsky, M. (1979). Brain function and language disabilities. *International Journal of Pediatric Otorhinolaryngology, 1,* 13–24.

Fleming, C. (1968). The verbal behaviour of hydrocephalic children. *Developmental Medicine and Child Neurology,* (Suppl. 15), 74–82.

Freedman, P., & Carpenter, R. (1976). Semantic relations used by normal and language-impaired children at stage 1. *Journal of Speech and Hearing Research, 19,* 784–795.

Friedman, D., Simon, R., Ritter, W., & Rapin, I. (1977). CNV and P300 experimental paradigms for the study of language. *Progress in Clinical Neurophysiology, 3,* 205–211.

Friedman, P., & Friedman, K. (1980). Accounting for individual differences when comparing the effectiveness of remedial language teaching methods. *Applied Psycholinguistics, 1,* 151–170.

Friel-Patti, S., Finitzo-Hieber, T., Conti, G., & Brown, C. (1982). Language delay in infants associated with middle ear disease and mild, fluctuating hearing impairment. *Pediatric Infectious Disease, 1,* 104–109.

Furth, H. (1966). *Thinking without language: Psychological implications of deafness.* New York: Free Press.

Gallagher, T. (1977). Revision behaviors in the speech of normal children developing language. *Journal of Speech and Hearing Research, 20,* 303–318.

Garvey, M., & Gordon, N. (1973). A follow-up study of children with disorders of speech development. *British Journal of Disorders of Communication, 4,* 227–241.

Goldman, S. (1976). Reading skill and the minimum distance principle: A comparison of listening and reading comprehension. *Journal of Experimental Child Psychology, 22,* 123–142.

Griffiths, C. (1969). A follow-up study of children with disorders of speech. *British Journal of Disorders of Communication, 4,* 46–56.

Grossman, H. (1977). *Manual on terminology and classification in mental retardation.* Washington, DC: American Association on Mental Deficiency.

Guttman, E. (1942). Aphasia in children. *Brain, 65,* 205–219.

Hadenius, A., Hagberg, B., Hyttnas-Bensch, K., & Sjogren, I. (1962). The natural prognosis of infantile hydrocephalus. *Acta Paediatrica, 51,* 117–118.

Hagberg, B. (1962). The sequelae of spontaneously arrested infantile hydrocephalus. *Developmental Medicine and Child Neurology, 4,* 583–587.

Hagberg, B., & Sjorgen, I. (1966). The chronic brain syndrome of infantile hydrocephalus: A follow-up study of 63 spontaneously arrested cases. *American Journal of Disabled Children, 112,* 189–196.

Hall, P., & Tomblin, J. (1978). A follow-up study of children with articulation and language disorders. *Journal of Speech and Hearing Disorders, 43,* 227–241.

Hammill, D., Goodman, L., & Wiederholt, J. (1974). Visual–motor processes: Can we train them? *The Reading Teacher, 27,* 469.

Holm, V., & Kunze, L. (1969). Effect of chronic otitis media on language and speech development. *Pediatrics,* 1969, *43,* 833–839.

Ingalls, R. (1978). *Mental retardation: The changing outlook,* New York: John Wiley.

Ingram, T., & Naughton, J. (1962). Paediatric and psychological aspects of cerebral palsy associated with hydrocephalus. *Developmental Medicine and Child Neurology, 4,* 287–292.

Inhelder, B. (1963). Observations sur les aspects operatifs et figuraifs de la pensee chez des enfants dysphasiques. *Problemes de Psycholinguistique, 6,* 143–153.

Jensema, C., & Trybus, R. (1978). *Communication patterns and educational achievements of hearing impaired children* (Series T, No. 2). Washington, DC: Gallaudet College, Office of Demographic Studies.

Johnson, D., & Myklebust, H. (1967). *Learning disabilities: Educational principles and practices.* New York: Grune & Stratton.

Johnson W., Anderson, V., Kopp, G., Mase, D., Schuell, H., Shover, J., et al. (1952). Speech disorders and speech correction. American Speech and Hearing Association Committee on the Midcentury White House Conference. *Journal of Speech and Hearing Disorders, 17,* 129–137.

Johnston, J., & Schery, T. (1976). The use of grammatical morphemes by children with communication disorders. In D. Morehead & A. Morehead (Eds.), *Normal and deficient child language.* Baltimore: University Park Press.

Jordan, T. (1967). Language and mental retardation. In R. Schiefelbusch, R. Copeland, & J. Smith (Eds.), *Language and mental retardation: Emperical considerations.* New York: Holt Rinehart & Winston.

Jordon, I., Gustason, G., & Rosen, R. (1967). Current communication trends in programs for the deaf. *American Annuals of the Deaf, 121,* 527–532.

Kamhi, A. (1981). Nonlinguistic symbolic and conceptual abilities of language-impaired and normally developing children. *Journal of Speech and Hearing Research, 24,* 446–453.

Kamhi, A., & Johnston, J. (1982). Towards an understanding of retarded children's linguistic deficiencies. *Journal of Speech and Hearing Research, 25,* 435–445.

Kanner, L. (1943). Autistic disturbances of affective contact. *The Nervous Child, 2,* 217–250.

Kanner, L. (1946). Irrelevant and metaphorical language in early infantile autism. *American Journal of Psychiatry, 103,* 242–246.

Kanner, L. (1971). Follow-up study of eleven autistic children originally reported in 1943. *Journal of Autism and Childhood Schizophrenia, 1,* 119–145.

Kanner, L. (1973). *Childhood psychosis: Initial studies and new insights.* Washington DC: V. H. Winston.

Karchmer, M., Milone, M., & Wolk, S. (1979). Educational significance of hearing loss at three levels of severity. *American Anuals of the Deaf, 124,* 97–109.

Kephart, N. (1960). *The slow learner in the classroom.* Columbus: Charles E. Merrill.

Kern, L., Koegel, R., Dyer, K., Blew, P., & Fenton, L. (1982). The effects of physical exercise on self-stimulation and appropriate responding in autistic children. *Journal of Autism and Developmental Disorders, 12,* 399–417.

King, R., Jones, C., & Lasky, E. (1982). In retrospect: A fifteen year follow-up report of speech–language disordered children. *Language, Speech and Hearing Serves in the Schools, 13*, 24–32.

Kinsbourne, M., & Swisher, L. (1977). Disorders of voice, speech, and language in children. *Practice of Pediatrics, 4*, 1–28.

Kirk, S. (1981). Comment on the term dyslexia. *Reading Instruction Journal, 24*, 8–9.

Kirk, S., & Kirk, W. (1971). *Psychological learning disabilities: Diagnosis and remediation.* Urbana, IL: University of Illinois Press.

Klein, D., & Pollack, M. (1966). Schizophrenic children and maternal speech facility. *American Journal of Psychiatry, 123*, 232.

Kriegsmann, E., Wulbert, M., Inglis, S., & Mills, B. (1975). Language delay and associated mother-child interactions. Developmental Psychology, 11, 61–70.

Landau, W., Goldstein, R., & Kleffner, F. (1960). Congenital aphasia: A clinico-pathologic study. *Neurology, 10*, 915–921.

Landau, W., & Kleffner, F. (1957). Syndrome of acquired aphasia with convulsive disorder in children. *Neurology, 7*, 523–530.

Laurence, K. (1969). Neurological and intellectual sequelae of hydrocephalus. *Archives of Neurology, 20*, 73–81.

Lenneberg, E. (1964). Language disorders in children. *Harvard Educational Review, 34*, 152–177.

Leonard, L. (1972). What is deviant language? *Journal of Speech and Hearing Disorders, 37*, 427–446.

Leonard, L. (1975). Facilitating linguistic skills in children with specific language impairment. *Applied Psycholinguistics, 2*, 89–118.

Leonard, L. (1982). The nature of specific language impairment in children. In S. Rosenberg (Ed.), *Handbook of applied psycholinguistics: Major thrusts of research and theory.* Hillsdale, NJ: L. Erlbaum.

Leonard, L., Bolders, J., & Miller, J. (1976). An examination of the semantic relations reflected in the language usage of normal and language disordered children. *Journal of Speech and Hearing Research, 19*, 371–392.

Lerner, J. (1981). *Learning disabilities: Theories, diagnosis, and teaching strategies.* Boston: Houghton Mifflin.

Leske, C. (1979). *Incidence and prevalence in panel communication disorders.* Report to the National Advisory Neurological and Communicative Disorders and Stroke Council, NIH Publication No. 79-1914.

Lewis, N. (1976). Otitis media and linguistic incompetence. *Archives of Otolaryngology, 102*, 387–390.

Lloyd, L., & Fulton, R. (1972). Audiology's contribution to communication programming with the retarded. In J. McLean, D. Yoder, & D. R. Schiefelbusch (Eds.), *Language intervention with the retarded–developing strategies.* Baltimore: University Park Press.

Lockyer, L., & Rutter, M. (1969). A five-to-fifteen year follow-up study of infantile psychosis. III. Psychological aspects. *British Journal of Psychiatry, 15*, 865–882.

Lovaas, O. (1966). A programme for the establishment of speech in psychotic children. In J. K. Wing (Ed.), *Early childhood autism.* Oxford: Pergamon.

Ludlow, C. (1980). Childrens language disorders: Recent research advances. *Annals of Neurology, 7*, 497–507.

Ludlow, C., Cudahy, E., Bassich, C., & Brown, G. (1982). The auditory processing skills of hyperactive, language impaired and reading disabled boys. In J. Katz & E. Lasky (Eds.), *Central auditory processing disorders: Problems of speech, language, and learning.* Baltimore: University Park Press.

Lyle, J. (1959). The effect of an institution environment upon the verbal development of imbecile children. I. Verbal intelligence. *Journal of Mental Deficiency Research, 3,* 122–128.

Mantovani, J., & Landau, W. (1980). Acquired aphasia with convulsive disorder: Course and prognosis. *Neurology, 30,* 524–529.

Maskarinec, A., Cairns, G., Butterfield, E., & Weamer, D. (1981). Longitudinal observations of individual infants vocalizations. *Journal of Speech and Hearing Disorders, 46,* 267–273.

Mattis, S., French, J., & Rapin, I. (1975). Dyslexia in children and young adults: Three independent neuropsychological syndromes. *Developmental Medicine and Child Neurology, 17,* 150–163.

McCauley, R., & Swisher, L. (1984a). Use and misuse of norm-referenced tests in clinical assessment: a hypothetical case. *Journal of Speech and Hearing Disorders, 49,* 338–348.

McCauley, R., & Swisher, L. (1984b). Psychometric review of language and articulation tests for preschool children. *Journal of Speech and Hearing Disorders, 49,* 34–42.

Menyuk, P. (1964). Comparison of grammer of children with functionally deviant and normal speech. *Journal of Speech and Hearing Research, 7,* 109–121.

Menyuk, P. (1979). Design factors in the assessment of language development in children with otitis media. *Annals Otology, Rhinology, and Laryngology, 88* (Suppl.), 78–87.

Meyers, D., & Goldfarb, W. (1961). Studies of perplexity in mothers of schizophrenic children. *American Journal of Orthopsychiatry, 31,* 551–564.

Miller, J. (1981, June). *Individual differences in the language acquisition of retarded children.* Paper presented at the Second Annual Symposium for Research in Child Language Disorders, University of Wisconsin at Madison.

Morley, M. (1965). *The development and disorders of speech in childhood.* Edinburgh: E. & S. Livingstone.

Morley, M., Court, D., Miller, H., & Garside, R. (1955). Delayed speech and developmental aphasia. *British Medical Journal, 2,* 436–467.

Needham, L. S., & Swisher, L. (1972). A comparison of three tests of audiology comprehension for adult aphasics. *Journal of Speech and Hearing Disorders, 37,* 123–131.

Needleman, H. (1977). Effects of hearing loss from early recurrent otitis media. In B. Jaffe (Ed.), *Hearing loss in children.* Baltimore: University Park Press.

Norlin, P., & Van Tasell, D. (1980). Linguistic skills of hearing-impaired children. *Monographs in Contemporary Audiology, 2,* 1–32.

O'Connor, N. (1975). Cognitive processes and language ability in the severely retarded. In E. H. Lenneberg & E. Lenneberg (Eds.), *Foundations of language development, Vol. 1.* New York: Academic Press.

Ogden, P. (1979). *Experiences and attitudes of oral deaf adults regarding oralism.* Unpublished doctoral dissertation, University of Illinois.

Paradise, J. (1981). Otitis media during early life: How hazardous to development? A critical review of the evidence. *Pediatrics, 68,* 869–873.

Parsons, J. (1968). An investigation into the verbal facility of hydrocephalic children, with special reference to vocabulary, morphology, and fluency. *Developmental Medicine and Child Neurology,* (Suppl. 16), 109–110.

Pascoe, D. (1975). Frequency responses of hearing aids and their effects on the speech perception of hearing-impaired subjects. *Annals of Otology, Rhinology, and Laryngology. 84,* 1–40.

Perkins, W. (1984). *Current therapy of communication disorders: Language handicaps in children.* New York: Thieme-Stratton.

Piaget, J. (1962). *Play, dreams, and imitation in childhood.* New York: Norton.

Pronovost, W. (1961). The speech behavior and language comprehension of autistic children. *Journal of Chronic Diseases, 13,* 228–233.

Quigley, S., & King, C. (1982). The language development of deaf children and youth. In S. Rosenberg (Ed.), *Handbook of applied psycholinguistics: Major thrusts of research and theory.* Hillsdale, N.J.: L. Erlbaum, Associates.

Rainer, J., Altschuler, K., & Kallmann, F. (Eds.). (1969). *Family and mental health problems in a deaf population* (2nd ed.). Springfield, IL: Charles C. Thomas.

Rapin, I. (1977). Language disability in children. In M. Blaw, I. Rapin, & M. K. Kinsbourne (Eds.), *Topics in child neurology.* Toronto: Spectrum.

Rapin, I., & Allen, D. (1983). Developmental language disorders: Nosological considerations. In U. Kirk (Ed.), *Neuropsychology of language, reading, and spelling.* New York: Academic Press.

Rawlings, B., & Jensema, C. (1977). *Two studies of the families of hearing impaired children* (Series R, No. 5) Washington, DC: Gallaudet College, Office of Demographic Studies.

Rees, N. (1973). Auditory processing factors in language disorders: The view from Procrustes' bed. *Journal of Speech and Hearing Disorders, 38,* 304–315.

Riese, W., & Collison, J. (1964). Aphasia in childhood reconsidered. *Journal of Nervous and Mental Disease, 138,* 293–295.

Rosenberg, S. (1982). The language of the mentally retarded: Development, processes, and intervention. In S. Rosenberg (Ed.), *Handbook of applied psycholinguistics: Major thrusts of research and theory.* Hillsdale, NJ: L. Erlbaum.

Ruttenburg, B., & Wolf, E. (1967). Evaluating the communication of the autistic child. *Journal of Speech and Hearing Disorders, 32,* 315–323.

Rutter, M. (1978). Language disorder and infantile autism. In M. Rutter & E. Schopler (Eds.), *Autism: A reappraisal of concepts and treatment.* New York: Plenum Press.

Rutter, M., Greenfeld, D., & Lockyer, L. (1967). A five to fifteen year follow-up study of infantile psychosis. II. Social and behavioral outcome. *British Journal of Psychiatry, 113,* 1183–1199.

Rutter, M., & Lockyer, L. (1967). A five to fifteen year follow-up study of infantile psychosis. I. Description of samples. *British Journal of Psychiatry, 113,* 1169–1182.

Rutter, M., & Bartak, L. (1971). Causes of infantile autism: Some considerations from recent research. *Journal of Autism and Childhood Schizophrenia, 1,* 20–32.

Sak, R., & Ruben, R. (1981). Recurrent middle ear effusion in childhood: Implications of temporary auditory deprivation for language and learning. *Annals of Otology, Rhinology, and Laryngology, 90,* 546–551.

Schaffer, H. (1964). The "too-cohesive" family. A form of group pathology. *International Journal of Social Psychiatry, 10,* 266–271.

Schlanger, B. (1973). *Mental retardation.* Indianapolis: Bobbs-Merrill.

Schlesinger, H., & Meadow, K. (1972). *Sounds and sign.* Berkeley: University of California Press.

Schopler, E., Brehm, S., Kinsbourne, M., & Reichler, R. (1971). Effects of treatment structure on development in autistic children. *Archives of General Psychiatry, 24,* 415–421.

Schopler, E., & Reichler, R. (1971). Parents as cotherapists in the treatment of psychotic children. *Journal of Autism and Child Schizophrenia, 1,* 87–102.

Schwartz, E. (1974). Characteristics of speech and language development in the child with myelomeningocele and hydrocephalus. *Journal of Speech and Hearing Disorders, 39,* 465–468.

Senf, G., & Feshbach, S. (1970). Development of bisensory memory in culturally deprived, dyslexia, and normal readers. *Journal of Educational Psychology, 61,* 461–470.

Silva, P. A. (1980). The prevalence, stability and significance of developmental language delay in preschool children. *Developmental Medicine and Child Neurology, 22,* 768–777.

Silverman, S. (1971). The education of deaf children. In L. E. Travis (Ed.), *Handbook of speech pathology and audiology.* New York: Appleton.

Snyder-McLean, L. (1984). Developmental therapy. In W. H. Perkins (Ed.), *Current therapy of communication disorders: Language handicaps in children.* New York: Thieme-Stratton.

Spain, B. (1974). Verbal and performance ability in pre-school children with spinal bifida. *Developmental Medicine and Child Neurology, 16,* 773–780.

Stark, R., & Tallal, P. (1981). Selection of children with specific language deficits. *Journal of Speech and Hearing Disorders, 46,* 114–122.

Stark, R., Tallal, P., & Mellits, E. (1982). Quantification of language abilities in children. In N. Lass (Ed.), *Speech and language: Advances in basic research and practice.* New York: Academic Press.

Stevenson, J., & Richman, M. (1976). The prevalence of language delay in a population of three-year-old children and its association with general retardation. *Developmental Medicine and Child Neurology, 18,* 431–441.

Swisher, L. (1976). Performance of the oral deaf. In H. Whitaker & H. Whitaker (Eds.), *Current trends in neurolinguistics.* New York: Academic Press.

Swisher, L., & Butler, R. (1984). Autism. In W. H. Perkins (Ed.), *Current therapy of communication disorders: Language handicaps in children.* New York: Thieme-Stratton.

Swisher, L., & Demetras, M. (1985). The expressive language characteristics of autistic children compared with mentally retarded or specific language-impaired children. In E. Schopler & G. Mesibov (Eds.), *Issues of autism, Vol. 3: Communication problems in autism.* New York: Plenum Press.

Swisher, L., Drzwicki, S., & Swisher, C. (1976). Language disorders of autistic children. In L. Lockman, K. Swaiman, J. Drage, K. Nelson, & H. Marsden (Eds.), *Workshop on the Neurobiological Basis of Autism.* Bethesda, MD: National Institute of Health.

Swisher, L., & Matkin, A. (1984). Specific language impairment. The method of L. Swisher and A. Matkin. In W. H. Perkins (Ed.), *Current therapy of communi-*

cation disorders: Language handicaps in children. New York: Thieme-Stratton.

Swisher, L., & Pinsker, J. (1971). The language characteristics of hyperverbal, hydrocephalic children. *Developmental Medicine and Child Neurology, 13,* 746–755.

Swisher, L., Reichler, R., & Short, A. (1976). Language development history and change in autistic children. In S. Hirsh, D. Eldredge, I. Hirsh, & S. Silverman (Eds.), *Hearing and Davis: Essays honoring Hallowell Davis.* St. Louis: Washington University Press.

Swisher, L., Wooten, N., & Thompson, E. (1977). Biological predictors of language development. In M. E. Blaw, I. Rapin, & M. Kinsbourne (Eds.), *Topics in Child Neurology.* New York: Spectrum.

Tallal, P., & Piercy, M. (1973). Developmental aphasia: Impaired rate of nonverbal processing as a function of sensory modality. *Neuropsychologia, 11,* 389–398.

Tallal, P. & Piercy, M. (1975). Developmental aphasia: The perception of brief vowels and extended stop consonants. *Neuropsychologia, 13,* 69–74.

Taylor, E. (1961). *Psychological appraisal of children with cerebral defects.* Cambridge, MA: Harvard University Press.

Tew, B. (1979). The "cocktail party syndrome" in children with hydrocephalus and spina bifida. *British Journal of Disorders of Communication, 14,* 89–101.

Tomblin, J. (1984). Specific abilities approach: An evaluation and an alternative method. In W. Perkins (Ed.), *Current therapy of communication disorders: Language handcaps in children.* New York: Thieme-Stratton.

Tonini, R. (1983). *The speech and language skills of four-year-old children with mild and severe histories of recurrent otitis media.* Unpublished master's thesis, University of Arizona, Tucson.

Treffert, D. (1970). Epidemiology of infantile autism. *Archives of General Psychiatry, 22,* 431–438.

Vellutino, F. (1979). *Dyslexia: Theory and research.* Cambridge, MA: MIT Press.

Vellutino, F. (1981) The mystique of dyslexia and other learning disabilities: A plea for common sense in remedial education.

Ventry, I. (1980). Effects of conductive hearing loss: Fact or fiction. *Journal of Speech and Hearing Disorders, 45,* 143–156.

Vernon, M. (1969). Sociological and psychological factors associated with hearing loss. *Journal of Speech and Hearing Research, 12,* 541–563.

Wiig, E., Semel, M., & Crouse, M. B. (1973). The use of English morphology by high-risk and learning disabled children. *Journal of Learning Disabilities, 6,* 457–465.

Wing, L. (1976). *Early childhood autism.* Oxford: Pergamon Press.

Woods, B. T., & Carey, S. (1979). Language deficits after apparent clinical recovery from childhood aphasia. *Annals of Neurology, 6,* 405–409.

Worster-Drought, C. (1971). An unusual form of acquired aphasia in children. *Developmental Medicine and Child Neurology, 13,* 563–571.

Zinkus, P., & Gottlieb, M. (1980). Patterns of perceptual and academic deficits related to early chronic otitis media. *Pediatrics, 66,* 246–253.

Zinkus, P., Gottleib, M., & Shapiro, M. (1978). Developmental and psychoeducational sequelae of chronic otitis media. *American Journal of Disabled Child, 132,* 1100–1104.

Linda Ewing-Cobbs
Jack M. Fletcher
Susan H. Landry
Harvey S. Levin

3
Language Disorders After Pediatric Head Injury

Acquired aphasia in children traditionally has been hypothesized to differ from aphasic disturbances in adults along three dimensions: (1) frequency of occurrence, (2) language symptoms, and (3) prognosis for recovery. In a critical review of these issues, Satz and Bullard-Bates (1981) concluded that the frequency of aphasic disorder is comparable in right-handed children and adults following unilateral lesions involving the language areas. Aphasic disturbance in children tends to be predominantly nonfluent. However, this pattern of symptoms is variable. As observed in adults, primary expressive disturbances may be associated with deficits of auditory comprehension, writing, reading, and arithmetic functions. Finally, the prognosis for recovery of expressive language functions appears to be more favorable in children. Despite the dramatic restitution of expressive language skills in the majority of pediatric cases, cognitive impairment and scholastic difficulties often persist.

The basis for developmental differences in aphasia symptoms and recovery has not been established. Age may be related to symptomatol-

This work was supported in part by Grant NS 21889-01, Neurobehavioral Outcome of Head Injury in Children, and by Grant NS 07377-14, Center for the Study of Central Nervous System Injury.

Speech and Language Evaluation in Neurology:
Childhood Disorders
ISBN 0-8089-1719-6

ogy and prognosis, but other factors such as etiology, lesion size, and lesion site influence the type and persistence of aphasic deficits (Satz & Bullard-Bates, 1981). Since these variables are often confounded in the major studies of childhood aphasia, the relative contribution of each variable to linguistic dysfunction remains obscure. Etiology appears to exert an important influence on both aphasia type and prognosis. Children with traumatic injuries characteristically exhibit expressive deficits and have a generally good prognosis, while vascular lesions may produce more varied and persistent symptoms (Guttman, 1942; van Dongen & Loonen, 1977). The few studies of aphasia secondary to vascular disease in children show striking parallels with adult patterns in terms of symptomalogy (Aram, Rose, Rekate, & Whitaker, 1983; Dennis, 1980).

To dissociate the effects of etiology and age on linguistic dysfunction, it is necessary to examine language disorders in more homogeneous samples. The purpose of this chapter is to examine acute linguistic disturbances associated with closed head injury (CHI) in children. A brief review of the nature of head injury in children is provided. Linguistic deficits in head-injured children are described and compared with disturbances commonly reported in adults. In addition, general principles related to the assessment and remediation of language disorders in the head-injured child will be discussed.

HEAD INJURY IN CHILDREN

Epidemiology and Pathophysiology

The epidemiology, mechanisms, and pathophysiology of CHI vary with development. Studies conducted in England and Wales suggest that accidents comprise 16 percent of all hospital admissions for children under 15 years of age; more than one third of all pediatric accident cases and 41 percent of pediatric mortalities were related to head injury (Craft, 1972; Field, 1976). In fact, the mortality associated with pediatric head injury is five times greater than leukemia, the second leading cause of death in children (Annegers, 1983).

The cause of injury differs in children and adults. While approximately one half of adult cases involve high-speed motor vehicle accidents, falls are responsible for half of the pediatric injuries (Levin, Benton, & Grossman, 1982). Even though vehicular accidents account for nearly one third of pediatric head injury cases, many of these are automobile/pedestrian accidents occurring at low speeds (Levin et al., 1982).

The primary mechanism producing brain injury following CHI is diffuse cerebral injury occurring at the time of impact (Adams, Mitchell, Graham, & Doyle, 1977; Strich, 1956). Rotational acceleration of the skull produces shear strains within the intracranial contents. Widespread injury to the cerebral white matter apparently results from shearing and stretching of nerve fibers (Adams et al., 1977). Since children are more likely to be injured as a result of falls or low-speed vehicular accidents, the rotational acceleration to which the brain is subjected may be lower and briefer than in high-speed vehicular accidents involving marked acceleration/deceleration. Injuries sustained by adolescents and adults in high-speed accidents presumably produce diffuse brain injury (Levin et al., 1982). Magnetic resonance imaging might demonstrate white matter lesions, which are seldom visualized by computed tomography (CT).

The pathophysiologic response of the brain to trauma varies with age. The incidence of intracranial mass lesions (i.e., contusions, hematomas) is significantly lower in children relative to adults (Jennett, 1972). Bruce and colleagues (1979) examined the nature of brain injury following severe CHI in 85 children and adolescents with Glasgow Coma Scale (GCS) (Teasdale & Jennett, 1974) scores of 8 or less. Scores in this range correspond to an inability to follow commands, the absence of eye opening, and failure to utter recognizable words. CT frequently disclosed general cerebral swelling, but focal mass lesions were rarely found. Based on regional cerebral blood flow studies, the investigators attributed the cerebral swelling to vascular congestion produced by increased blood volume and flow. In adults, however, swelling is often associated with edema, or the accumulation of excess fluid in the brain parenchyma. Cerebral blood flow may be decreased (Zimmerman, Bilaniuk, Bruce, Dolinskas, Obrist, & Kohl, 1978).

Because of these differences, studies comparing outcome in children and adults must be interpreted cautiously. It is clear that many factors associated with CHI, including the cause of injury, mechanisms of impact, and the pathophysiologic response of the brain, vary with development. The extent to which these variables influence outcome measures is unclear.

Long-Term Outcome

Despite the high incidence of pediatric CHI, there are few studies of cognitive recovery. Recent reviews of research concerning neuropsychologic recovery from CHI in children indicate that cognitive impairment frequently persists after severe injury despite impressive resolution of focal motor and sensory deficits and resumption of daily activities (Levin, Eisenberg, & Miner, 1983). An evaluation of recovery based solely on the resolution of acute deficits and focal neurologic signs is likely to underestimate the disability produced by head injury (Miner, 1984). Failure to appreciate the severity of long-term neuropsychologic deficits may perpetuate the general view that recovery from brain injury is enhanced in children. Follow-up studies of pediatric CHI suggest that residual deficits are at least as severe in children as in adolescents or adults (Brink, Garrett, Hale, Woo-Sam, & Nickel, 1970; Lange-Cosack, Wider, Schlesner, Grumme, & Kubicki, 1979; Levin, Eisenberg, Wigg, & Kobayashi, 1982).

Consequently, children need careful, long-term monitoring well after the acute stage of injury. This monitoring is especially important for linguistic skills. Language is a crucial skill for learning in school and interactions with other people. Although children typically recover language skills after head injury, their subsequent linguistic development and scholastic achievement may be affected.

LANGUAGE FOLLOWING PEDIATRIC CLOSED HEAD INJURY

Previous Studies

In a classic study, Hecaen (1976) described 26 cases of childhood aphasia, including 16 cases of head trauma, ranging in age from 3 to 15 years. Four of the head-injured children had primary right hemisphere damage; the presence of bilateral injury could not be excluded, particularly in view of the unavailability of CT in this study. Aphasic disturbance was initially manifested by a period of mutism that existed for as long as 3 months. Expressive language disorders were the most common and were often characterized by decreased initiation of speech. Paraphasias and logorrhea were uncommon. Naming disorders, dyscalculia, and dysgraphia were frequent and persistent. Receptive language disturbances were apparent in one third of the children. Resolution of auditory comprehension deficits, however, was usually rapid. Hecaen (1976) inferred that the prognosis for acquired aphasia in children was better than in adults.

Levin and Eisenberg (1979a) examined posttraumatic language dysfunction following pediatric CHI using the Neurosensory Center Comprehensive Examination for Aphasia (NCCEA) (Spreen & Benton, 1969). Sixty-four children and adolescents were evaluated within 6 months of injury. Linguistic deficits were observed in 31 percent of the sample. The most common deficits were dysnomia for objects presented visually (13 percent) or tactually to the left hand (12 percent). Auditory comprehension was impaired in 11 percent of the sample while verbal repetition was affected in only 4 percent. A higher incidence of linguistic disturbance was identified in head-injured adults receiving similar evaluations. One half of the adults exhibited dysnomia and/or decreased verbal fluency while one third were impaired on measures of auditory comprehension

(Levin & Eisenberg, 1979b). Levin and Eisenberg (1979b) concluded that their findings were consistent with previous studies of acquired aphasia that suggest more rapid and complete recovery in children. These findings are also compatible with studies indicating better linguistic recovery following head injury than other etiologies (Guttman, 1942; van Dongen & Loonen, 1977).

Recent findings converge in identifying subtle language processing deficiencies that persist following pediatric head injury. Chadwick, Rutter, Shaffer, and Shrout (1981) reported that object-naming latency was impaired 1 year after severe head injury. By 2 years, 3 months postinjury, performance of severely injured children was in the normal range. However, Gaidolfi and Vignolo (1980) identified residual impairment of oral expression, which was characterized by a reduction in spontaneous speech, in four of 21 children evaluated approximately 10 years following severe head injury.

A Recent Study

We recently examined linguistic performance shortly after head injury in 24 children (ages 5–10) and 33 adolescents (ages 11–16) who sustained CHIs. The severity of injury was categorized as mild or moderate–severe. Mild injuries (n = 25) had negative neurologic findings and were unconscious for less than 15 minutes, while moderate–severe injuries (n = 32) exhibited positive CT scan findings, neurologic deficits, and/or coma persisting for at least 15 minutes. The severity of injury, as assessed by the duration of impaired consciousness and the GCS score, did not differ statistically in the child and adolescent groups. However, a trend indicating that the children sustained more severe injuries was apparent. In patients with moderate–severe injuries, the mean duration of unconsciousness was 8.8 days in the child group and 3.6 days in the adolescent group. CT findings were used to categorize the moderate–severe injuries into left hemisphere (n = 9) right hemisphere (n = 6), bilateral hemispheric (n = 4), or diffuse (n = 13) groups.

The NCCEA was administered to each individual within 5 months of injury following resolution of posttraumatic amnesia. A striking percentage of the total sample exhibited clinically significant language impairment on the NCCEA subtests. A score was regarded as impaired if it fell below the sixth percentile obtained by the normative child sample. Thirty percent of the sample was impaired on measures of writing to dictation. At least eighteen percent of the children and adolescents performed in the impaired range on subtests examining object description, sentence repetition, auditory comprehension of syntactically complex sentences, verbal fluency, and/or copying sentences. The subtests least affected by CHI evaluated auditory comprehension of single words (2 percent), construction of sentences containing target words (9 percent), and visual confrontation naming (9 percent). The mean percentiles obtained by the mild and moderate–severe injury groups on each subtest are provided in Table 3-1.

The NCCEA subtests were grouped into naming, expressive, receptive, and graphic categories based on the face validity of the subtest content (see Table 3-1). The age-adjusted percentiles obtained on the subtests within each of the composite groupings were averaged to yield a total score. To examine the effect of age and severity of injury on language skills, a 2 (Age) × 2 (Severity) analysis of variance was completed on the averaged percentiles from the naming, expressive, receptive, and graphic subtest groupings.

Severity of injury effects

As compared with mild injuries, moderate–severe CHI was most likely to be associated with poorer performance on the naming and graphic subtest groupings. Neither the expressive nor the receptive composite scores were significantly affected by CHI. While no severity group differences were anticipated on the receptive measures, it was expected that moderate–severe injury would negatively impact expressive functions. Given the small sample size and concomitant reduction in power, it is difficult to determine whether these null findings reflect the robustness of expressive language or insufficient power to detect group differences.

Age effects

The severity of acute linguistic disturbance was comparable in children and adolescents on the composite measures of naming, expressive, and receptive skills. Written language skills were significantly more affected in children than in adolescents. Examination of the component graphic subtests revealed that children were impaired relative to the adolescents on writing to dictation; however, no age effects were obtained for copying sentences. Similarly, Hécaen, Perenin, and Jeannerod (1984) indicated that dysgraphia was more prevalent in children less than 10 years of age than in older children. Written language skills develop most rapidly between the ages of 6 and 8. The finding that graphic skills were disporportionately affected in children implies that skills that are in a rapid stage of development may be more affected by cerebral injury than well-consolidated skills. This is consistent with Hebb's (1942) suggestion that brain injury may predominantly affect the acquisition of new skills.

At the present time, our explanation for this age effect is admittedly conjectural, and further research is necessary to confirm this postulation. Older children and adolescents have received extensive formal instruction and practice in writing. As this skill becomes overlearned and au-

Table 3-1

Mean Percentiles on the Neurosensory Center
Comprehensive Examination for Aphasia

	Severity of Injury*	
Subtest	Mild	Moderate–Severe
Naming functions		
Visual naming		
Mean	65.4	43.2
SD	23.6	30.7
Tactile naming—right		
Mean	62.9	48.8
SD	24.8	28.8
Tactile naming—left		
Mean	65.6	53.2
SD	25.4	31.2
Expressive functions		
Description of use		
Mean	68.6	42.3
SD	29.8	34.4
Sentence repetition		
Mean	47.3	38.8
SD	30.1	33.6
Word fluency		
Mean	35.4	25.6
SD	24.9	24.4
Sentence construction		
Mean	49.2	47.6
SD	31.9	31.0
Receptive functions		
Identification by name		
Mean	61.0	62.1
SD	14.1	14.0
Identification by sentence		
Mean	46.6	38.3
SD	25.6	33.0
Graphic functions		
Writing to dictation		
Mean	42.5	26.8
SD	27.0	28.6
Writing to copy		
Mean	47.1	36.9
SD	28.9	27.4

* Based on the Glasgow Coma Scale score, duration of coma,
and CT findings (see text).

tomatized, it may be more resistant to disruption. Moreover, writing is an extremely complex task composed of many subskills (Gibson & Levin, 1975). Impairment of a component skill such as phonemic segmentation or visual–motor integration may disrupt writing abilities. Further research is needed to isolate the source and neuropsychologic correlates of posttraumatic dysgraphia.

Conclusions

The results of our study are consistent with previous studies of acquired language disturbances in children. These studies also describe a high frequency of naming disorders, dysgraphia, and reduced verbal productivity in children (e.g., Alajouanine & L'hermitte, 1965; Hecaen, 1976). It is interesting to note that head injury represents a major etiology of many of the available studies of acquired aphasia in children (Woods & Teuber, 1978). These studies have often been interpreted to show differences in symptomatology and recovery rate between children and adults. Head injury in children and adults, however, seems to produce a wide range of deficits involving both expressive and receptive functions. Due to the lack of information regarding recovery from posttraumatic linguistic disorders in children, it is not possible to compare the recovery rate across age-groups.

As the few available studies show, classic aphasic syndromes occur infrequently after CHI in adults (Heilman, Safran, & Geschwind, 1971). Sarno (1980) observed that the linguistic deficits following head trauma in adults differed considerably from the classical syndromes identified in stroke patients. Similarly, Levin, Grossman, and Kelly (1976) reported that linguistic disturbances in adults tended to be general and nonspecific, particularly when associated with prolonged coma. Although several instances of specific dysnomia or word-finding difficulties were observed by Levin et al. (1967), language profiles consistent with other classical aphasic syndromes were infrequently identified. Children also show a broad range of deficits after CHI and rarely exhibit classic aphasic syndromes. At the same time, many children (and adults) show subtle language problems that Sarno (1980) described as "subclinical aphasia." Subclinical aphasia refers to impaired language processing apparent upon standardized assessment in patients with intact conversational speech. The majority of adults and children with language problems after CHI are best characterized as exhibiting subclinical language disorders.

In our study, aphasic disturbance was present in less than 10 percent of the sample. Consistent with adult studies (Levin et al., 1976), acute linguistic difficulties after pediatric CHI were nonspecific in nature and did not vary consistently with the type of cerebral involvement. The severity of diffuse brain injury, as opposed to the presence or lateralization of a focal lesion, appeared to be the overriding determinant of linguistic performance.

In contrast to previous studies (Lenneberg, 1967), we found no evidence for sparing of linguistic function in children as compared with adolescents. Moreover, the types of deficits observed in our sample were similar to those described by Levin et al. (1976), who studied a group of adult CHI patients from the same geographic region with a comparable range of injury severity. The adults were evaluated using the Multilingual Aphasia Examination (Benton, 1967) and selected NCCEA subtests. In both the pediatric and adult samples, linguistic disturbance was most common on measures of verbal fluency and auditory comprehension of syntactically complex sentences. Approximately 30 percent of each sample exhibited written language deficits. Neither adults nor children were significantly impaired on measures of auditory comprehension for single words or phrases. Age-based differences were apparent, however, on two of the subtests examined. Collapsing across severity in each sample, 40 percent of the adults and 9 percent of the children and adolescents performed in the impaired range on measures of visual confrontation naming. These findings suggest that the incidence of modality-specific naming deficits is higher in adults. Interestingly, while only 4 percent of the adults performed below expected levels when repeating sentences, 21 percent of the pediatric sample exhibited difficulty. The high percentage of repetition disturbances in younger individuals may reflect a greater susceptibility to disruption of attentional processes.

These age differences are consistent with Rutter's (1982) hypothesis that the effects of brain injury may be influenced by the stage of development of the cognitive function being evaluated. Since children are in the process of developing skills, brain injury may produce deficits that reflect the degree to which a skill has been acquired. Skills that are in a rapid stage of acquisition could be more vulnerable to injury than skills that are more fully developed. Our finding of greater written language impairment in children as compared with adolescents may reflect the rate of development of these skills.

Many language skills develop rapidly prior to age 6. Language development after head injury in children under 6 has rarely been studied; language problems could potentially be more pervasive and show a different pattern than in children over 6. Also, few studies of long-term outcome of language skills after pediatric CHI have been completed. Since some studies suggest that problems with other aspects of language (e.g., reading) typically emerge after a delay following the acute stage of head injury in children (Shaffer, Bijur, Chadwick, & Rutter, 1980), long-term follow-up is needed. Given the prevalence of subtle language problems after CHI, children will benefit from individualized language evaluation and remediation because of the impact of the injury on later language development and school performance.

ASSESSMENT AND REMEDIATION OF LANGUAGE DEFICITS

Effective assessment procedures and language training programs are important not only for the child's language development but also for cognitive, social, and affective development. The failure to develop an adequate linguistic system has been reported to have its most serious impact during adolescence in nonlinguistic areas of development (de Ajuriaguerra et al., 1976). In addition to changing language behaviors, language training programs can have a positive effect on other behaviors such as self-regulation skills, self-confidence, and attentional behaviors. Children with head injuries are frequently observed to have additional problems such as distractibility, lack of task persistence, and impulsivity. In general, all language training of CHI children must take place in the context of their attentional and memory deficits. The type of skills that are trained in language programs would give a child better control over these behaviors.

Although children with head injuries are most frequently reported to have expressive language disorders such as decreased oral word fluency, a thorough evaluation of the child's entire language system will be important because of the lack of specificity of linguistic disturbance after CHI. Language can be evaluated with both formal and informal assessment instruments. In most cases the use of both types of measures provides the most complete description of the child's language abilities. Both types of assessment should be used only as tools for gathering information about the way a child understands and uses language.

Formal or standardized assessments are usually highly structured observations of a child's language. Observations are taken of a single instance of behavior and often recorded as either right or wrong, or present or absent. If a child's language abilities are only evaluated with standardized instruments, it will be difficult to observe how a child actually uses and understands language as a means for communication.

Informal assessment techniques usually involve engaging the child in activities that provide opportunities to initiate interactions with other people concerning objects and situations that are similar to communication experiences the child might actually encounter. In addition, the clinician has the opportunity to observe how the child responds to the language of others. However, Chapman (1978) cautions clinicians using informal assessment techniques to carefully evaluate the child's comprehension skills. Children of all ages can appear to understand more language than they actually do. Gestural and contextual cues can provide sufficient information for the child to respond appropriately without actually understanding the linguistic structure being used. This suggests that assessment procedures must consider the specific conditions under which particular language behaviors do and do not occur. Highly structured standardized assessment instruments can overestimate the consistency with which a child uses and responds to language as well as the range of contexts in which particular language behaviors occur.

A child may appear to have pervasive word-finding difficulties when in fact these problems are only present in the absence of any contextual cues. When the language is presented in a meaningful context and used with appropriate gestural cues, a child's word-finding skills may be much improved (Meyuk & Looney, 1976). This type of qualitative assessment provides valuable descriptive information for planning effective language training programs (Muma, 1978). Since children with head injuries can have language comprehension difficulties, training them to be aware when a message is not clear and stressing effective strategies for obtaining additional contextual information could be very beneficial.

The evaluation and remediation of language deficits in children with CHI must be made in the context of the child's level of functioning in other cognitive and behavioral areas. Assessment procedures need to be appropriate to the child's level of cognitive, fine motor, and perceptual abilities. Responses to language tasks should not require other abilities that are inappropriate to the child's overall developmental level. In particular, procedures that emphasize attentional or memory skills may suggest the presence of language problems when the child is simply unable to perform the required task because of these confounding sequelae.

Treatment procedures will also need to be sensitive to the child's level of functioning. The type of language behaviors included in a treatment program, such as word-retrieval skills and comprehension abilities, are appropriate at any age. Specific syntactical structures and expressive vocabulary, however, must be taught according to the child's degree of development in these areas. Recent findings concerning normal language acquisition can be very useful when devising assessment and treatment programs for children with language disorders. Treatment programs for children with expressive semantic deficits must first delineate the nature of the child's general cognitive development in order to understand the kinds of cognitive discriminations the child is capable of making (Bowerman, 1976). Linguistic input will not be helpful to children if it is not consistent with their overall pattern of cognitive strengths and weaknesses (Taylor, Fletcher, & Satz, 1984).

Finally, differences in the success of remedial procedures for children with cognitive and linguistic deficits may be explained in part by the family's ability to develop effective teaching skills. Parental involvement is especially important for pediatric CHI because of the disruptive effects of severe injury on the family (Fletcher, Ewing-Cobbs, McLaughlin, & Levin, 1985). Clinicians need to help parents understand their child's problems. In addition, parents will require training in order to assist in the child's treatment program. Parents can provide the essential carryover from language sessions to everyday experiences. This will facilitate children's ability to generalize what they have learned in the context of a treatment activity to other situations.

CONCLUSIONS

Children are at substantial risk for subtle language disturbances and related disorders after CHI. Previous studies suggesting differences in the nature and extent of impairment may have exaggerated the degree of recovery after head injury in children. In fact, the nature of language impairment in school-aged children, adolescents, and adults shows many similarities. These similarities may reflect a common etiology (CHI). Comparisons of recovery in cases with varying etiologies may be limited because of differences in the occurrence of neurologic syndromes in children and adults. There are also important differences in outcome after CHI that may be related to the degree and rate of development of language skills in children. In order to fully understand these potential differences, children under 6 years of age must be studied. In addition, follow-up studies with baseline and long-term evaluations are needed to determine how well children recover language skills after CHI. Because of the prevalence of subclinical language deficits and the importance of linguistic skills for learning and interacting within the environment, careful evaluation and remediation of language skills is required. Language programs can also be effective for remediating the attentional and memory problems that characterize many children who sustain CHI (Levin et al., 1982, 1983). With careful focus on the child's long-term recovery after CHI, it is possible to maximize adaptive potential and minimize the cognitive and behavioral problems for which these children are at high risk.

REFERENCES

Adams, J. H., Mitchell, D. E., Graham, D. I., & Doyle, D. (1977). Diffuse brain damage of the immediate impact type. *Brain, 100,* 489–502.

Alajouanine, T., & L'hermitte, F. (1965). Acquired aphasia in children. *Brain, 88,* 653–662.

Annegers, J. F. (1983). The epidemiology of head trauma in children. In K. Shapiro (Ed.), *Pediatric head trauma* (pp. 1–10). Mount Kisco, NY: Futura.

Aram, D. M., Rose, D. F., Rekate, H. L., & Whitaker, H. A. (1983). Acquired capsular/striatal aphasia in childhood. *Archives of Neurology, 40,* 614–617.

Benton, A. L. (1967). Problems of test construction in the field of aphasia. *Cortex, 3,* 32–58.

Bloom, L., & Lahey, M. (1978). *Language development and language disorders.* New York: John Wiley.

Bowerman, M. (1976). Semantic factors in the acquisition of rules for word use and sentence construction. In D. M. Moorehead & A. E. Morehead (Eds.), *Normal and deficient child language.* Baltimore: University Park Press.

Brink, J. D., Garrett, A. L., Hale, W. R., Woo-Sam, J., & Nickel, V. L. (1970). Recovery of motor and intellectual function in children sustaining severe head injuries. *Developmental Medicine and Child Neurology, 12,* 565–571.

Bruce, D. A., Raphaely, R. C., Goldberg, A. I., Zimmerman, R. A., Bilaniuk, L. T., Schut, L., et al. (1979). Pathophysiology, treatment and outcome following severe head injury in children. *Child's Brain, 5,* 174–191.

Chadwick, O., Rutter, M., Shaffer, D., & Shrout, P. E. (1981). A prospective study of children with head injuries: IV. Specific cognitive deficits. *Journal of Clinical Neuropsychology, 3,* 101–120.

Chapman, R. (1978). Comprehension strategies in children. In J. Kavanaugh & W. Strange (Eds.), *Speech and language in the laboratory, school, and clinic.* Cambridge: MIT Press.

Craft, A. W. (1972). Head injury in children. In P. D. Vinken & G. W. Bruyn (Eds.), *Handbook of clinical neurology* (Vol. 23, pp. 445–458). New York: Elsevier.

de Ajuriaguerra, J., Jaeggi, A., Guignard, F., Kocher, F., Maquard, M., Roth, S., et al. (1976). The development and prognosis of dysphasia in children. In D. M. Morehead & A. E. Morehead (Eds.), *Normal and deficient child language.* Baltimore: University Park Press.

Dennis, M. (1980). Language acquisition in a single hemisphere: Semantic organization. In D. Caplan (Ed.), *Biological studies of mental processes* (pp. 159–185). Cambridge: MIT Press.

Field, J. H. (1976). *Epidemiology of head injury in England and Wales: With particular application to rehabilitation.* Leicester: Printed for H. M. Stationery Office by Willsons.

Fletcher, J. M., Ewing-Cobbs, L., McLaughlin, E. J., & Levin, H. S. (1985). Cognitive and psychosocial sequelae of head injury in children: Implications for assessment and management. In B. Brooks (Ed.), *The injured child* (pp. 30–39). Austin: University of Texas Press.

Gaidolfi, E., & Vignolo, L. A. (1980). Closed head injuries of school aged children: Neuropsychological sequelae in early adulthood. *Italian Journal of Neurological Sciences, 1,* 65–73.

Gibson, E. J., & Levin, H. (1975). *The psychology of reading.* Cambridge: MIT Press.

Guttman, E. (1942). Aphasia in children. *Brain, 65,* 205–219.

Hebb, D. O. (1942). The effect of early and late brain injury upon test scores, and the nature of normal adult intelligence. *Proceedings of the American Philosophical Society, 85,* 275–292.

Hecaen, H. (1976). Acquired aphasia in children and the ontogenesis of hemispheric specialization. *Brain and Language, 3,* 114–134.

Hecaen, H., Perenin, M. T., and Jennerod, M. (1984). The effects of cortical lesions in children: Language and visual functions. In C. R. Almli and S. Finger (Eds.), *Early brain damage, volume 1: Research orientations and clincial observations* (pp 277–298). New York: Academic Press.

Heilman, K. M., Safran, A., & Geschwind, N. (1971). Closed head trauma and aphasia. *Journal of Neurology, Neurosurgery, and Psychiatry, 34,* 265–269.

Jennett, B. (1972). Head injuries in children. *Developmental Medicine and Child Neurology, 14,* 137–147.

Lange-Cosack, H., Wider, B., Schlesner, H. J., Grumme, T., & Kubicki, S. (1979). Prognosis of brain injuries in young children (one until five years of age). *Neuropaediatrie, 10,* 105–127.

Lenneberg, E. (1967). *Biological foundations of language.* New York: John Wiley.

Leonard, L. B. (1984). Normal language acquisition: Some recent findings and clinical implications. In A. Holland (Ed.), *Language disorders in children.* San Diego: College-Hill Press.

Levin, H. S., Benton, A. L., & Grossman, R. G. (1982). *Neurobehavioral consequences of closed head injury.* New York: Oxford University Press.

Levin, H. S., & Eisenberg, H. M. (1979a). Neuropsychological impairment after closed head injury in children and adolescents. *Journal of Pediatric Psychology, 4,* 389–402.

Levin, H. S., & Eisenberg, H. M. (1979b). Neuropsychological outcome of closed head injury in children and adolescents. *Child's Brain, 5,* 281–292.

Levin, H. S., Eisenberg, H. M., & Miner, M. E. (1983). Neuropsychologic findings in head injured children. In K. Shapiro (Ed.), *Pediatric head injury* (pp. 223–240). Mount Kisco, NY: Futura.

Levin, H. S., Eisenberg, H. M., Wigg, N. R., & Kobayashi, K. (1982). Memory and intellectual ability after head injury in children and adolescents. *Neurosurgery, 11,* 668–673.

Levin, H. S., Grossman, R. G., & Kelly, P. J. (1976). Aphasic disorder in patients with closed head injury. *Journal of Neurology, Neurosurgery, and Psychiatry, 39,* 1062–1070.

Menyuk, P., & Looney, P. L. (1976). A problem of language disorder: Length versus structure. In D. M. Morehead & A. E. Morehead (Eds.), *Normal and deficient child language.* Baltimore: University Park Press.

Miner, M. E. (1984, May). *Recovery vs. outcome after brain injury.* Paper presented at the Houston Conference on Neurotrauma, Houston.

Muma, J. R. (1978). *Language handbook: Concepts, assessment, intervention.* Englewood Cliffs, NJ: Prentice-Hall.

Rutter, M. (1982). Developmental neuropsychiatry: Concepts, issues, and problems. *Journal of Clinical Neuropsychology, 4,* 91–115.

Sarno, M. T. (1980). The nature of verbal impairment after closed head injury. *Journal of Nervous and Mental Disorders, 168,* 685–692.

Satz, P., & Bullard-Bates, C. (1981). Acquired aphasia in children. In M. T. Sarno (Ed.), *Acquired aphasia* (pp. 399–426). New York: Academic Press.

Shaffer, D., Bijur, P., Chadwick, O., & Rutter, M. (1980). Head injury and later reading disability. *Journal of the American Academy of Child Psychiatry, 19,* 592–610.

Spreen, O., & Benton, A. L. (1969). *Neurosensory Center Comprehensive Examination for Aphasia: Manual of directions.* Victoria, BC: University of Victoria, Neuropsychology Laboratory.

Strich, S. J. (1956). Diffuse degeneration of the cerebral white matter in severe dementia following head injury. *Journal of Neurology, Neurosurgery, and Psychiatry, 19,* 163–185.

Taylor, H. G., Fletcher, J. M., & Satz, P. (1984). Neuropsychological assessment of children. In M. Hersen & G. Goldstein (Eds.), *Handbook of Psychological assessment* (pp. 211–234). New York: Pergamon.

Teasdale, G., & Jennett, B. (1974). Assessment of coma and impaired consciousness: A practical scale. *Lancet, 2,* 81–84.

van Dongen, H. R., & Loonen, M. C. B. (1977). Factors related to prognosis of acquired aphasia in children. *Cortex, 13,* 131–136.

Woods, B. T., & Teuber, H. L. (1978). Changing patterns of childhood aphasia. *Annals of Neurology, 3,* 273–280.

Zimmerman, R. A., Bilaniuk, L. T., Bruce, D., Dolinskas, C., Obrist, W., & Kuhl, D. (1978). Computed tomography of pediatric head trauma: Acute general cerebral swelling. *Radiology, 126,* 403–408.

Thomas P. Marquardt
Carla Dunn
Barbara Davis

4
Apraxia of Speech in Children

Apraxia of speech in children has been known by a number of labels including developmental verbal dyspraxia (Edwards, 1973), childhood verbal apraxia (Chappell, 1973), and developmental apraxia of speech (Rosenbek & Wertz, 1972). The disorder most frequently is described as a neurogenically based deficit in the ability to carry out coordinative movements of the respiratory, laryngeal, and oral muscles for articulation in the absence of impaired neuromuscular function (Morley, Court, & Miller, 1954). Alternately, it has been defined as an ". . . impairment of sensory processing and in particular of proprioceptive input, with an ensuing failure to programme, to organise and to carry out movements necessary for expressive speech" (Edwards, 1973, p. 65). Since, as Walton, Ellis & Court (1962) have observed, ". . . it is never possible to distinguish completely apraxia from agnosia, for defects of recognition almost invariably lead to defects of execution" (p. 46), we will not make a distinction between sensory and motor bases of the disorder.

Serious concern has been voiced as to whether apraxia of speech in children is an objectively identifiable syndrome or a "label in search of a population" (Guyette & Diedrich, 1981, p. 39). This concern apparently has arisen from two major shortcomings of experimental research: (1) distinctive characteristics and patterns of impairment sufficient for differential diagnosis have not been clearly identified, and (2) the neurologic basis for the disorder has not been adequately documented.

Speech and Language Evaluation in Neurology:
Childhood Disorders
ISBN 0-8089-1719-6

In the following sections we will review the characteristics and etiology of apraxia of speech in children. We also will summarize assessment
and treatment procedures for the disorder. Since the heterogeneity of
children studied to date precludes our making unequivocal descriptive
statements, we will provide a synthesis of the information available indicating, where appropriate, areas of poor agreement.

CHARACTERISTICS

Apraxia of speech is a recognized clinical entity and has been included within pediatric syndromes of cerebral palsy and childhood aphasia (e.g., Rosenbek & Wertz, 1972). However, is it a symptom or a unique
syndrome separate from these disorders? In a review of the literature,
Guyette and Diedrich (1981) concluded that these children could not be
clearly distinguished from other children with communication disorders.
Other investigators (Rosenbek & Wertz, 1972; Yoss & Darley, 1974a)
studied children who purportedly demonstrated such a syndrome. This is
not a new debate. The controversy arises because there are few, if any,
behaviors that are unique to a neurogenic communication disorder syndrome. For example, almost all adult aphasics demonstrate deficits in
oral expression, auditory comprehension, reading, and writing. What sets
the syndromes of adult aphasia apart is the relative degree of impairment
of various speech and language abilities and the overall pattern of deficits. A unique pattern of impairment for apraxia of speech in children has
not been firmly established.

A number of speech and nonspeech characteristics have been included in the syndrome of apraxia of speech. Many of these factors are
based on clinical observation, most are not fully agreed upon, and few
have been documented experimentally. Moreover, not all children with
apraxia of speech would be expected to present with the full range of
symptoms.

Speech

Speech Sound Production

Children with apraxia of speech demonstrate a restricted repertoire
of phonemes (Chappell, 1973; Edwards, 1973). Their speech sounds are
limited to those that occur early in development and contain simple combinations of distinctive features (e.g., nasals, plosives). Speech sounds
that require complex articulatory adjustments such as fricatives and af-

fricates frequently are produced incorrectly (Smartt, LaLance, Gray, & Hibbet, 1976). Omission errors predominate (Rosenbek & Wertz, 1972), but substitutions, distortions, and additions comprise a significant portion of the total errors produced. Vowel errors also are a part of the pattern of deficits (Rosenbek & Wertz, 1972; Smartt et al., 1976) although this characteristic has not been consistently demonstrated (Yoss & Darley, 1974a).

Apraxic children demonstrate perseverative, anticipatory assimilative, and metathetic errors (Smartt et al., 1976) that may be related to problems in the sequencing of sound elements and to reductions in the complexity of word shapes. The speech sound errors of these children are inconsistent (Rosenbek, Hansen, Baughman, & Lemme, 1974), although not necessarily unsystematic. The inconsistency of their productions may be related to contextual effects. For example, /d/ may be substituted for /k/ in *duke* because of consonant harmony while it is omitted in the word *shake* because it is preceded by a word initial fricative that is difficult to produce.

Speech production deficits are most apparent on longer units of output. Initiation of utterances is difficult, speech sound errors increase with increases in the length of the utterance (Smartt et al., 1976), and intelligibility is reduced on polysyllabic words and on phrases. Additional characteristics include more errors on sounds occurring in the initial compared with the final position of words (Yoss & Darley, 1974a), reduced diadochokinetic rates for syllables (Nicolosi, Harryman, & Kresheck, 1978), and retrials and oral rehearsals during attempts by the older child to imitate speech sounds (McClumpha & Logue, 1972).

Prosody

Prosodic disturbances are characteristic of children with apraxia of speech. Yoss and Darley (1974a) described an overall slowness of rate and monotony of stress patterns, particularly in older children. McClumpha and Logue (1972) suggested that prosodic disturbances increase with utterance length, citing longer than normal segmental duration, unsteady pitch, and the lack of sound blending.

These observations are consistent with the previously noted increase in speech sound errors with increases in utterance length. A higher incidence of errors and frequent syllable omissions and transpositions might be expected to have a cumulative effect in altering the intonational contour of the child's utterance. Behaviors such as durational lengthening, monotony of stress, and lack of speech sound blending could be interpreted as conscious attempts to compensate for severe production problems, or they may be an intrinsic component of the articulatory deficit.

Nonspeech

Volitional Nonspeech Movements

A frequently noted feature of children with apraxia of speech is the normal functioning of the speech production apparatus for vegetative activities such as chewing and swallowing. In contrast, volitional movements of these structures in the performance of nonverbal tasks (e.g., smiling, tongue protrusion) are impaired (Rosenbek & Wertz, 1972). Several investigators (Smartt et al., 1976; Yoss & Darley, 1974a) considered the presence of an oral apraxia of this type to be so distinctive that it was used as a diagnostic criterion for assignment of children to an apraxic group. Other (Court & Harris, 1965; Morley & Fox, 1969) have found that volitional oral movements are normal in some of these children.

Limb apraxia also has been proposed as an associated symptom of children with apraxia of speech. Logue & McClumpha (1970) noted that these children have difficulty in integrating both sides of the body into sequential movements, planning sequential movement patterns, and fine motor coordination. Gubbay, Ellis, Walton, and Court (1965) concluded that fine coordination problems were responsible for an almost universal difficulty with handwriting in apraxic children. Kools and Tweedie (1975), however, in an investigation of praxis in normal children, did not find a "strong" relationship within any age interval between articulatory ability and oral and limb praxis. Whether the same findings would have resulted from study of children with apraxia of speech is not known.

Cognition

Intellectual ability does not appear to be a distinctive variable in distinguishing apraxia of speech since the disorder has been identified in mentally retarded (Ferry, Halls, & Hicks, 1975) and nonretarded (Yoss & Darley, 1974a) children. However, Gubbay et al. (1965) and Walton et al. (1962) noted a marked superiority of performance compared with verbal intelligence quotient (IQ) scores for these children, which may be an additional characteristic of the syndome.

Language Skills

Children with apraxia may have a developmental delay in language acquisition (Aram, 1979; Edwards, 1973). Rosenbek and Wertz (1972) proposed that the delay is characterized by receptive language skills decidedly superior to expressive skills. Snyder, Marquardt, and Peterson (1977) found significantly higher receptive than expressive scores on the Northwestern Syntax Screening Test (Lee, 1971) for children with apraxia and for children with functional articulation disorders, but not for normal children. These results suggest that expressive language impairment is a corollary of apraxia of speech, just as it is an element of other communication disorders of children such as functional articulation disorders and childhood aphasia.

Sensation

Orosensory deficits (two-point discrimination, oral stereognosis) have been included as a symptom of apraxia of speech (Chappell, 1973; Macaluso-Haynes, 1978). However, deficits in oral perception are a pervasive finding in studies of other organically based disorders of children such as cerebral palsy and are by no means limited to children with apraxia of speech.

Neurologic findings

Positive neurologic signs are characteristic of children with apraxia. Included, among others, are decreased alternate motion rates of the tongue and extremities, difficulty with gait and coordination, and electroencephalogram (EEG) abnormalities. Apraxic children also have a history of delay in walking along, sitting alone, and onset of the first word (Palmer, Wurth, & Kinchloe, 1964), and they demonstrate clumsiness in dressing, feeding, writing, and walking (Walton et al., 1962).

Sex

Apraxia of speech effects males more often than females. The apraxic subjects of Rosenbek and Wertz (1972) included 38 males and 12 females. The "clumsy" group of children studied by Gubbay and colleagues (1965) contained 38 males and 12 females. Ferry and associates (1975) investigated 49 males and 20 females. The ratio of males to females is approximately 3:1.

Incidence

The incidence of apraxia of speech in children has not been established because of the heterogeneity of the groups studied. Rosenbek and Wertz (1972), for example, did not exclude children with language delay, aphasia, mental retardation, or neuromuscular disorders. Yoss and Darley (1974), in contrast, excluded children with an apparent organic basis for the disorder. Palmer et al. (1964) investigated the incidence of apraxia and agnosia in 1000 consecutive cases of children with functional articulation disorders. They found that 10.7 percent demonstrated "lingual apraxia" and 2.4 percent demonstrated apraxia and agnosia. However, their subjects were not selected on the basis of apraxia of speech. Results from available studies suggest that no statistically acceptable incidence figures are currently available.

Summary

A large number of symptoms have been included in the syndrome of apraxia of speech in children. None of the deficits have been demonstrated to be unique to the disorder; they are shared with other communication disorders such as childhood aphasia, developmental dysarthria, and functional articulation disorders. This does not mean that a symptom complex sufficient for differential diagnosis cannot be established—only that there is a need to investigate more fully the unique pattern of impairment for this group of children.

ETIOLOGY

In adults with acquired brain damage, apraxia of speech typically results from an objectively measurable lesion of known etiology to Broca's area and contiguous tissue of the language-dominant left hemisphere. No analagous statement can be made for children with apraxia of speech. Rather, it has been observed that "We are not justified at this time in concluding anything but the fact that these cases do have neurological involvement" (Palmer et al., 1964, p. 8).

In the following discussion of etiology, it should become apparent that we do not know whether the disorder is due to early acquired neuropathology or a congenital (developmental) failure in brain maturation. We also do not know whether the neural dysfunction is bilateral or unilateral, focal or diffuse. Even if this information were available, the fact that the brain dysfunction/damage is congenital or occurs early in childhood would necessitate exploration of the effects of cortical plasticity, since the infant brain is capable of substantial compensation for impaired function (Lenneberg, 1967). No such research has yet been undertaken with this population of children.

There are two general views of etiology. Each utilizes similar data to arrive at different conclusions. The data are limited to EEG and neurologic examination findings. Neither of these forms of evidence is conclusive in isolating the type and extent of neural involvement. Abnormal EEG may be found in normal children (Myklebust, Bosher, Olson, & Cole, 1969), and children with significant nervous system impairment may have EEG results interpretable as normal. Similarly, soft neurologic signs (e.g., gait problems, positive Babinski reflex, poor gross motor skills) are found in children without communication disorders and in children with apraxia of speech. A related problem is that a circular argument is sometimes used to establish a neurologic basis for observed deficits. The presence of apraxia is used to infer brain dysfunction which in turn is used to account for the presence of the disorder.

The first perspective on etiology proposes specific neuroanatomical deficits. Rosenbek and Wertz (1972) investigated 50 children diagnosed as demonstrating apraxia of speech by a neurologist and a speech–language pathologist. No specific subject selection criteria were reported. Neurologic examination was completed on 36 of the children. Twenty-two of the children had essentially normal examinations with the exception of either generalized apraxia or apraxia confined to the orofacial structures. For the remaining 14 subjects, apraxia was associated with other neurologic deficits including muscle weakness, hyperreflexia, spasticity, hyporeflexia, and/or hyperkinesia. EEG findings from 26 of the 50 children revealed that 58 percent had either focal or generalized abnormalities. Based on this evidence, it was concluded that children with apraxia of speech are "brain damaged." This conclusion was reached even though 61 percent of the neurologic examinations were normal with the exception of a finding of apraxia, and 42 percent of the EEG results were interpreted as normal. Although the data were not provided, it would appear safe to conclude that some of the children had normal EEG results and no abnormal neurologic examination findings with the exception of apraxia.

A second perspective proposes a disturbance in normal neurologic maturation. Yoss and Darley (1974a) investigated 30 children with moderate to severe articulation disorders. None of the children had an apparent organic basis for the disorder. Each was administered a battery of auditory, oral movement, and speech production tests and received a neurologic examination. Division of the children at the median score on an isolated volitional movement task yielded a subgroup who demonstrated deficits consistent with earlier descriptions of apraxia of speech in children. Neurologic soft signs were found in 15 of the 16 children in the apraxic subgroup and in four of the 14 children in the functional articulation disorder subgroup. The most frequent findings were decreased alternate motion rates of the tongue and extremities and difficulty with gait and coordination. The neurologic ratings, when combined with articulatory variables, were the best predictor in differentiating the 2 groups of children. Yoss and Darley concluded that "Soft neurologic signs of uncertain significance or equivocal clinical importance do not imply minimal cerebral dysfunction or a *pathologic* [emphasis added] condition of the central nervous system" (p. 411). They interpreted the neurologic evidence as consistent with a developmental immaturity of "some degree." However, since children with an apparent organic basis for the disorder were excluded from the study, it would not be expected that brain damage would arise as a supportable etiology for the observed deficits.

Gubbay and colleagues (1965) attempted to bridge the gap between propositions of CNS damage and developmental delay by postulating heterogeneity of underlying causality. Based on a study of 21 clumsy children, they proposed that disordered cerebral anatomy (e.g., a focal lesion) was the primary etiologic factor in the majority of cases, whereas fundamentally disordered physiology (e.g., defective establishment of physiologic dominance) was the basis for the minority.

In summary, maturational and/or acquired CNS deficits appear to be responsible for apraxia of speech in children. No other etiologies have been proposed. However, the children studied have been heterogeneous and the neurologic evidence presented for many of these children has been weak. There is a definite need to investigate CNS integrity in groups of children with apraxia of speech selected on the basis of consistently applied criteria. Until such research has been completed, neurologic bases of the disorder will remain obscure.

ASSESSMENT

Evaluation of the child with apraxia will include neurologic, psychological, and speech and language examinations. The neurologic examination is undertaken to determine if there is evidence of brain damage or developmental delay. Whether specialized testing (EEG, computerized axial tomography, etc.) is appropriate will depend on the results of the initial examination. The psychological evaluation should (1) address the possibility of associated mental retardation, (2) explore emotional reactions of the child to his or her inability to produce speech, and (3) determine whether a discrepancy exists between verbal and performance intellectual abilities.

Assessment of communicative functioning will include administration of hearing, speech, and language tests. Audiometric testing is used to rule out hearing loss as a basis for the disorder. Administration of language tests aids in determining whether receptive skills are clearly superior to expressive abilities, a reported characteristic of the disorder. The examination of the speech mechanism is used to document the speed, range of motion, and strength of the mobile articulators, and it should prove useful in identifying possible neuromuscular impairment of the speech production apparatus. Volitional oral movements typically are assessed utilizing an adaptation (Kools et al., 1971) of the DeRenzi et al. (1966) measure for adults with apraxia. An articulation battery and spontaneous speech sample are required to evaluate speech production abilities. The articulation test (e.g., Templin-Darley Tests of Articulation) provides information on the types of errors produced and the phonetic inventory of the child. Differences in the frequency and type of errors produced within single words and longer utterances and ratings of prosody and intelligibility are obtained from evaluation of the speech sample.

Blakeley (1983) has developed a screening test for apraxia of speech in children. The first subtest uses results from measures of language comprehension and language expression to rule out mental retardation and to investigate discrepancies between receptive and expressive language skills. Other subtests are used to evaluate (1) vowel and diphthong production, (2) volitional oral movements, (3) verbal sequencing, (4) speech sound development, (5) imitation of motorically complex words, (6) production of multisyllabic words that frequently result in sound and syllable transpositions, and (7) prosody in connected speech. Weighted scores for the examination are used to determine the likelihood that the child demonstrates apraxia of speech. This screening instrument is useful in identifying those children who require further exploration of their disorder.

There is no assurance that results from a battery of tests will allow reliable differential diagnosis since, as noted earlier, many of the characteristics of apraxia are shared with other communication disorders. However, these tests should provide information on the types of deficits the child presents with and a framework for treatment.

TREATMENT

A primary reason for evaluating a communicative disorder is to provide direction for clinical intervention. Treatment procedures for apraxia in children are based on the characteristics of the speech behavior and therapy principles for functional articulation disorders. There are few reports which carefully document therapy procedures or progess. Instead, treatment principles are based on descriptive follow-up of children with widely differing speech characterisitics who have been diagnosed as apraxic. The following discussion will integrate these principles according to the following framework: (1) goals of treatment, (2) structure of treatment sessions, (3) sound stimuli, (4) teaching hierarchy, and (5) treatment strategies. Several reports provide the basis for the review (Chappell, 1973; Rosenbek et al., 1974; Yoss & Darley, 1974b). More recent discussions have drawn from these sources and are included when they provide unique information.

Goals of Treatment

A primary difficulty of children with apraxia of speech is the inability to combine sound into words and sentences of increasing length and complexity. A breakdown often occurs between single sound or monosyllabic word production and more complex sequences required for phrases and sentences. Chappell (1973) indicated that treatment must assist the child in establishing volitional control over sensorimotor experiences by building " . . . imagery, memory, and motor plans for highly selective motor activity" (p. 366). This statement reflects the general goal of treatment: to establish complex, volitional sensorimotor production patterns that the child has failed to develop independently.

Structure of Treatment Sessions

Intensive, systematic, drill-oriented sessions apparently are most successful. Drill provides repeated practice of the motor patterns of the sound selected for training. Daily therapy (Blakeley, 1983; Morley & Fox, 1969) and short periods of intense drill appear most beneficial.

Sound Stimuli

One reported characteristic of children with apraxia of speech is the inability to produce vowels accurately. If the child produces vowel errors, it is suggested that these speech sounds be established before consonants are attempted (Blakeley, 1983; Chappell, 1973). Chappell recommended beginning with the vowels /o,a,i,æ/, probably because they represent highly contrastive tongue positions.

Teaching visible sounds is a frequent recommendation (Blakeley, 1983; Macaluso-Haynes, 1978; Rosenbek et al., 1974; Smartt et al., 1976; Yoss & Darley, 1974b). In contrast, Chappell (1973) proposed teaching consonants with markedly different points of articulation and patterns of movement, namely, /p, t, k, f, s/. The rationale provided was that the movements required for producing these sounds are highly distinguishable and, once established, are available for combination, shaping, and modifying into other consonants.

No guidelines have been proposed beyond these recommendations for initial training of vowels and consonants and the suggestion that the departure point for treatment should be the sounds the child is capable of producing. There appears to be little information regarding which sounds will provide the basic movement patterns needed for maximal success in therapy.

Teaching Hierarchy

Very specific information is provided about the order in which linguistic structures are to be taught. The typical sequence begins with single nonsense syllables, usually of a consonant–vowel (CV) structure (e.g., *ba*). Gradually more complex structures (e.g., CVCV, *baba*) are taught. Syllables are followed by monosyllabic words, which are often very salient to the child and which contain the sounds that have been established at the syllable level. Multisyllabic words are gradually introduced in order to increase the length and complexity of the sounds to be sequenced. The next step is the production of the trained words in phrases and sentences.

The most controversial aspect of the hierarchy is whether sounds should first be taught in isolation or in syllables. With few exceptions (Chappell, 1973; Yoss & Darley, 1947b), it is recommended that work should begin at the syllable level followed by training at the word level as soon as possible. Severely impaired children, however, may require that sounds be established in isolation before progressing to a syllable level.

Treatment Strategies

The most distinguishing characteristics of treatment for apraxia are the cuing strategies used for establishing sound patterns. In training children with functional articulation disorder, auditory cues are the primary input modality. Apraxic children, however, seem unable to learn sensorimotor patterns through primarily auditory cues. Intense visual cues are recommended in addition to auditory cues. These cues include working in front of a mirror in order to see placement of the articulators and written cues that pair the sound with the written symbol. Several clinicians imply that visual cuing is essential for successful training (Blakeley, 1983; Rosenbek et al., 1974; Yoss & Darley, 1974b).

Apraxic children may have reduced orosensory awareness (Macaluso-Haynes, 1978). Tactile cues, therefore, are recommended. These cues take the form of stimulating the articulators involved in producing the desired sound. Stimulation includes application of various textures or pressure and swabbing or probing the lips and tongue at the site of desired contact. The success of these procedures has not been documented.

Rosenbek and colleagues (1974) suggested a strategy that incorporates the use of rhythm, stress, and intonation into the production of speech patterns. For children who can produce sentences, rhymes and songs are used as stimulus materials. The natural stress and intonation patterns ". . . apparently assist in facilitating motor sequencing" (Macaluso-Haynes, 1978, p. 247). The production of songs and rhymes is paired with physical movement such as beating time or squeezing a bean bag with each syllable. Children are urged to slow their rate of speech in order to achieve an even stress pattern. This strategy apparently aids in maintaining the sounds in the target sequences. Although Rosenbek and colleagues (1974) reported success with these approaches in a case study of a nine-year-old girl, there is no empirical documentation as to which factors are critical for success. Additionally, these strategies appear most useful for children who are able to produce phrases and sentences. They would not be applicable for the severely impaired child who produces sounds only at the single syllable or word level.

One of the greatest problems in treating an apraxic child is developing retention of a movement pattern so that it can be used repeatedly in longer and more complex words and sentences. Chappell (1973) recognized this problem and made suggestions for gradually increasing the time spent practicing a particular movement pattern so that accuracy could be maintained for the duration of the task. He also suggested gradually providing increasingly longer time periods between practice of a particular pattern in order to help the child maintain the memory for these movements. He identified the need for children to monitor their own productions so that they could determine the accuracy of the productions and attempt self-correction, if necessary. Aside from these suggestions, development of self-monitoring, retention, and transfer skills that may be critical for successful treatment of apraxic children have been largely ignored.

Summary

The treatment approaches described for apraxic children are primarily descriptive summaries of procedures that have been used clinically. There are virtually no experimental data to support the descriptions. The approaches are eclectic in nature and include a variety of techniques. The factors that seem to make the most difference for success are as follows:

- Frequent, systematic, drill-oriented therapy that provides much repetition of sound patterns
- A program based on the individual child's entry skills and response to different types of cues
- Frequent use of cues that reinforce the movement patterns, particularly visual and tactile cues
- Development of self-monitoring, retention, and transfer skills

It is important to recognize that each child presents with a unique group of characteristics (e.g., one child labeled apraxic will have few consonant or vowel sounds while another will have many sounds but not be able to sequence them in complex words). There is no single approach that is likely to be satisfactory for all children. Rather, clinicians " . . . must rely upon the frequency, consistency and motivation of their instruction for success with . . . apraxia" (Blakeley, 1983, p. 27).

PROGNOSIS

Children with apraxia of speech appear to improve very slowly. Although improvement with treatment has been reported (Rosenbek et al., 1974), these children often remain in therapy for several years and sometimes never achieve normal intelligible speech (Blakeley, 1983). In a follow-up investigation 12–16 months after their initial study, Yoss and Darley (1973) noted that only one of ten children enrolled in therapy had been discharged, and only after 139 hours of individual, intensive, speech therapy. A year later, one additional child had been dismissed from treatment. Significant improvement with treatment appears to occur only after an enormous expenditure of time and effort.

CASE STUDY

A case summary may be helpful in demonstrating how faithfully our discussion of apraxia of speech has captured important elements of the disorder. A 3-year-old boy was referred for evaluation. His mother reported that her health was "poor" during the pregnancy. She was hospitalized for hypertension during the eighth month of the term at which time the infant was delivered by Caesarean section. He was placed in a moderate care unit for 1 week due to low birth weight and jaundice. Motor developmental milestones for sitting, walking, and so forth were within normal limits. Speech development was characterized as "slow." The mother reported that he talked infrequently and was seldom intelligible. She estimated that his oral vocabulary was 35 words.

Administration of the Sequenced Inventory of Communication Development (Hedrick, Prather, & Tobin, 1975) yielded a receptive language age of 32 months and an expressive age of 16 months. Phonetic inventory was limited to vowels, stops, nasals, and glides. Final consonant deletion was the most consistently used process identified from phonological analysis (Hodson, 1980). Cluster reduction, stopping, velar fronting, and unstressed syllable reduction were also noted. Initial consonant deletion also was used, most often for /w/ and /h/. Although the patient used all vowels, they were frequently incorrect. Inconsistent vowel and consonant errors occurred in repeated productions of the same words. Speech sound production was not noticeably improved by repeated auditory and visual stimulation, and regardless of context, /d/ was typically substituted for target consonants. His preferred word shape was a (CV) form. More complex canonical shapes were attempted, but they were also reduced to these CV combinations.

Conversational speech was severely reduced in intelligibility and attempts at communication included use of a well-developed gestural system. Auditory acuity was within normal limits bilaterally. Examination of the speech mechanism did not reveal evidence of neuromuscular impairment although alternating movements of the tongue and lips were performed slowly, diadochokinetic rates were reduced for /pʌ/ and /kʌ/, and multisyllabic sequences (pʌtʌkʌ) could not be imitated. A psychological evaluation found that cognitive functioning on nonverbal tests was in the high average to superior range and that receptive vocabulary and visual integration abilities were average.

During the 2 years following the initial evaluation, the patient received 100 hours of therapy, which was directed toward using auditory, visual, and tactile cues to establish imitative and spontaneous productions of consonants in monsyllables and disyllables. Progress was very slow, and he continued to demonstrate numerous misarticulations and remained highly unintelligible.

When the patient was 5 years old, additional testing was completed to evaluate further the type and severity of his oral expression problems. Cognitive development was judged to be within the average range from results obtained on the McCarthy Scales of Children's Abilities (McCarthy, 1972). Administration of the Carrow Elicited Language Inventory (Carrow, 1974) revealed frequent omissions of articles, pronouns, verbs, negatives, and conjunctions. However, adjectives, adverbs, and nouns were almost always retained.

Imitative production of sentences from the Carrow Inventory was characterized by variable, context-dependent speech sound errors. Variability in sound production was reduced on more complex sentences, with frequent substitution of /d/, /b/, and /w/ for target sounds. Longer utterances were highly unintelligible due to sound and syllable omissions and transpositions. Word shapes were primarly CV combinations.

The patient received a score of 32 on the Templin-Darley Diagnostic Articulation Test (Templin & Darley, 1969). The mean for male children his age is 106. Results of a phonological analysis (Hodson, 1980) were similar to those of the first evaluation completed 2 years earlier. Phonetic inventory was limited to vowels, stops, nasals, glides, and infrequent liquids. No fricatives or affricates were noted. Commonly occurring phonological processes included consonant deletion, cluster reduction, and stridency deletion. In conversational speech, avoidance behaviors were noted on words containing fricative sounds. Prosody was abnormal on longer utterances and was characterized by inappropriate loudness dynamics.

Several additional measures were used to explore the type and extent of apraxic involvement. Based on the results from the Screening Test for Developmental Apraxia of Speech (Blakeley, 1980), the probability of the patient's correct assignment to an apraxic diagnostic category was greater than 99 percent. Perseveration, avoidance, and grouping behaviors frequently were noted during testing. On the Boston Verbal Agility subtest (Goodglass & Kaplan, 1972), his productions of multisyllabic stimuli were characterized by transpositions of sounds and syllables and reductions in word complexity. Six of 10 items of the Kools et al. (1971) adaptation of the DeRenzi et al. (1966) test of oral apraxia were scored as incorrect on the basis of defective amplitude, accuracy, and force. He also demonstrated difficulty in rapidly producing six of the seven tasks (e.g., alternating tongue movements, mouth opening and closing) from the Boston Oral Agility subtest (Goodglass & Kaplan, 1972). Administration of the Bruininks-Oseretsky Test of Motor Proficiency (Bruininks, 1978) found fine and gross motor coordination to be within normal limits. On the adapted version (Kools et al., 1971) of the DeRenzi et al. (1966) test of limb apraxia, however, he correctly completed only five of 10 items.

Is the patient apraxic? We think so. There is no evidence of mental retardation, severe personality disorder, hearing loss, or neuromuscular impairment that could account for his speech production deficits. He also does not demonstrate auditory perception/integration deficits that have been cited as important elements of childhood aphasia (Benton, 1964; Eisenson, 1972). It could be argued that he demonstrates a functional articulation disorder. Since evidence of specific brain damage was not found, we cannot verify an organic basis for the disorder. However, the presence of a severe articulatory deficit, vowel errors, severely reduced intelligibility, oral and limb apraxia, and other characteristics of apraxia of speech previously described suggests that he would be an unusually atypical example of a child assigned a diagnosis of functional articulation disorder. We believe that his pattern of deficits is sufficiently unique to be considered an example of a child with apraxia of speech.

CONCLUSION

A large number of characteristics have been proposed as symptomatic of apraxia of speech in children. No single symptom appears to be sufficient to distinguish the disorder from other communication problems of children with which it shares important elements. Attempts to establish a pattern of impairment have been hampered by marked differences in the selection criteria used to identify children for study. We believe a group of children can be identified who have a neurogenically based inability to program volitional movements as a primary feature of their disorder. Additional investigations of behavioral characteristics and etiology are needed, however, before reliable differential diagnosis can be accomplished in clinical settings.

REFERENCES

Aram, M. (1979, November). *Developmental apraxia of speech.* Paper presented at the Annual Convention of the American Speech and Hearing Association, Atlanta.

Benton, A. (1964). Developmental aphasia and brain damage. *Cortex, 1,* 40–52.

Blakeley, R. (1980). *Screening test for developmental apraxia of speech.* Tigard, OR: C. C. Publications.

Blakeley, R. (1983). Treatment of developmental apraxia of speech. In W. Perkins (Ed.), *Dysarthria and apraxia* (pp. 25–33). New York: Thieme-Stratton.

Bruininks, R. (1978). *Bruininks-Oseretsky test of motor proficiency.* Circle Pines, MN: American Guidance Service.

Carrow, E. (1974). *Carrow elicited language inventory.* Lamar, TX: Learning Concepts.

Chappell, G. (1973). Childhood verbal apraxia and its treatment. *Journal of Speech and Hearing Disorders, 38,* 362–368.

Court, D., & Harris, M. (1965). Speech disorders in children—Part II. *British Medical Journal, 11,* 409–411.

Edwards, M. (1973). Developmental verbal dyspraxia. *British Journal of Disorders of Communication, 8,* 64–70.

Eisenson, J. (1972). *Aphasia and language disorders in children.* New York: Harper & Row.

Ferry, P., Hall, S., & Hicks, J. (1975). Delapidated speech: Developmental verbal apraxia. *Developmental Medicine and Child Neurology, 17,* 749–756.

Goodglass, H., & Kaplan, E. (1972). *The assessment of aphasia and related disorders.* Philadelphia: Lea & Febiger.

Gubbay, S., Ellis, E., Walton, J., & Court, S. (1965). Clumsy children: A study of apraxic and agnosic defects in 21 children. *Brain, 88,* 295–312.

Guyette, T., & Diedrich, W. (1981). A critical review of developmental apraxia of speech. In N. Lass (Ed.), *Speech and language: Advances in basic research and practice, Vol 5* (pp. 1–49). New York: Academic Press.

Hedrick, D., Prather, E., & Tobin, A. (1975). *Sequenced inventory of communication development.* Seattle: University of Washington Press.

Hodson, B. (1980). *The assessment of phonological processes.* Danville, IL: Interstate Printers and Publishers.

Kools, J., & Tweedie, D. (1975). Development of praxis in children. *Perceptual and Motor Skills, 40,* 11–19.

Kools, J., Williams, A., Vickers, M., & Caell, A. (1971). Oral and limb apraxia in mentally retarded children with deviant articulation. *Cortex, 7,* 387–400.

Lee, L. (1971). *Northwestern Syntax Screening Test.* Evanston, IL: Northwestern University Press.

Leeneberg, E. (1967). *Biological foundations of language.* New York: John Wiley.

Logue, R., & McClumpha, S. (1970, November). *Apraxia of speech: A case description.* Paper presented at the Annual Convention of the American Speech and Hearing Association, New York.

Macaluso-Haynes, S. (1978). Developmental apraxia of speech: Symptoms and treatment. In D. Johns (Ed.), *Clinical management of neurogenic communication disorders* (pp. 243–250). Boston: Little, Brown.

McCarthy, D. (1972). *McCarthy scales of children's abilities.* New York: Psychological Corp.

McClumpha, S., & Logue, R. (1972, November). *Approaches to children with motor programming disorders of speech.* Paper presented at the Annual Convention of The American Speech and Hearing Association, San Francisco.

Morley, M., Court, D., & Miller, H. (1954). Developmental dysarthria. *British Medical Journal, 1,* 8–10.

Morley, M., & Fox, J. (1969). Disorders of articulation: Theory and therapy. *British Journal of Disorders of Communication, 4,* 151–165.

Myklebust, H., Bosher, B., Olson, D., & Cole, C. (1969). *Minimal brain damage in children.* Washington, DC: Department of Health, Education and Welfare, National Institute of Health.

Nicolosi, L., Harryman, E., & Kresheck, J. (1978). *Terminology of communicative disorders: Speech, language, hearing.* Baltimore: Williams & Wilkins.

Palmer, M., Wurth, C., & Kinchloe, J. (1964). The incidence of lingual apraxia and agnosia in "functional" disorders of articulation. *Cerebral Palsy Review, 25,* 7–9.

Rosenbek, J., Hanson, R., Baughman, C., & Lemme, M. (1974). Treatment of developmental apraxia of speech: A case study. *Language, Speech, and Hearing Services in Schools, 5,* 13–22.

Rosenbek, J., & Wertz, R. (1972). A review of 50 cases of developmental apraxia of speech. *Language, Speech, and Hearing Services in Schools, 3,* 23–33.

Smartt, J., LaLance, L., Gray, J., & Hibbert, P. (1976). Developmental apraxia of speech: A Tennessee Speech and Hearing Association subcommittee report. *Journal of The Tennessee Speech and Hearing Association, 20,* 21–39.

Snyder, D., Marquardt, T., & Peterson, H. (1977). Syntactical aspects of developmental apraxia. *Human Communication, 2,* 151–158.

Templin, M., & Darley, F. (1969). *The Templin-Darley tests of articulation 2nd ed.* Iowa City: The University of Iowa.

Walton, J., Ellis, E., & Court, S. (1962). Clumsy children: Developmental apraxia and agnosia. *Brain, 85,* 603–612.

Yoss, K., & Darley, F. (1973, November). *What happens to children with developmental apraxia of speech? A follow-up of fifteen cases.* Paper presented at the Annual Convention of The American Speech and Hearing Association, Detroit.

Yoss, K., & Darley, F. (1974a). Developmental apraxia of speech in children with defective articulation. *Journal of Speech and Hearing Research, 17,* 399–416.

Yoss, K., & Darley, F. (1974b). Therapy in developmental apraxia of speech. *Language, Speech, and Hearing Services in Schools, 5,* 23–31.

II. DYSARTHRIA

J. Keith Brown

5
Dysarthria in Children: Neurologic Perspective

Children suffering from disorders of speech are seen by many different professionals as part of what is often described as a multidisciplinary team approach that may include pediatrician, pediatric neurologist, speech pathologist, speech therapist, psycholinguist, psychologist, bioengineer, and teacher. All these people may offer advice to the parent who in some instances may be receiving opinions from a minimum of 15 professionals. The president of the American Academy of Cerebral Palsy pointed out in his presidential address of 1982 that a multidisciplinary approach produces overlap, and it is a well-known principle of physics that there is a tendency for friction to occur at interfaces and that friction is notorious for producing more heat than light.

One frequent cause for misunderstanding is the use of terminology that is interpreted differently by different professional groups. The prefix *dys* is used in medicine simply to indicate that a person has difficulty with a particular physiologic function; e.g., dyspnea simply means difficulty in breathing and says nothing at all about the underlying pathophysiology or the many possible causes. Unfortunately there has been a tendency to use terms such as dyslexia, dysphasia, or dyspraxia as a specific diagnosis. This is illustrated by the use of the term *dyslexia,* which medically means that the child has difficulty reading, and says nothing about the very many potential causes or whether this is a specific learning difficulty or part of a global learning difficulty (Brown, 1981).

Speech and Language Evaluation in Neurology:
Childhood Disorders
ISBN 0-8089-1719-6

Similarly, *dysarthria* has been interpreted, for the purpose of this article, as meaning simply that the child has difficulty with articulation. This may be due to anatomical or neurologic factors, i.e., an anatomical dysarthria or a neurologic dysarthria (Brown, 1984).

CLASSIFICATION OF SPEECH DISORDERS IN CHILDHOOD

The clinical classification of speech disorders in children proposed by Ingram (1959) is shown in Table 5-1. He proposes two major divisions of disorders of spoken speech: (1) primary disorders of speech, in which the predominant difficulty is producing speech sounds and sequencing them into words with syntactically correct sentences; and (2) speech disorders secondary to an abnormality in inner language. Confusion often arises over the use of the term *language,* which can be defined (1) as a specific type of language being spoken (e.g., English, French, German; (2) as a study of the grammatical structures of the language, i.e., the syntax; (3) in the computer sense (e.g., basic, Fortran, Pascall); and (4) in the psycholinguistic sense of the study of words and their meanings. (Crystal, 1980; Martlew, 1981).

The syntactical aspects of speech, i.e., the grammatical construction of sentences, usually parallels the motor development of speech (in which case inner language may or may not be completely normal). The child may have abnormal inner language but normally pronounced speech as seen in echolalia or in the so-called cocktail party personality in which the child speaks in well-articulated grammatically correct sentences but has no idea of the meaning of the sentence. It is not necessary to be able to speak in order to develop inner language, as is evidenced in children with so-called locked-in syndrome in which alternative communication systems illustrate that the child has well-developed inner language. The same observations apply to spelling, which tends to be associated with the motor aspects of writing. In this chapter the term language will be used with the same meaning as a computer language, i.e., a system of symbols used by the brain to code or classify information into groupings, subroutines, or concepts. Inner language may involve the use of symbol systems apart from words, e.g., musical notations, chemical symbols, electronic symbols, mathematical symbols, Blissymbols, or sign language. The deaf child, for example signs to himself or herself; there is evidence that the child taught Blissymbols thinks pictographically. The musically literate can write music on a musical stave with the same ease that most of us would write sentences in our native tongue. The motor learning engrams of speech and writing are localized in Broca's area for speech or in the graphomotor area for writing. Words and language symbols tend to be localized in the region of the angular gyrus in the left

Table 5-1
Classification of Speech Disorders in Children

Primary Speech Disorders		
Dysphonia	Acute	Acute laryngitis
(Anatomical, neurological)	Chronic	Familial Congenital laryngeal abnormalities Nodules, laryngeal tumours Brain stem lesions Recurrent laryngeal palsy
Dysrhythmias	Physiological	Stutter/stammer/clutter
	Pathological	Cerebellar and Basal Ganglia disease
Dysarthria	Anatomical	Cleft palate
	Neurological	Flaccid bulbar palsy Pseudo bulbar (spastic) palsy Extrapyramidal hyperkinetic/hypokinetic Ataxic
Dyspraxia		Developmental in 10% of population Familial speech retardation Articulatory dyspraxia due to mild brain damage Acquired frontal lobe damage
Secondary Speech Disorders		High tone and central deafness Congenital sensory and expressive dysphasia Acquired sensory and expressive dysphasia (CVA, embolus, trauma, tumour, epilepsy, meningitis, encephalitis, encephalopathy, e.g. scalds) Mental retardation Psychosis (autism, schizophrenic word salad)

hemisphere while spatial and musical symbols are localized on the opposite side. Although the lexicon or word store is usually localized in Wernicke's area, "language" itself is not localized as such. The word *orange,* for example, is a structured symbol system that links together a concept of memories relating to size, shape, smell, taste, feel, color, etc. The word, therefore, allows memories at different "addresses" within the brain to be linked together into a concept as well as being the basic unit of spoken speech. This concept then allows us to say that "we understand" or "know" the meaning of the word.

Clinical Grouping of Speech and Language Disorders

Many of the pathologies seen in children are much more diffuse than the focal pathology seen in the adult. In the adult, vascular lesions, tumors, and trauma will produce localized discreet lesions within the brain, while in children it is more likely that asphyxia, jaundice, infection, and trauma will produce more diffuse lesions (Brown, 1976). For this reason one often sees a mixed picture and cannot classify a child as suffering simply from dysarthria as he or she may have associated deafness, mental handicap, or autistic features. The child with congenital rubella syndrome may have deafness or a mental handicap with a high-tone deafness. Certain chromosome disorders can be associated with a specific speech problem such as the marked expressive dysphasia and cortical dysarthria seen in children with Klinefelter's syndrome and the XYY syndrome. (Ratcliffe, 1982) Although this chapter focuses on dysarthria, it should be taken as mandatory that a detailed profile of all aspects of hearing, language development, and general intelligence will be assessed in every child. (Ardan & Kemp, 1970; Mutton & Lea, 1980; Rutter & Martin, 1972).

CLINICAL TYPES OF DYSARTHRIA

Anatomical Causes of Dysarthria

The most common cause of dysarthria in children due to an anatomical defect is the cleft palate syndrome. (Nylen, 1961) Improvements in plastic surgery in recent years have resulted in acceptable cosmetic results in the treatment of the harelip, but children with severe anatomical dysarthria from the cleft palate are still seen. Drillien and Ingram (1966) reported 40 percent with unintelligible speech at 3 or more years of age. Research is now being directed to achieve better repair of the palate. The use of palatal obturators to improve alveolar alignment and to prevent turning out at the edge of the cleft while awaiting repair may be helpful. Some surgeons suggest early closure at 4 months of age rather than waiting until 18 months of age. Modern techniques of nasal endoscopy and video-fluoroscopy may help to give a more dynamic view of palatal function to assess whether a pharyngoplasty would improve the speech. If the palate is not intact or is short, the soft palate does not completely close off the nasal cavity from the oral cavity (Subtelny, Koepp-Baker, & Subtelny, 1961), so that intrabuccal pressure cannot be increased to produce certain sounds such as *p, t,* or those which require a sustained flow of air, e.g., *s-s-s-s.* When the child tries to regulate the air flow and so increase intrabuccal pressure, air escapes through the nose and may be heard during speech as nasal escape. In the normal child, making a noise such as *e-e-e-e* elevates the soft palate and all the air escapes through the mouth, so that covering the mouth occludes the sound but pinching the nose does not cause any modulation. The opposite is the case with a sound such as *m-m-m-m* where covering the mouth makes no difference while occlusion of the nose obliterates the sound completely. In the child with nasal escape one may hear air escaping through the nose during speech, but in making a sound such as *e-e-e-e* pinching the nose will cause a marked change in volume and pitch with modulation of noise. The palate itself may be congenitally short in isolation or as part of the malformation of cleft palate. The palatal repair may have become infected with subsequent contraction due to scar tissue formation with fibrosis. Acquired palatal disorders such as injury from falling on a sharp object while holding it in the mouth or chronic infection of the palate as used to be seen with syphilis could result in a fistula of the hard or soft palate with scarring and contraction. If the palate is congenitally short without an obvious cleft there may be a submucous cleft if a bifid uvula is seen (Fig. 5-1).

There is also a syndrome in children where the maxilla is very long, which is associated with scaphocephalic heads so that the soft palate only approximates to the posterior pharyngeal wall, provided there is a pad of adenoids against which it can approximate. Removal of the adenoids in these cases can result in deterioration of the speech with hypernasality. (Birrell, 1966) This condition is often referred to as *palatal disproportion syndrome.* The opposite of hypernasal speech, i.e., hyponasal speech or hyporhinophonia, occurs when there is obstruction to the nasopharyngeal air passage. The most obvious cause is enlargement of the adenoids causing mouth breathing, snoring, poor resonance to the voice, eustachian obstruction with secretory otitis, and hyponasal speech. Palatal disproportion in conditions such as the Treacher Collins syndrome is the oppo-

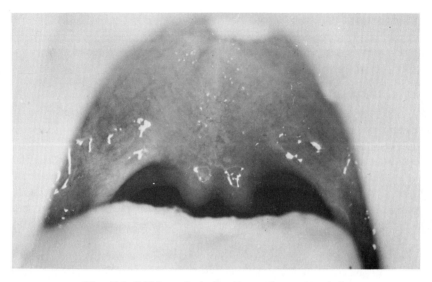

Fig. 5-1. Bifid uvula indicating submucous cleft.

site to that found in scaphocephaly when there is maxillary hypoplasia and a very narrow nasopharynx so that everything is crowded together. Tumors of the nasopharynx such as rhabdomyosarcoma, angiofibroma, or even carcinomas occur in children and are often missed for long periods of time until infiltration of the lower cranial nerves occurs or the tumors track upward into the orbit causing proptosis.

A fashionable cause of dyslalia years ago was tongue-tie. There is no evidence that simple tongue-tie causes speech difficulty, and recognition of the characteristic pattern of consonant substitution, omission, and reversal should prevent unnecessary operations on children. The importance of the tongue in speech has been overemphasized. It is possible to have clear speech and yet be an aglot, and we have seen children with hemiglossectomy for tumors of the tongue who have had perfectly normal speech. (Fig. 5-2) The tongue may be infiltrated in cases of neurofibromatosis or enlarged in cases of hypothyroidism.

More recently, the effect of the enlarged tongue in the relatively small mouth of the child with Down's syndrome has been suggested as a cause of speech difficulty rather than the CNS disorder. This has led to a renewed vogue in operating on the tongue to improve speech.

Dental malocclusion, especially with hypomandibulosis when the jaw is too short or prognathism when it is too long, results in a gap between the teeth, and there is a tendency for the tongue to protrude between the gap causing an interdental *s,* or sigmatism. These anatomi-

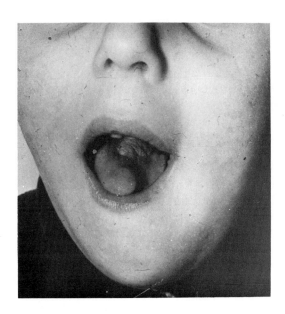

Fig. 5-2. Abnormality of the tongue following hemiglossectomy for an infiltrating tumor in a child with normal speech.

cal variations may interfere with accurate bilabial and alveolar articulation but more often cause lisping. Chronic thumb sucking has also been suggested as a cause of malocclusion with a lisp. The small infant does not suck in the sense of creating a negative pressure but milks the mother's nipple with a stripping movement of the tongue. When he or she swallows the milk, the tongue is often protruded between the alveolar ridges. After 7 months of age when the infantile feeding reflexes have disappeared, the teeth have erupted and biting and chewing develop. The tongue is kept behind the teeth and approximated to the roof of the mouth during swallowing. A few children maintain this infantile tongue-thrusting type of sucking and swallowing. This pattern persists in some children with neurologic abnormalities and may also occur in isolation as a dominantly inherited condition. The tongue thrust often pushes saliva forward and so drooling accompanies the tongue thrust and lisping. In the past it was thought that this was a sign of chronic nasal obstruction and adenoidectomy was usually recommended, but persisting tongue thrust can occur in the absence of any nasopharyngeal obstruction. Cleft palate or any midline defect in the facial structures can be associated with corresponding abnormalities in the brain, which may be gross as in holoprosencephaly, arrhinencephaly, and absence of corpus callosum, or microscopical as with cortical dysplasia. Mental handicap or other neurologic signs can then complicate the anatomical speech abnormality.

Neurologic Causes of Dysarthria

Anatomy & Physiology

The larynx developed in evolutionary terms first as a sphincter in order to protect the respiratory tract from aspiration of food. It subsequently developed a secondary function in phonation. The same muscles used in articulation also have important functions in feeding, i.e., biting, chewing, and swallowing. Control of breathing forms the third important parameter; phonation usually occurs on expiration, which has to be interrupted for phoneme production and sustained (i.e., inspiration is inhibited) according to the punctuation of speech. It is not surprising that disorders of biting, chewing, swallowing, phonation, and respiratory control often accompany a dysarthria. The amount of air expelled from the lungs determines the volume of the voice, and the vocal cords vibrate only when they are approximate and contracted. The voice is not produced by a free vibration of loose cords in an airstream. The tension in the cords will vary according to the contraction of the laryngeal muscles, and this in turn will vary the pitch.

The cricothyroid muscle is the main muscle to cause lengthening of the vocal cord; the thyroarytenoid (which includes the vocalis muscle) shortens the cords. Other muscles of the larynx that are important are (1) those that dilate the glottis in order to allow an increase in air flow during breathing (e.g., posterior cricoarytenoid muscles); and (2) closure of the glottis and approximation of the vocal cords, which produces the sphincter action in order to prevent aspiration. This is achieved by the lateral cricoarytenoid and the aryepiglottic muscles. The vocal cords themselves produce a rather weak, reedy sound, if not modified by resonation of the nasal cavity, sinuses, and skull bones.

The muscles of the larynx together with the other bulbar musculature (i.e., the muscles of the face, lips, tongue, and palate) are supplied from the brainstem (pons and medulla). Facial movements (e.g., lip pursing) have their own representation in the large facial nuclei on each side of the midline in the upper part of the fourth ventricle while tongue movements are represented by the hypoglossal nucleus on each side of the midline in the bottom half of the fourth ventricle. Closely related developmentally to these nuclei is the nucleus ambiguous, which is responsible for control of movement of the pharynx and larynx. The nucleus ambiguous is odd in that it uses parasympathetic fibers to supply striated muscle. The nucleus ambiguous supplies the muscles of the larynx and pharynx via several cranial nerves, in particular the 9th (glossopharyngeal), 10th (vagus), and 11th (accessory nerves).

Another motor nucleus, the vagal motor nucleus, sends all of its motor impulses via the parasympathetic component of the 10th vagus

Table 5-2
Clinical Aspects of Bulbar Function

Normal Function	Abnormal Function
Articulation	Imprecise consonants, slow, slurred, labored
Phonation	Harsh voice, breathy, aphonia, monotone, loss of high frequencies, low amplitude
Airway protection	Asphyxiate (adducted cords), aspirate, absent gag or cough
Mastication	Spastic jaw, no bite, no chew
Salivation	Drooling
Taste	Dysgeusia/ageusia
Swallow	Dysphagia—liquidized or semisolids only; aphagia—need tube feeding or gastrostomy; drooling
Palatal closure of nasopharynx	Nasal escape, poor intrabuccal pressure, recurrent otitis media
Respiratory control	Inspire when swallowing and aspirate
	Rhythm speech erratic, explosive, and no stress
Oral sensation	Anesthesia, burns, mutilation

nerve and is responsible for esophageal and gastric motility. There must obviously be close cooperation between the nucleus ambiguous and the dorsal vagal nucleus so that swallowing is a coordinated and continuous action. Biting and chewing depend more on the powerful pincer effects resulting from contraction of the masseter, temporalis, and pterygoid muscles. These muscles receive their motor nerve supply separately via the motor subdivision of the mandibular branch of the trigeminal nerve, and their central connection is to the masticatory nucleus and not the nucleus ambiguous. These muscles are the ones involved in the jaw jerk and are not important in articulation. Sensation from the larynx, pharynx, and the gut is transmitted via afferent fibers in the 7th, 9th, and 10th nerves, which go to the main sensory nucleus for the bulbar region, i.e., the nucleus of the tractus solitarious. Another important brainstem nucleus is the salivary nucleus, which projects visceral motor afferent nerves via several different cranial nerves to the salivary glands.

It can be seen, therefore, that mastication, salivation, taste, swallowing, and articulation may share common cranial nerves but have already been sorted into separate functions at brainstem level (Tables 5-2 and 5-3). Each nucleus may make connections with other nuclei in the brainstem allowing development of the so-called brainstem reflexes and will have rostral connections to different parts of the brain (e.g., the connection via the cortical bulbar pathways of Broca's area to the nucleus am-

Table 5-3
Clinical and Anatomical Comparison of Bulbar Function

Bulbar Function	Cranial Nerve	Nucleus in Bulb
Tongue movement	(12) Hypoglossal	Hypoglossal nucleus (lower half of 4th ventricle—medullary level)
Pharyngeal movement	(10) Vagus	Nucleus ambiguous
	(9) Glossopharyngeal	Nucleus ambiguous (central medulla above olive)
Mastication (bite and jaw jerk)	(5) Trigeminal (motor)	Masticatory nucleus
Lip closure	(7) Facial	Facial nucleus (upper half floor of 4th ventricle—pontine level)
Touch (lips, jaw, and lower teeth)	(5) Trigeminal (lingual branch)	Trigeminal nucleus
Taste	(7) Facial via chorda tympani (lingual)	Tractus solitarius
	(9) Glossopharyngeal	Tractus solitarius (lateral medulla above inferior cerebellar peduncle)

biguous). The importance of considering these anatomical structures is that in a child with dysarthria there may be different combinations of these associated abnormalities.

Each individual cranial nerve can convey motor, sensory, or autonomic information. Some are fairly single minded and specialized in their function such as the hypoglossal nerve, which is the main motor nerve to the tongue. Alternatively, the vagus nerve, for example, contains all types of fiber. It is evident from this rather sketchy anatomical description, however, that a lesion of one cranial nerve may cause a disorder localized to a particular anatomical segment (e.g., wasting or fasciculation of the tongue in a hypoglossal nerve lesion) or it may result in loss of sensation, salivation, and taste in a particular anatomical distribution. When we reach a brainstem level of integration, specialization of function is already taking place so that disorder of function such as salivation, mastication, taste, swallowing, phonation, or articulation is more likely to occur.

Brainstem Reflexes

Brainstem reflexes can be divided into three main groups: (1) Protective reflexes that are present in early life and persist throughout life; (2) a group of primitive reflexes that are present at birth in relationship to breast feeding and are subsequently inhibited; and (3) a group of developmental reflexes that may be present in utero, may or may not persist postnatally, but may become obligatory in disease states.

Protective reflexes. These are reflexes that protect (1) against aspiration and obstruction of the airway as with coughing; (2) against ingestion of harmful material as with vomiting; and (3) the upper airway as in sneezing and the gag reflex. The gag reflex consists of contraction of the pharyngeal wall and expulsion of whatever is in the mouth and pharynx with sensation of choking. Stimulation of the pharyngeal wall results in impulses traveling via the ninth nerve to the tractus solitarius. Connections between this nucleus and the nucleus ambiguous complete the reflex arc allowing muscular contraction of the pharynx to be initiated via the 10th vagus nerve. (Brodal, 1981) The cough reflex is similar in that stimulation of the larynx or bronchi results in afferent stimuli via the vagus passing to the solitary tract, but this time they are transferred to the respiratory center and result in a sudden forced expiration. It should be remembered that the respiratory center that is formed from part of the brainstem reticular formation is in essence another brainstem nucleus that is closely linked with the nuclei discussed previously. Control of respiration has been emphasized in articulation, but inspiration must be accompanied with dilatation of the glottic ring, swallowing is normally associated with inhibition of respiration, and vomiting is also accompanied by inhibition of respiration. Vomiting is considered briefly as this forms a rather more complex brainstem reflex pattern. (Gilman & Winans, 1982) Afferent stimuli may consist of an objectionable smell, a horrible taste, or stimulation anywhere in the gastrointestinal tract of the visceral afferent fibers that travel via the vagus nerve. These feed into the nucleus of the tractus solitarius, one part of which must be specifically oriented to form what is generally called a *vomiting center.* This center may also be acted upon by certain drugs such as opiates by raised intracranial pressure, and it also receives stimuli from the vestibular nuclei as in motion sickness. The output from this center is to several brainstem nuclei, e.g., to the dorsal motor nucleus of the vagus, which causes dilatation of the cardiac sphincter at the gastroesophageal junction and contraction of the stomach. Fibers of the nucleus ambiguous will close the glottis and fibers of the reticular formation will arrest respiration and cause contraction of the abdominal muscles and diaphragm via the reticulospinal pathways. We now have, therefore, a more sophisticated pattern of response than a simple reflex, and we have a built-in committed computer circuit with a preprogrammed behavioral response, at an even more sophisticated level this is seen in coordination of all the different feeding reflexes into feeding behavior.

Development of primitive feeding reflexes.   The perioral muscles and tongue have well-differentiated muscle spindles by 12 weeks after conception. The peripheral nerves, although poorly myelinated, are well developed; the brainstem shows differentiation of neurons but no myelination of any long tracts except for a small amount in the medial lemniscus and the posterior columns of the spinal cord. If the face is stroked the lips purse, and if the cheek is pricked the head turns away (i.e., there are avoidance reactions). By 14 or 16 weeks gestation the mouth will open on stimulation of the lips and turn toward stimulation of the cheek (rooting). As the fetus enters the first extensor phase of development, the mouth will open on stimulation of the lower lip (i.e., cardinal point reflex) and also will open as part of mass extensor activity. The fetus at 20 weeks shows significantly more extensor activity with stretching responses in the arms and legs, and the mouth may open as part and parcel of these tonic extensor movements. Spontaneous sucking and swallowing movements occur and the fetus is, by this time, swallowing amniotic fluid.

The small fetus born round about 25 weeks gestation will show so-called ingesting reflexes. On stroking the cheek the mouth will move toward the stimulus; the mouth will open on stimulation of the lower lip; and spontaneous sucking movements and tongue rolling are initiated by pressure over the lip or upon introduction of an object into the mouth. Avoidance, lip pursing, tongue rejection, coughing, gagging, and the negative or rejecting reflexes are also present. These individual reflexes are not integrated into what one could call feeding behavior until about 34 weeks gestation. The mouth turns to the nipple as soon as it touches the cheek; the lower lip causes the mouth to open; the tongue makes sucking movements; the nipple is drawn into the mouth and is milked by the stroking movements of the tongue rather than sucking with a negative pressure as an older child will when drinking through a straw. The milk is channeled on either side of the epiglottis and the infant may breathe while sucking. In addition, the protective reflexes that inhibit respiration and cause coughing and spluttering are well developed, should there be any tracheal overspill.

The full-term infant will show ingesting reflexes (e.g., rooting, cardinal points, and sucking reflexes) when aroused or alert through hunger or thirst, as well as rejecting reflexes (e.g., pursing, tongue rejection, coughing, gagging, vomiting in response to asphyxia, drugs, raised intracranial pressure, or a noxious taste). Taste is well developed in the neonate and will increase ingesting reflexes as will hunger, thirst, mild hypoglycaemia (causes hunger drive), mild hypernatraemia (causes thirst drive), or a high state of arousal from any other cause (e.g., drug withdrawal or recovery phase of asphyxia). (Brown, 1969).

In a normal child, by 7 months postnatal these reflexes have become progressively inhibited so that the child does not have to open his or her mouth obligatorily or start sucking once something touches the lower lip: biting is voluntary. Teeth erupt and thus the tongue would be at risk if the primitive sucking pattern of tongue thrust persisted. The mature swallowing pattern develops so that the tongue is kept behind the teeth, pushed against the roof of the mouth when swallowing occurs. By the end of the first year, the child can bite and chew voluntarily, has inhibited all the primitive reflexes, and has a mature swallowing pattern with no overspill or physiologic gastroesophageal reflux.

Miscellaneous brainstem reflexes. The third group of reflexes consists of a mixed bag. The jaw jerk is a simple monosynaptic reflex through the temporalis and masseter muscles in which tapping the semiopened jaw results in a brisk contraction or, if the reflex is uninhibited, jaw clonus. In severely brain-damaged children with brainstem release, tapping the facial muscles (e.g., the lips) causes reflex pursing due to tonic contraction. Several other reflexes exist (Bosma, 1973): (1) grimacing in response to a bad taste (gustato facial reflex); (2) salivation in response to a particular taste such as lemon juice; (3) the tongue tip may rise when the mouth is passively opened due to a stretch reflex through the pterygoid muscles; (4) pressure on the nose causes the mouth to open, sucking movements, doggy paddling of the upper limbs, and neck retraction (snout reflex); and (5) the tongue will deviate toward a unilateral stimulus whether tactile or chemical.

LOWER MOTOR NEURON BULBAR PALSIES

In this article we are going to include in the lower motor neuron the various motor nuclei in the medulla, the cranial nerves, and the bulbar muscles themselves. Dysarthria may result from a lesion in any one site, i.e., in the muscle itself, the neuromuscular junction, the cranial nerve, or its nucleus in the brainstem. The pattern of neurologic abnormality and the effect on speech will vary according to the site of the lesion. It will cause the least trouble with speech when one isolated cranial nerve not intimately involved in articulation such as facial nerves is involved. Dysarthria or even anarthria will be most profound in bilateral lesions of the brainstem itself, a true flaccid bulbar palsy. The types of lesion that result in dysarthria can be categorized as either congenital or acquired. The acquired group can be subdivided further into progressive and nonprogressive (Table 5-4).

Table 5-4
Causes of a Lower Motor Neurone, Hypotonic, True Bulbar Palsy

Myopathic
  Infant of mother with dystrophia   Oculopharyngeal dystrophy
    myotonica
  Nemaline myopathy   Central core disease
  Myotubular myopathy   Whistling face syndrome

Neuromuscular Junction
  Neonatal myasthenia gravis   Botulism
  Congenital myasthenia gravis   Diphtheria
  Juvenile myasthenia gravis

Peripheral nerve
  Polyneuritis cranialis   Juvenile Paget's disease
  Leukemia   Osteopetrosis
  Sarcoidosis   Glomus jugular tumors
  Nasopharyngeal tumors

Anterior horn cells
  Werdnig-Hoffman disease   Pontine glioma
  Fazio–Londe syndrome   Rhombencephalitis
  von Laere syndrome   Dandy–Walker malformation
  Motor neuron disease   Birth injury (vertebral artery,
  Porphyria   postfossa hemorrhage)
  Neonatal asphyxia   Head injury
  Brainstem dysplasias   Syringobulbia
  Mobius' syndrome   Basilar, AVM, embolus, aneurysm

Metabolic diseases
  Malignant hyperphenylalaninemia   Nonketotic hyperglycinemia
  Proprionic acidemia   Zellwegger syndrome
  Leigh's encephalopathy   Infantile Gaucher's disease
  Hypersarcosinemia

Disorders of Muscle Causing Dysarthria in Children

The bulbar muscles may be very severely affected in the congenital form of dystrophia myotonica (Fig. 5-3). It is always the mother and not the father who has the disease, which often has not been diagnosed at the time of birth and may not be diagnosed for many years unless one is aware of the possibility of the condition. The diagnosis rests upon electromyographic study of the small muscles of the hand in the mother, looking for the classical myotonia. The infant presents as a floppy baby who may

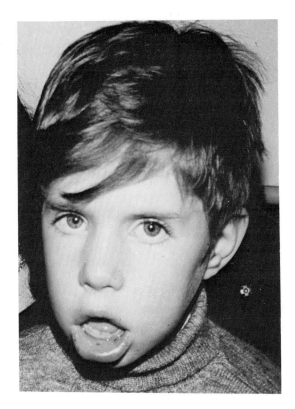

Fig. 5-3. Classical droopy facies in a child with dystrophia myotonica.

have evidence of deformity of the feet or hips as a result of immobility in utero. There is droopy face and a complete bulbar paresis, and the infant may not be able to suck or swallow for many months after birth, thus requiring tube feeding.

The bulbar muscles are not usually affected in the progressive form of Duchenne muscular dystrophy, the severe form of muscular dystrophy affecting boys. Some difficulty swallowing and some pseudohypertrophy of the tongue may be seen in advanced cases but it is rare that speech or swallowing are significantly affected. In the fascio–scapulae humoral type of muscular dystrophy the face is markedly affected, droopy, expressionless, and the child cannot purse the lips or whistle. There is also a rare form of ocular pharyngeal muscular dystrophy that is not usually seen in childhood but causes progressive deterioration in speech with a neuromuscular dysarthria in the adolescent and older patient. The so-called whistling face syndrome may also be associated with facial muscle involvement, a nonprogressive or slowly progressive myopathy.

Disorders of the Neuromuscular Junction

The neuromuscular junction is classically affected in myasthenia gravis. This may be congenital when the baby gets a transient form of muscle weakness that is thought to be due to passage of the antiacetylcholine receptor antibodies across the placenta. There is a more persistent infantile form but the usual type is the onset in childhood of what may be an insidious disorder or a relatively acute one following an infection. Abnormal eye movements or drooping of the eyelids is common. The palate, swallowing, and respiration may be involved early in the course of the disease. The weakness need not be symmetrical and one eye may be affected with drooping of the eyelid, squint, and abnormal eye movements; one side of the palate may be affected with deviation of the tongue suggesting a more central lesion. The whole picture rapidly reverts to normal after injection of intravenous edrophonium. A condition that may mimic myasthenia can follow infection, and some children appear to get a type of bulbar polyneuritis that may result in a similar picture lasting several months. Neuromuscular junction is also affected by toxins such as *botulinum,* and both botulism and diphtheria may present with deterioration in speech, palatal paralysis, and a bulbar palsy as a result of neurotoxins produced by the organism.

Cranial Nerve Lesions

The muscular disorders described previously tend to affect muscles equally on both sides and therefore resemble the central bulbar types of bulbar palsy. The same applies to the toxic bulbar palsies (e.g., diphtheria or botulism) when the circulating toxin will affect the palatal and pharyngeal muscles symmetrically. Lesions of cranial nerves tend to produce a much more discreet, easily identifiable type of lesion.

Seventh, facial nerve lesion

Facial palsy is not uncommon in children. It may be of the idiopathic type due to a virus infection, e.g., Bell's palsy. This is only rarely due to a recognized virus such as mumps virus. It is seen bilaterally in disorders such as sarcoidosis and polyneuritis cranialis, an allergic polyneuritis secondary to infection (e.g., Epstein–Barr virus). Facial nerve palsy may also be the presenting feature of leukemia or hypertension in children and thus should be taken seriously and investigated. Infection of the geniculate ganglion with herpes is not as commonly seen in children as adults. The face is affected in the upper and lower halves; the child cannot wrinkle the forehead or close the eye properly. There is a risk of exposure keratitis, the cheek tends to blow in and out with respiration, and saliva may drip from the corner of the mouth. Food tends to lodge between the gum and the cheek, and there is difficulty with lip movement so that bilabial sounds such as *p* and *b* are selectively affected with a *labial dysarthria*.

Tenth, Vagus Nerve Lesions

In unilateral lesions of the vagus nerve the child has difficulty clearing mucous and saliva from the throat, which may be frothy due to a mixture with air. There is difficulty with coughing and clearing the throat and there may be overspill into the trachea. The palatal arch droops on the side of the lesion and the uvula deviates to normal side upon saying *ah*. The inability to elevate the palate results in nasal escape, hypernasality, and difficulty with palatal sounds such as *k* and *g*, i.e., a *palatal dysarthria*.

Recurrent Laryngeal Nerve Lesion

The recurrent laryngeal nerve may be injured during neck surgery, e.g., during surgery on the thyroid gland or for removal of a cystic hygroma. It may be injured in chest surgery, being especially vulnerable on the left side where it runs around the aortic arch. It can be trapped in supurating lymph nodes or tumor. Lesions of the recurrent laryngeal nerve cause paralysis of the abductor muscles of the larynx (Semon's law), which results in the vocal cord on the affected side moving toward the midline. Hoarseness, dysphonia, and stridor then occur. As the palsy becomes complete the cord becomes situated in the so-called cadaveric or half abducted position. If the lesion is unilateral the opposite cord will gradually manage to oppose the paralyzed cord so that the hoarseness will disappear, but if the paresis is bilateral aphonia may be permanent and severe respiratory obstruction can occur. Loss of volume of voice is also a usual accompaniment of recurrent laryngeal nerve lesion.

Twelfth Hypoglossal, Nerve Lesion

The hypoglossal forms the main motor nerve supply to the muscles of the tongue. A unilateral lesion results in the tongue wasting with coarse fasciculation movements (Fig. 5-4). The genioglossus muscle normally pulls the root of the tongue forward and enables the tip of the tongue to be protruded in the midline. If there is a unilateral hypoglossal nerve lesion then the tongue will deviate to the paralyzed side, i.e., the side of the lesion. There will be difficulties with such sounds as *d* and *l* and hence this has been described as a *lingual dysarthria*. Hypoglossal nerve lesions are uncommon in children and are usually seen as a result of lesions of the hypoglossal nucleus rather than a peripheral nerve itself. Isolated

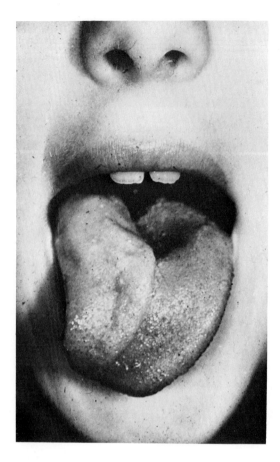

Fig. 5-4. Wasting of the tongue in hypoglossal nerve lesion.

lesions may be seen, e.g., after trauma to the tonsillar fossa caused by the child falling with an object in his or her mouth.

Jugular Foramen Lesions

Three cranial nerves, the glossopharyngeal (ninth), the vagus (tenth), and the spinal accessory nerves leave the base of the skull through the jugular foramen. They are particularly vulnerable at this point and thus a so-called jugular foramen syndrome may arise. The difficulty in diagnosing nasopharyngeal tumors, which tend to infiltrate upward into the base of the skull, has already been stressed. Other malignancies such as leukemia in children may present with meningeal infiltration, neuroblastoma may present with metastasis into the base of the skull, and sarcoidosis may also cause strangulation neuropathies. One can also get a tumor within the jugular foramen i.e., a glomus jugular tumor. The result is a unilateral lesion affecting palate, pharynx, and larynx. The lower cranial nerves have functions other than simply supplying the muscles of articulation and are involved in (1) the sensation from lips, tongue, and palate; (2) the sense of taste; (3) the secretion of saliva; (4) biting; and (5) chewing. These functions will be considered in more detail in the following section of this chapter.

Disorders of the Brainstem

True bulbar palsy

In lesions of the pons or medulla (i.e., the bulb) in which the nuclei supplying the bulbar musculature are primarily involved, there will be a lower motor neuron paralysis with resultant weakness, wasting, fasciculation and a complete absence of monosynaptic, primitive, and protective reflexes. The clinical presentation of a flaccid bulbar palsy is that the child has a lax open mouth with no nasolabial creases, i.e., a droopy, sad-looking face (Fig. 5-5). There is drooling. The lower lip is often everted and saliva runs over the everted lip. Biting and chewing will be difficult if the masticatory muscles are involved. Tongue will be wasted with fasciculation in severe cases. The child is unable to swallow saliva or food and there will be a complete aphagia. Laryngeal protective reflexes are lost and overspill into the chest with repeated chest infections together with the risk of aspiration and death is ever present. In severe cases anarthria would be the rule with difficulties in phonation, respiration, and articulation. Tube feeding or a gastrostomy will be required to aid feeding. A tracheotomy will be required to maintain the airway and an alternative communication system to overcome the anarthria. In milder cases there will be dysphagia with a slurred dysarthria, and food will tend to come down the nose and regurgitate up into the nasopharynx. The voice will lack power and will be forced, monotonous, and breathy. There will be no cough reflex, gag reflex, or jaw jerk, and the palate will not move on saying *ah*. There will be marked nasal escape.

The causes of true bulbar palsy in childhood are shown in Table 5-4. Many of these are progressive so that the child will progress from a mild dysarthria to total anarthria and aphagia. The nerve cells of the motor nuclei may be selectively involved in a similar way to the progressive bulbar palsy that is seen in motor neuron disease in the adult. The acute infantile form of anterior horn cell degeneration (Werdnig–Hoffman's disease) is associated with wasting and fasciculation of the tongue, progressive bulbar involvement, and death, usually as a result of respiratory

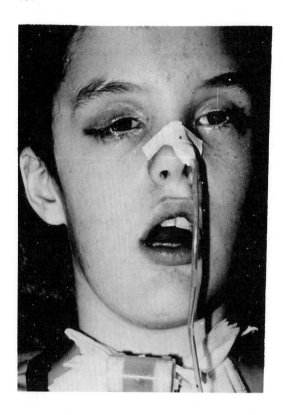

Fig. 5-5. Complete bulbar palsy with ophthalmoplegia bulbar palsy that includes aphagia and bilateral vocal cord paresis.

failure and pneumonia. The later-onset anterior horn cell degenerative diseases such as type II spinal muscular atrophy of Kugelberg–Welander disease do not usually affect the motor neurones of the brain stem nuclei. There are, however, familial progressive diseases such as von Laere syndrome and the Fazio–Londe syndrome, both of which are associated with progressive wasting and weakness of the bulbar muscles from degeneration of the corresponding nuclei. (Gomez, Clermont, & Bernstein, 1962) The anterior horn cells in the medulla that form the cranial nerve nuclei may be involved in bulbar polio myelitis or acute intermittent porphyria. There is an odd condition of Rhombencephalitis occasionally seen in association with mumps virus when there may be extensive inflammatory damage. The not uncommon tumour of childhood of pontine glioma usually presents either with isolated cranial nerve lesions or a progressive dysarthria and bulbar palsy (Fig. 5-6).

There may be congenital dysplasia of the brainstem and the baby may be born with a complete bulbar palsy that never recovers so that oral feeding is impossible as there is continuous overspill into the trachea, and bronchi or permanent anarthria would then be the rule. In addition, these children are often mentally retarded. A more restricted form of

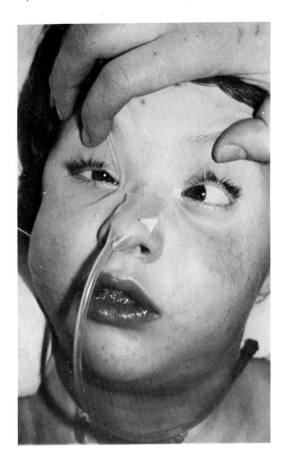

Fig. 5-6. Total bulbar palsy and ophthalmoplegia secondary to a pontine glioma.

dysplasia of the brainstem nuclei seen in the Mobius syndrome, which usually affects the sixth and seventh nerves so that there is facial paralysis and paralysis of abduction of the eyes (Fig. 5-7). Occasionally in the extended Mobius syndrome (Meyerson, 1978), however, there may be involvement of the palate or even of the limbs, causing associated conditions such as talipes. Vascular lesions of the brainstem are less common than in adults. Secondary brainstem hemorrhages occur following a head injury or raised intracranial pressure from any cause. Emboli into the vertebral–Basilar system may occur in children with congenital heart disease. Hemorrhage may occur into the cerebellum and brainstem from a microvascular malformation. Other than the congenital dysplasias and the Mobius syndrome, most of the conditions discussed are progressive diseases; onset of a hypotonic true bulbar palsy in childhood will usually be associated with progressive deterioration in speech and feeding and is always a mandatory indication for full neurologic investigation. There

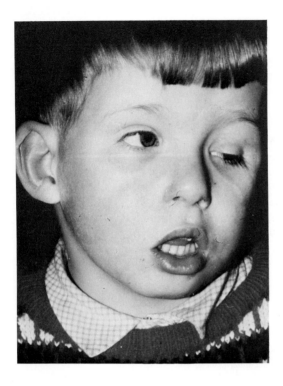

Fig. 5-7. Mobius syndrome.

are exceptions in that it is possible for the baby to be born with what appears to be a very severe bulbar palsy and yet make a surprising recovery. The infant of the mother with dystrophia myotonica was discussed previously. The child with Prader–Willi syndrome may have profound generalized hypotonia, poverty of movement, a mask-like face with no emotional responses, and a total bulbar palsy with no gag or cough reflexes, total inability to feed, and necessity to tube feeding for many weeks or even months. This may gradually improve, however, so that one is worried by the time the child is 2 or 3 years old about overeating and obesity, which may then complicate the picture. These children often speak slowly, with a developmental speech problem later rather than persisting with a lower motor neuron bulbar paresis.

Another odd form of congenital bulbar palsy is seen in Pfeiffer's syndrome in which large thumbs and toes are associated with bulbar difficulties from birth and a severe dysarthria that persists through life. Apart from those diseases that select only the neurons of the brainstem nuclei, it is more likely that in structural diseases such as encephalitis, tumor, and infarcts, an area of brainstem will be destroyed and so a more mixed picture results with abnormal eye movements, hearing deficits, sensory problems, and a combination of lower motor neuron, upper motor neuron, and cranial nerve abnormalities. Some of these give rise to defined syndromes: Avelli's syndrome, Schmidt's syndrome, Jackson's syndrome, Tapia's Syndrome, Bonnier's Syndrome, and Wallenberg's syndrome. These are well described in adults, but the rarity of discreet vascular lesions of the brainstem in children makes these less important; identical syndromes, however, will be seen in children with Rhombencephalitis or pontine glioma. Avelli's syndrome is caused by a lesion of the nucleus ambiguous, tractus solitarus, and the adjacent spinothalamic tract so that there is paralysis of the soft palate, pharynx, and larynx on the same side of the lesion with resultant dysarthria, dysphagia, and anesthesia of the pharynx and larynx. It is associated with loss of pain and temperature on the opposite side of the body. Jackson's syndrome is when the 10th, 11th, and 12th nuclei are affected together, which causes paralysis of the muscles that elevate the shoulder (i.e., trapezius and the sternomastoid) as well as paralysis and wasting of the tongue on the same side. The importance of grouping these signs together is that it indicates that the lesion must be in the brainstem and is not a result of a lesion in the peripheral nerve.

Pseudobulbar palsy in Children

The primitive brainstem reflexes and simple preprogrammed behavioral responses that have been discussed are normally inhibited by a variety of pathways coming from higher parts of the brain. Feeding, behavior, and respiratory control all have override from higher centers. In a pseudobulbar palsy, these higher pathways are disrupted but the lower motor neuron is left intact along with the brainstem reflexes. Thus the protective reflexes such as cough and gag are preserved so that the risk of aspiration in the bronchial tree and death from airways obstruction is far less than with the true bulbar palsy. Pharyngeal reflexes are normal and oral feeding is usually possible. The muscles of mastication are spastic so that they show increased resistance to stretch and increased reflexes, hence the jaw jerk is brisk and jaw clonus is common. The jaw does not open fully, and the tongue is small and bunched. In several cases there will be obicularis oris spasticity and dermatone to myotone responses with oral pursing, as already described. Biting, chewing, and swallowing solids are difficult, although spoon feeding with a semifluid diet will usually be feasible.

It is important to note that all muscles, other than those of the lower face, have bilateral representation in the cerebral cortex and thus unilateral lesions of the cerebral cortex result only in paralysis of the lower face. (The face can move unilaterally under voluntary control, but the palate cannot move unilaterally.) Bulbar palsy is not seen in association with an uncomplicated cortical hemiplegia. (A combined Hemiplegia and

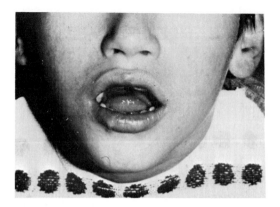

Fig. 5-8. Bulbar palsy with facial involvement and drooling in a child with cerebral palsy secondary to intrapartum asphyxia.

bulbar palsy may be seen as a result of perinatal asphyxia, but this is due to two lesions, one in the cortex and one in the brainstem.) The tongue also has bilateral representation, but there seems to be slightly stronger lateralization so that after an acute unilateral lesion of the cerebral cortex the tongue will deviate, but this is nearly always transitory and recovers. There is no wasting of the muscles and no fasciculation; the tone is increased as opposed to the decrease in the lower motor neuron lesion. Drooling is a frequent and distressing symptom (Worster-Drought, 1968).

Speech is slow and labored with little variation in pitch. It is hypernasal, the voice is harsh, and the rhythm may be explosive. Pronounciation of consonants is imprecise, slurred, and inconsistent. (Farmer & Lenicione, 1977) Emphasis is absent or applied incorrectly, and the child finds it difficult to control breathing, thus interfering with normal phrasing (Darley, 1975; Rosenbeck & LaPointe, 1978).

Causes of a psuedobulbar palsy.

The more learning involved in any movement, the more lateralized it is. Hand manipulative skills and speech, therefore, are strongly lateralized and are affected by unilateral cerebral hemisphere lesions while walking, trunk control, feeding, biting, chewing, and swallowing are bilaterally represented. Spastic dysarthria, therefore, is more likely to be seen in children with a double hemiplegia or a tetraplegic cerebral palsy (Fig. 5-8), or in the very severe form of diplegia of prematurity (Ingram, 1961) Hypoxic ischemic encephalopathy usually due to intrapartum asphyxia in the newborn period is by far the most common cause although severe anoxic brain damage may result at any time in the same clinical picture. Disseminated sclerosis, which is a common cause of pseudobulbar palsy and dysarthria in adolescents and young adults, is not common in prepubertal children. Brainstem ischemia with infarction from embolization in association with congenital heart disease can also result in a pseudobulbar palsy or, as discussed earlier, a true bulbar palsy. Degenerative brain diseases not uncommonly present with dysarthria in a spastic bulbar palsy, especially in conditions such as subacute sclerosing encephalitis, metachromatic leukodystrophy, Alexander's disease, Batten's disease, or the adolescent form of GM2 gangliosidosis. The onset of a dysarthria in children in association with a pseudobulbar palsy and jaw spasticity has the same implications for investigation as other forms of bulbar palsy. Children who have sustained head injuries with raised intracranial pressure and a midbrain or upper brainstem shearing injury (as a result of a deceleration/acceleration type of injury) may have a severe dysarthria, which is made worse if there has been secondary brainstem hemorrhage due to tentorial herniation (Fig. 5-9). Although the dysarthria is often extremely severe in children after head injury, recovery is usually surprisingly good.

There is an unusual form of psuedobulbar palsy that presents in the neonatal period with feeding difficulties and then appears to recover. This is followed by a delay in speech development with a dysarthria that is accompanied by drooling, poor fast tongue movements, poor palatal movements, and a very brisk jaw jerk. By this time (3–4 years of age), however, there are few feeding difficulties. This occurs in isolation without any obvious pyramidal involvement or spasticity in any other muscles (e.g., arms and legs). It must be differentiated from bulbar palsy secondary to perinatal asphyxia and is often known as the Worster-Drought syndrome and is thought to be a developmental, probably genetically determined condition.

Spastic Dysarthria and Cerebral Palsy

The commonest type of pseudobulbar palsy seen in childhood is that associated with the various spastic forms of cerebral palsy in which 20–40 percent may have no speech at all. The brainstem of the newborn infant is particularly susceptible to hypoxia so that perinatal asphyxia is likely to be associated with spastic types of cerebral palsy associated with dysarthria. Most other forms of spastic cerebral palsy will be associated with extensive bilateral lesions of the cerebral hemispheres. This may be the result of intracerebral hemorrhage as with massive intraventricular hemorrhage of the low-birth-weight infant, or it may be due to factors before birth such as infection with cytomegalovirus during pregnancy or the various genetic syndromes associated, in particular, with microcephaly and cortical dysplasia.

Cerebral palsy, in the past, has tended to be treated as a disease entity. In fact, cerebral palsy is simply the name given to the motor

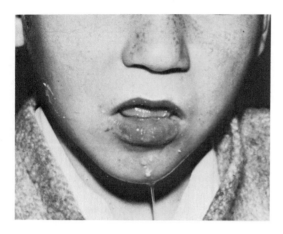

Fig. 5-9. Isolated pseudo-bulbar paresis without gross motor involvement of the limbs.

manifestations of nonprogressive brain damage sustained during the phase of active brain growth. This means that the picture changes as the brain develops even though the pathology is static. Furthermore, because the child is brain damaged, associated problems such as mental handicap, perceptual problems, specific cognitive defects, epilepsy, organic behavior problems, and learning difficulties will occur. These are not necessarily complications of the cerebral palsy but rather complications of the same pathology that caused the cerebral palsy. Most children with bilateral spasticity will also be profoundly mentally retarded. Children with the encephalopathy of low birth weight have spasticity involving primarily the lower limbs with relative preservation of intelligence, and they have reasonable language development but can suffer from a spastic dysarthria. Cerebral palsy is a common condition in childhood; many speech therapists may spend their entire professional career seeing only children suffering from cerebral palsy, and one must try to avoid a very narrow view of causes and types of dysarthria in childhood (Ingram, 1961).

EXTRAPYRAMIDAL BULBAR PALSY

The problems in the severely dysarthric child with an extrapyramidal cerebral palsy who is locked in but with normal intelligence has continued to be one of the greatest clinical challenges. In Malaysia where glucose 6 phosphate dehydrogenase deficiency is a major cause of jaundice in the newborn, kernicterus is extremely common and schools are full of children with choreoathetosis, severe dysarthria, and varying degrees of deafness. In the Western World where this condition is less

Table 5-5
Clinical Classification of Dyskinesias in Children

Hyperkinetic Dyskinesias	Chorea
	Tic
	Hemiballismus
	Orofacial
Hypokinetic	Parkinsonian syndrome
Rigidities	Flexor
	Extensor
	Hemiplegic
	Fluctuant (athetosis)

Dyskinesias are further classified according to their type of presentation; acute dyskinesia, chronic non-progressive dyskinesia (cerebral palsy), or chronic progressive dyskinesia.

common and where the major causes of kernicterus such as rhesus isoimmunization and prematurity have been conquered, dyskinetic cerebral palsy now forms only a very small percentage of the total number of cerebral palsy children. Improvements in our knowledge of neurochemistry has led us to more satisfactory classification and understanding of the dyskinesias of childhood. More careful investigations of children with various types of dyskinesia, avoiding the obvious label of dyskinetic cerebral palsy, has produced a very wide differential diagnosis (Table 5-5).

Hypokinetic Dyskinesia

Hypokinetic dyskinesia is identical to the syndrome of parkinsonism seen in the adult and is due to a low dopamine production by the substantia nigra or blocking of dopamine receptors in the basal ganglia. It is a rare form of dyskinesia in children but may occur as a progressive familial pallidonigral degeneration (Hunt's disease), and it has been suggested that familial cases could be due to a block in the biosynthesis of dopamine. Involuntary movements with a dyskinesia are seen in phenylketonuria due to the secondary deficiency in tyrosine, and this can be lessened by the administration of L-dopa. Drug-induced parkinsonism can occur at any age and postencephalitic parkinsonism was common in children in the days of epidemic encephalitis lethargica. Subacute encephalitis such as that seen with measles may present with a parkinsonian picture. Batten's disease, one of the degenerative diseases, can also present at puberty with a picture of parkinsonism appearing in a blind child. The clinical picture consists of three components: tremor, bradykinesia, and flexor rigidity. The component most obviously affecting speech is the difficulty in starting and stopping a movement, combined with slowness in movement (bradykinesia), so that speech is slow, the voice is of low amplitude, there is difficulty in starting, and once started the speech may come faster and faster, i.e., festination in speech (Darley, 1975). The voice is a monotone and all prosodic features in speech may be lost. In very severe cases the bradykinesia may amount to akinesia so that the patient cannot initiate any movement at all although not paralyzed. The facial movements are affected so that the impression is often one of misery, sadness, or totally impassive. The child may not be able to respond quick enough to shake hands when someone offers theirs, the arms do not swing, and there is no spring in the gait. It is therefore easy to misinterpret emotional states of the child since he or she may appear unduly sad and withdrawn. This contrasts with the hyperkinetic dyskinesias where inappropriate emotion and risus may make the child appear bright and sociable, but again this may be an apparent emotion and may not mirror the true feelings of the person.

Hyperkinetic Dyskinesia

Whereas the hypokinetic dyskinesias are due to deficiency in dopamine with the basal ganglia of the brain, the hyperkinetic dyskinesias are due to excess dopamine. They may again be chronic and static, chronic and progressive, or acute in onset (Table 5-6). The typical abnormality is a random sudden contraction of a muscle group as in the choreas, hemiballismus, stereotypies, tics, and orofacial dyskinesias (Brown, 1984). The movements disappear in sleep and differentiation of the different types is not as easy as standard textbooks would have us believe. The simple repetetive tic, common in normal children, is easy to define. Some of the wild, flinging movements of the convulsive tics, however, may resemble hemiballismus. Videotapes of children suffering from the multiple tic syndrome (Gilles de la Tourette) may be very difficult to differentiate from the choreiform movements of kernicterus or the resolving case of Sydenham's chorea.

Clinical features

The child is exactly the opposite to the one suffering from hypokinetic dyskinesia. He or she is restless, fidgety, cannot sit still, jumps up and down, grimaces, shakes the head, grunts, makes clucking noises, and shows irregular respiratory movement. The movements vary from blinking of an eye or shaking of the head to wild flinging movements of the arms and legs so that standing, sitting, walking, feeding, or speaking becomes absolutely impossible. True choreiform movements tend to be jerky, unpredictable, and random, differing from tics in that they have no

Table 5-6

Dyskinesias

Acute dyskinesias in children
  Carbon monoxide poisoning
  Cardiac bypass surgery
  Hemophilus influenza meningitis
  Encephalitis lethargica, mumps encephalitis
  Familial paroxysmal choreoathetosis
  Postdialysis dyskinesia
  Burns encephalopathy, scalds shakes
  Hypernatremic dehydration
  Heavy-metal poisoning—manganese, thallium, etc.
  Drug-induced dyskinesias
  Extrapyramidal epilepsy
  Tumors of the third ventricle
  Convulsive tics
  Gilles de la Tourette's syndrome
  Familial striatal necrosis
  Leigh's encephalopathy
  Intermittent maple syrup urine disease
  Subacute sclerosing panencephalitis
  Sydenham's chorea
  Chorea gravidarum

Chronic nonprogressive dyskinesias (cerebral palsies)
  Asphyxia
  Hyperbilirubinemia
  Familial nonprogressive dyskinesia
  Autosomal recessive nonprogressive dyskinesia
  Familial (dominant) nonprogressive dyskinesia
  Familial striatonigral dysplasias

Chronic progressive dyskinesias of childhood
  Huntington's chorea
  Hallevorden–Spatz disease
  Wilson's disease
  Ataxia telangiectasia
  Fahr's syndrome
  Pelizaeus–Merzbacher disease
  Encephalitis lethargica
  Creutzfeldt–Jakob disease
  Subacute sclerosing panencephalitis
  Striatonigral degeneration (Hunt's, juvenile
    parkinsonism)
  Hunt's pallido/cerebellar degeneration
  Lesch–Nyhan syndrome
  Late infantile or juvenile Leigh's disease
  Glutaric aciduria
  Dystonia musculorum deformans
  Piloid astrocytoma basal ganglia
  Sulfite oxidase deficiency
  Familial striatal necrosis

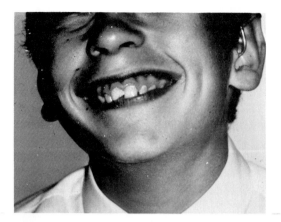

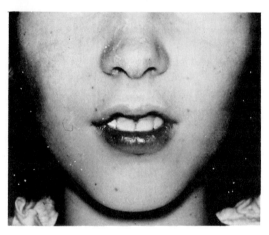

Fig. 5-10. (A) The classical risus, happy smiling facies of a child with hypokinetic dyskinesia. (B) Fixed rigid smile (risus) in a young woman presenting with Wilson's disease.

stereotyped pattern of repetition. The sudden wild flinging of an arm may be made semipurposive by the child pretending to scratch the head or straighten hair. The child may sit on a hand or hold the tongue between the teeth to try and lessen the movement. The face may be drawn up into a grimace with a risus sardonicus so that the child seems happy and constantly smiling (Fig. 5-10). There may be random twitching of the mouth, sudden deviation of the eyes, quivering of the chin, rolling of the tongue, repeated tongue protrusion (Fig. 5-11), sudden mouth opening (Fig. 5-12), titubation of the head, pursing of the lips, and mouthing movements as if the child was speaking. Some of these facial contortions are so grotesque that the child's life is made a misery due to being teased at school. In the Gilles de la Tourette syndrome, the clucking and respiratory noises are further exacerbated by forced utterances that are often copralalic four-letter words. The tongue and facial muscles are in a chronic state of jerking and grimacing so that speech becomes suddenly

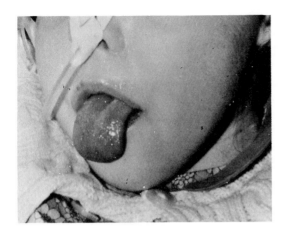

Fig. 5-11. Tongue rolling and protrusion (lingual dyskinesia) in a child with Lennox–Gastaut syndrome.

arrested or mutilated. Dyskinetic cerebral palsy constitutes one type of chronic static hyperkinetic dyskinesia and is usually due to one of two main causes, i.e., intrapartum asphyxia or kernicterus. Children who have suffered intrapartum asphyxia have a more mixed picture with mental handicap, epilepsy combined with spasticity, and a dyskinesia (which typically has a major athetoid/dystonic component).

The purest form of dyskinesia is that seen following jaundice in the newborn as a result of kernicterus. In these children intelligence is well preserved; there may be a high-tone deafness. There is no spasticity, and underneath the involuntary movements the child often has normal voluntary patterns, i.e., there is no dyspraxia. The movements are choreiform in the older child, but dystonia and athetosis are mixed in the younger child. The tragedy of these children is that they may be completely locked in and unable to communicate. Their gross involuntary

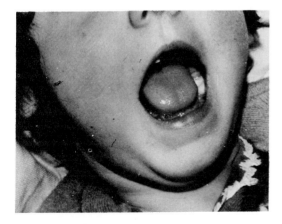

Fig. 5-12. Tonic mouth opening as part of a mass extensor movement in a child with rigid dystonic cerebral palsy.

movements of the hands makes writing, typing, or any use of a structured gesture system such as Paget–Gorman or Makaton impossible. The total disruption of lips, tongue, and palate by involuntary movements makes speech incomprehensible, and these are the children who, par excellence, benefit from an alternative communication system and for whom Blissymbols or some of the modern computer aids are ideal. Fortunately for the children, and unfortunately for the development of alternative communication systems, these children are now in a small minority of cases of cerebral palsy in the western hemisphere. Huntington's chorea in childhood is more likely to be manifested by fits or mental deterioration compared with a simple chorea. Hyperkinetic dyskinesias may be a feature of several other inborn errors of metabolism such as glutaric aciduria, Leigh's encephalopathy, Hallervorden–Spatz syndrome, Wilson's disease, Farr's syndrome, and Lesch–Nyhan syndrome (Table 5-6).

Athetosis

It is common to classify chorea and athetosis together as choreoathetosis. Athetoid movements are slower then choreiform ones and are less random. Because of changes in muscle tone and posture, they represent in essence a flip-flop between different primitive postures, i.e., the avoiding extended posture versus the flexed or forced grasping posture (hemiplegic dystonia) (Denny-Brown, 1966). These children are very stiff babies showing marked extensor hypertonus and retention of all their primitive reflexes, i.e., walking, stepping, and feeding reflexes (Table 5-7). The marked distortions of posture only appear several years later. Both chorea and athetosis are due to basal ganglia disease and, therefore, often coexist. There are several types of dystonia (Fig. 5-13;) flexor dystonia seen in parkinsonism, extensor dystonia, hemiplegic dystonia, and athetosis (a combination of extensor and hemiplegic dystonias). Retention of the primitive reflexes is one of the hallmarks of an extrapyramidal cerebral palsy. The tonic and asymmetrical tonic neck reflexes are obligatory. A severe extensor hypertonus affecting the neck trunk together with the upper and lower limbs is released if the child is placed flat on his or her back in contact with a firm surface. If the child is suspended under the armpits and his head allowed to extend, rigid extension of the legs and arching of the back will occur again. Any change in the relationship of the head to the body either by flexion/extension, or by turning the head to the right or the left, will enhance this pattern of muscle tone. Pressure over the snout or perineum will also cause the child to go into rigid extension and will stimulate doggy-paddling movements of the arms whilst the legs tend to remain rigidly extended.

The mouth will open in a tonic fashion if the grasp reflexes in the hands are elicited and then traction applied to them (Palmomental re-

Table 5-7
Types of Primitive Reflexes Seen in Children with Dyskinetic Cerebral Palsy

Feeding reflexes
  Avoiding
    Facial avoidance
    Pursing lip rejection
    Tongue rejection
    Tongue rolling
    Gag reflex
    Vomiting
    Tonic mouth opening
    Spastic bite
  Ingesting
    Rooting reflex
    Cardinal points reflex
    Tongue furling
    Sucking
    Swallowing
    Cricopharyngeal relaxation

Progression reflexes
  Walking/cycling
  Stepping
  Positive supporting
  Crossed extensor
  Crawling reflex
  Bauer response
Primitive postural reflexes
  Asymmetrical tonic neck reflex
  Tonic neck reflex
  Trunk incurvation reflex
  Snout reflex

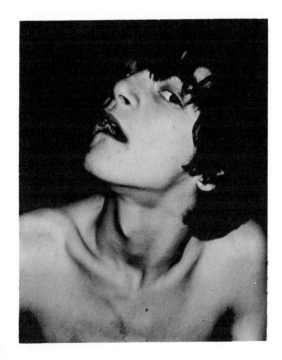

Fig. 5-13. Torticollis due to muscle rigidity in a boy with a positive family history of the same condition and presenting with severe dysarthria.

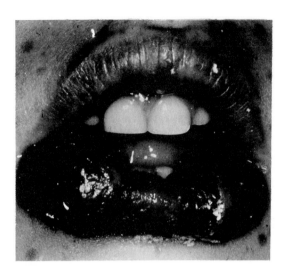

Fig. 5-14. Self mutilation in a case of Lesch–Nyhan syndrome.

flex). If the lower lip is stroked with a firm object and then pressure applied, the cardinal points reflex is elicited in which there is opening of the mouth, extension of the neck, and a rhythmic rolling movement of the tongue. This is ineffective from the point of view of feeding, since the movements merely push the food off the spoon. Metal spoons are more likely to trigger reflexogenic zones, causing either a bite reflex or tonic mouth opening and rhythmic sucking with tongue thrust. It can be seen, therefore, that the position of the child in space, the relationship of the head to the body, and trigger zones around the mouth may all cause an increase in muscle tone, which would then inhibit speech and feeding. Any pressure over the region of the trigeminal nerve distribution to the face, especially pressure over the nose, may not only cause tonic mouth opening but will also cause neck retraction and the upper limbs to go into rigid extension with doggy paddling movements of the outstretched arms. Even if the position of the body and head is adjusted to minimize the amount of tone in the bulbar muscles, stimulation of bulbar proprioception may change the whole pattern of body tone so that the child arches out of the chair or goes into opisthotonos. In some cases (e.g., Lesch Nyhan syndrome) self-mutilation may further compound the clinical picture (Fig. 5-14).

The child suffering from the classical type of extrapyramidal bulbar palsy will show retention of all the baby feeding reflexes (rooting, sucking, lip reflexes). There will be a tendency for mass movements to produce tonic contraction of the bulbar muscles, particularly causing mouth opening. There is no weakness or wasting of any muscle group. The muscles are not weak as can be shown by the power of the involuntary movements or dystonic movements. Protective reflexes are present and thus oral feeding is usually possible without any tracheal overspill. The child may be able to bite, and even in the presence of marked choreiform movements and severe dysarthria, may be able to chew. Voice shows variation in pitch and at times may sound rather high pitched with variation in the loudness. The speech is slow or explosive. The rhythm is disrupted by the choreiform movements and tic-like movements of lip, tongue, and palate.

In relatively mild cases there is a gross dysarthria as shown by change in voice, intonation, imprecise articulation of consonants, and disrupted rhythm. There also may be difficulties of the later-acquired consonants. Children with high-tone deafness and mental handicap will have additional language problems that may prevent the development of any speech at all. In severe cases of dyskinesia the child may be of normal intelligence but completely anarthric. Feeding may be extremely messy, but oral feeding is safe and possible in the majority of children due to the normal protective reflexes.

Ataxic Dysarthria

It is thought that in the adult the cerebellum is concerned predominantly with coordination and that in disease states adults present with the classical symptoms of nystagmus, dysarthria, intention tremor and dysmetria, and an ataxic gait. Speech is explosive, staccato, and slurred. The cerebellum is a major subcortical computer center that adjusts the speed, force, and direction of any movement that is planned by the cerebral cortex, and it is an integral part of the motor learning circuit. It is usual to divide ataxic diseases in children into truncal ataxia (which consists of a floppy baby syndrome associated with slowness in sitting, crawling, walking, and balance reactions) and a volitional ataxia (incoordination of speech, gaze, and hand manipulation). Nystagmus (incoordination of voluntary gaze) is not seen in congenital ataxia and is always a sign of an acquired ataxia. Speech development in congenital ataxia is more likely to show a developmental pattern, i.e., slow motor learning of the engrams required for the positioning of lips, tongue, and palate and the sequencing of these into words (i.e., a form of articulatory dyspraxia rather than staccato explosive and dysrhythmic speech). Acquired cerebellar disease, on the other hand, is more likely to show the trio of nystagmus, true dysarthria, and limb incoordination. Severe forms of congenital ataxia, however, will be associated with intention tremor and dysmetria as well as with difficulty in learning hand skills. Clinically ataxic children are hypotonic; the mouth tends to be kept open and drools. They may be misdiagnosed as having a flaccid bulbar palsy. The protective reflexes, however, are normal as is the swallowing pattern, and the child can usually eat solids, bite, and chew without any choking, regurgitation, or aspiration. The primitive reflexes are inhibited unlike the child with the extrapyramidal type of bulbar paresis. The jaw is often lax and there is no spasticity. The tongue may appear flat and large rather than the small, bunched spastic tongue.

The causes of ataxia are shown in Table 5-8 and 5-9. Congenital ataxia is more likely to be genetic in origin and may be associated with malformations of the cerebellum such as agenesis, hypoplasia, or vermis aplasia. It may also be complicated by mental retardation or deafness. Children with congenital hydrocephalus often show an ataxic syndrome as may children who have suffered from intrapartum asphyxia. Hypothyroidism is also complicated by long-term ataxic syndromes if there has been delay in diagnosis. There are many causes of acquired ataxia, most of which have a sinister prognosis, e.g., the posterior fossa tumors such as medelloblastoma, cerebellar astrocytoma, or haemangioblastoma, the various degenerative diseases such as Friedreich's ataxia or ataxia-telangiectasia, and the degenerative diseases such as metachromatic leukodystrophy.

Cortical Dysarthria

A major cause of confusion and disagreement among different professionals is the use of synonyms (Martin, 1974). This is easily appreciated if one considers the term cortical dysarthria, which is used synonymously with articulatory dyspraxia, speech dyspraxia, dyspraxic dysarthria, Broca's ephymia, speech–sound muteness, aphasic anarthria, syndrome with phonetic disintegration in aphasia, phonetic paraphasia, apraxia of vocal expression, and literal aphasia (Blair & Jones, 1983; Chappell, 1973). By definition, if a speech disorder is of cortical origin then it involves learning, and since it is a specialized type of learning we would expect it to be a lateralized cortical function. As discussed previously, the bulbar muscles have bilateral cortical representation from the point of view of feeding, for example, so that if the cerebral cortex is intact on one side only this is sufficient to inhibit brainstem reflexes and spasticity and to allow normal feeding. In cortical dysarthria due to a unilateral cortical lesion, one expects no anatomical or neurologic abnormality of bulbar function; i.e., the protective reflexes (cough, sneeze, gag, vomit) will be completely normal. The airways are protected. There is no regurgitation or risk of aspiration into the bronchial tree. Bite and chew are completely normal. There is no wasting, weakness, fasciculation, spasticity, or hypotonia of the bulbar muscles. The primitive reflexes are inhibited. The only abnormality seen on examination is variable nasal escape during consecutive speech as well as difficulty in performing alternating movement patterns such as putting the tongue in different positions (Table 5-10. In the pure form of cortical dysarthria, hearing, comprehension, auditory discrimination, and inner language will also be normal.

Table 5-8
Causes of Chronic Progressive Ataxia in Childhood

Friedreich's ataxia
Marie's ataxia
Olivo–Ponto cerebellar degeneration
Fazio–Londe syndrome
Hunt's cerebellar degeneration with myoclonus
Leigh's encephalopathy
Pyruvate dehydrogenase deficiency
Lipoamide deficiency
Abetalipoproteinemia
Metachromatic leukodystrophy
Late infantile Batten's disease
Adult type GM1 gangliosidosis
Type 3 GM2 gangliosidosis
Menke's cerebral and cerebellar degeneration
Dejerine–Sottas proprioceptive ataxia
Roussy–Levi syndrome
Refsum's syndrome
Pelizaeus–Merzbacher syndrome
Central pontine myelinosis
von Hippel–Lindau syndrome with hemangioblastoma
Ataxia telangiectasia
Progressive neuraxonal dystrophy with spheroids
Juvenile tabes dorsalis
Lennox–Gastaut syndrome

Neuroanatomical basis of Cortical Dysarthria

The brain at birth weighs around 350 g and by 4 years of age has added an additional 1000 g. Growth of the cerebellum is slow compared with the growth of other parts of the brain so that motor skills always lag behind sensory skills and comprehension. Speech is one of the most sophisticated motor skills in a normal 2- or 3-year-old child. The brain develops more slowly in the male, in whom all developmental disorders are up to five times more common than in the female. Males also appear to show slow maturation of the dominant left hemisphere; this is even more apparent in chromosome disorders (e.g., XYY syndrome). Conversely, females (e.g., with Turner's syndrome) show gross developmental delay in normal right hemisphere function (visuospatial problems). Even genetically determined disorders of speech will be more apparent in the male members of the family.

The motor learning involved in speech development involves not only motor areas of the brain such as the cortical speech area of Broca but also the circuits to the cerebellum and the basal ganglia. A developmen-

Table 5-9
Causes of Chronic Nonprogressive Ataxia in Childhood (Cerebral Palsies)

Genetic
  Biemond's syndrome, short 3rd and 4th metacarpals, proprioceptive ataxia,
    and nystagmus (autosomal dominant)
  Flynn–Aird syndrome—ataxia, cataracts, deaf, epilepsy, dementia, ulcerated
    skin, and bone cysts (autosomal dominant)
  Aniridia, ataxia, and mental deficiency
  Cerebellar and renal cystic disease
  Marinesco Sjogren—cataracts, ataxia, and mental deficiency
  Hypogonadism and ataxia (sex linked)
  Ataxia, ocular dyspraxia, and mild mental retardation (dominant)
  Cerebellar ataxia with myotonia and cataracts
  Dandy–Walker and Arnold–Chiari malformations
  Occipital encephalocele and cerebellar hypoplasia
  Ataxia, retinitis pigmentosa, deafness, and mental retardation (Francois
    Descempas)
  Joubert—absent vermis, abnormal eye movement, and hyperventilation
  Disequilibrium syndrome
  Familial paroxysmal ataxias
  Primary cerebellar atrophy—vermis dysplasia and hemisphere dysplasia
  Ataxia with macular degeneration
Nongenetic
  Asphyxia
  Hydrocephalus
  Head injury with "stem" syndrome
  Cerebellar hemorrhage—congenital heart disease with embolism,
    thrombosis, germinal layer, tight bands around occiput, and postbypass
  Hypothyroidism
  Congenital trauma to vertebral arteries
  Vertebral artery trauma

tal speech disorder need not indicate slow maturation or damage to Broca's area but rather maturation delay to the motor learning circuits. For this reason the term *articulatory dyspraxia* is preferable to *cortical dysarthria* since the latter suggests that more is known of the cause than is usually the case (Geschwind, 1975; Mohr, 1978).

When considering that the engram of the message to be conveyed is transformed into a pattern of motor impulses to the bulbar muscles that will result in a certain spoken sequence, it must not be forgotten that this process will require sensory feedback not only from hearing the word spoken but also the proprioceptive feedback relating to the position of lips, tongue, and palate. Cortical aspects of speech have thus been divided into an afferent and efferent type of dyspraxia (Luria, 1970). The cerebellar circuits are responsible for setting the force, speed distance, and direc-

Table 5-10
Comparison of the Various Types of Bulbar Dysfunction

Bulbar Dysfunction	Protective Reflexes	Primitive Reflexes	Jaw Tone	Jaw Jerk	Face	Swallow Dysphagia	Voluntary Bite	Respiration Risk of Aspiration	Dysarthria
Lower motor neuron true bulbar palsy	−	−	Hypotonic	−	Droopy	+++	−	+++	+++
Supranuclear bulbar palsy	++++	−	Spastic	++++	Fixed immobile	+++	Spastic bite ++ Voluntary −	+	+++
Hyperkinetic bulbar palsy	++	++++	Rigidity fluctuates with position of head and contact	−	Grin	++	+ or −	−	+++
Hypokinetic bulbar palsy	++	+	Rigid	−	Sad immobile	− or +	++	−	+ or ++
Ataxic bulbar palsy	++	−	Hypotonic	++	Droopy open mouthed	− or +	++	−	+
Dyspraxia	++	−	Normal	++	Normal	−	++	−	Developmental pattern Developmental or deviant substitution pattern

tion involved in the muscle movement while the basal ganglia circuits are involved in starting, stopping and dampening the movement. Damage to these subcortical circuits in the very young child will produce a more generalized disruption of motor learning (Yoss & Darley, 1974).

Skilled movements are first learned by making the movements in isolation and then by sequencing them into skill. Speech is gradually acquired and the movement is then said to be overlearned until it becomes a subconscious act. At this point one may add in prosodic features (emotional overtones) as the motor activities are no longer occupying consciousness. This is seen not only in speech but also in learning to play the piano or learning to dance. If one still has difficulties remembering where to put the fingers or interpret the musical symbols one is not likely to be able to put emotional feeling into a performance of Mozart. If one is still having to consciously think about steps it is equally unlikely that emotional satisfaction and rhythm will easily come in the case of learning to dance. The pattern of learned movement is often spoken of as an engram and can be considered similar to the subroutine in computer terminology. If an individual wants to execute a certain pattern of properly learned movements, he or she can in effect follow a subconscious routine. The learning of speech is no different from the learning of other motor skills.

Learning of Speech in the Normal Child

The 5-month-old infant can make in isolation all the speech sounds that are required in the English language. It may be another 7 years before he or she can actually put each sound into a sequence. Certain sounds such as b, t, and d, are acquired early along with the vowels so that the normal baby talk of "baba," "pappa," "tata," "mamma," "boo," and "poo" are easily explicable. Any sounds that can be prolonged, especially the fricative sounds in speech, are among the last consonants to be learned so that s, th, sh, f, ch, j, l, and r may not be produced by some children until school age. The child will omit sounds he or she cannot yet make, substitute others, reverse within words, and may use similar sounding phonemes (e.g., led for red, poon for spoon, odilay for holiday).

The child may be able to make a particular sound (e.g., s-s-s-s) in isolation perfectly adequately but will not be able to put it into certain consonant blends and thus will say poon and find it absolutely impossible to say spoon. This is often interpreted by the parents as laziness because the normal mechanisms of motor learning are not appreciated. A further point is that syntax appears to be learned in parallel with the spoken speech as well as the ability to sequence words not only into sentences but also into groups (e.g., days of the week, nursery rhymes, months of the year, numbers, etc.). The child with slow development of speech will have a shorter mean length of utterance, and the longest utterance will also be shorter than that of a normal child of the same age. He or she will tend to be slower in developing pronouns, (e.g., the use of *I* for *me*) and will use primitive tenses such as always applying *ed* to produce a past tense construction (e.g., *comed, goed,* and *wented*). The ability to make sounds in isolation but not put them into words (word dumbness), to pronounce simple but not compound words (e.g., *wheel* but not *wheelbarrow*), or to pronounce words in isolation but not within a phrase or sentence is characteristic of cortical dysarthria. Certain words may be overlearned and pronounced well. It is apparent why it may be difficult to differentiate this from an expressive aphasia in which there is difficulty in selecting the word from the lexicon rather than actually saying it.

The strategy of the brain in learning motor skills is the same whether it is delayed in a specific way or in a more global way as with mental handicap or in association with sensory deprivation or abnormal feedback as in a child with glue ears.

Etiology of Articulatory Dyspraxia

There is a severe form of isolated articulatory dyspraxia that is more common in boys and may be seen in certain chromosome disorders such as the XYY or XXY syndromes. It has been suggested in other cases that there may be excessive heterochromatin, or inactivated DNA, on certain chromosomes. All severe cases of isolated articulatory dyspraxia should have a full chromosome analysis performed. There is also a severe genetically determined type of articulatory dyspraxia. The genetic form, those associated with chromosome disorders, and a severe idiopathic form are all associated with a poor prognosis and the child may have persisting difficulties with articulation throughout life.

Another area of disagreement and confusion arises as to whether the common specific developmental slow speech syndrome (Dyslalia) should be regarded as a type of developmental articulatory dyspraxia (Ingram 1959). As a neurologist it is more appealing to regard this as a developmental dyspraxia rather than as a separate entity. There is no good reason not to accept a spectrum of articulatory dyspraxia, ranging from the normal children in any population who will be slower in development of speech than their peers simply because they form the lower tenth centile of a normal distribution curve. Mild brain damage, as is seen in association with perinatal asphyxia, prematurity, hypothyroidism, or hydrocephalus, will have a slowing effect upon the rate of brain development and consequential slowing of speech development. There are some families in which slow speech development is inherited as a dominent characteristic, but as a result of the differing rates of brain development in boys and girls, it may appear five times more commonly in boys. There may also be an association with left handedness or ambilaterality, and in a high percentage of cases this is followed by reading retardation, and then specific difficulties in spelling (word blind aphasia syndrome). This group of children with familial slow speech development followed by specific learning difficulties constitutes one of the most important groupings, whether one is considering a developmental articulatory dyspraxia or a learning disabled child. Finally, in the group of developmental articulatory dyspraxias is a very severe form with persistent disruption of speech which may last throughout the child's life and certainly will result in a major communication problem up to the ages of 10 or 11. This is the condition which speech therapists would normally consider as a typical articulatory dyspraxia, and may be associated with chromosome damage. There is a form of acquired articulatory dyspraxia which is rare in children and may follow damage to Broca's area (Schiff et al., 1983).

This is not to say that speech development will not be equally retarded for other reasons such as environmental deprivation, sensory deprivation from chronic ear problems, or anything else that slows the rate of brain development such as slow acquisition of dominance or hormone abnormalities. In these cases, however, the speech problem is not likely to be a specific disorder of motor learning but rather part of a more generalized disorder. Forty percent of children with a hemiplegia have slow development of articulation, which corresponds more to the overall IQ than to the side of the hemiplegia.

PROSODIC FEATURES OF SPEECH

Prosody is the name given to the emotional features of speech, i.e., the intonation, stress, and change in volume that is added to basic articulation in order to convey emotional information as opposed to the factual information within the sentence structure. In addition to the prosodic features of speech there are many body movements, gestures, and in particular facial expressions that also convey meaning. For example, it is thought that the mentally handicapped child who is word-deaf may be able to perceive communication cues from intonation and nonverbal communication. We are all familiar with how stressing one word in the middle of a sentence completely changes the meaning of that sentence. Prosodic features of speech change or add to the meaning and tell a lot about how the person feels about what he or she is saying. They are thought to depend on the opposite (right) hemisphere to that used in the other aspects of speech. This is not surprising since we are literally singing while we speak, and true singing merely adds a proscribed prosodic pattern of intonation to the words.

The child can communicate many feelings to parents long before he or she has developed any meaningful speech. The limbic system of the brain is a primary area and is relatively well developed at birth. The child learns that the mother signals her feelings to him or her through smell, taste, and facial expression and so he develops a repertoire of responses. Shortly after birth the child will diminish the amount of movement and will change respiratory pattern and heart rate in response to the mother speaking to him or her. The child will turn to the mother's breast pad and will selectively prefer the taste of his or her own mother's milk within a day or two of birth. Full-term infants already have visual fixation and very soon learn to fix on a face rather than any other object. By 6 weeks the infant has developed a social smile and will look the mother in the eyes, will smile, and will move the eyes in order to follow her when she moves. By 4 months of age, the infant excites at the sight of a familiar person or food, stops crying, and smiles at the sight of the mother. The mother's eyes and face already are recognized as a source of signals, of pleasure or displeasure. From very early days, the infant will imitate tongue protrusion and lip movements; by a few months of age he or she will take great delight in imitating sounds after the mother. No mother is in any doubt that her child is alert, aware of her as a person, likes to see her, is excited, shows pleasure and displeasure, and that this communication system develops a year before the child communicates by spoken speech. Absence of this communication system is the basis of autism.

A prosodic dysarthria is when one loses emotional cues in speech due to monotone and monopitch. This in conjunction with incorrect signaling of facial expression in children suffering from dyskinesia will give false emotional signals. There is also a type of cortical prosodic dysarthria.

INVESTIGATION OF CHILDREN WITH DYSARTHRIA

It is most important to take a careful history that includes family history, details of the pregnancy, birth, delivery, and any postnatal problems. A detailed neurologic examination is also mandatory. Acquired dysarthrias are always much more sinister than congenital abnormalities of speech. The pitfalls of the diagnosis of cerebral palsy must always be borne in mind as this is not a diagnosis but merely a mixed group of brain-damaged children. Some of them will be found to have genetic disorders; progressive disorders may easily be missed and therefore one should aim at a diagnostic classification (e.g., cerebral palsy secondary to hypoxic ischemic encephalopathy or cerebral palsy secondary to prematurity and intraventricular hemorrhage). Diagnosis will be followed by assessment of all areas of the child's development and not limited just to motor difficulties either in speech, hand manipulation, or mobility. It is necessary to get an overall picture of the child's developmental level from the psychometric point of view using either a standardized preschool test or a formal intelligence test so that one can get some idea as to whether the child's difficulties are specific or part of a global retardation syndrome. The child with an onset progressive dysarthria will require multiple investigations including computerized tomography (CT) scans, degenerative enzymes, and a full metabolic work-up that can be determined easily from the list of various causes that are given in association with each neurologic grouping. The speech work-up will also have to include assessment of hearing when brainstem evoked responses may be useful in evaluating the possibility of brainstem pathology. A full speech therapy assessment is necessary including assessment of auditory discrimination, auditory memory, active and passive vocabulary, comprehension, and documentation of syntactical development, which apart from standardized tests should include the longest utterance, mean length of utterance, use of personal pronouns, and use of grammar such as verb tense and plurals (Enderby, 1980; Ingram & Henderson, 1972). The standardized articulation tests such as the Edinburgh Articulation Test will tell whether the speech is patterned and has a developmental (i.e., slowed motor learning pattern) or whether it is deviant or inconsistent. Analysis of speech by a skilled speech therapist will be able to detect hyporhinophonia, specific defects, and palatal, lingual, and labial function (Ingram & Henderson, 1972; Renfrew, 1972).

One may not immediately get a family history of slow speech development, but other areas of linguistic competence such as reading and spelling should be investigated in the parents and siblings. Most children with a severe dysarthria will probably be subjected to a CT scan.

Tests for cerebral dominance such as injection of sodium amytal into the carotid artery (Wada test) are not applicable in young children, but the use of less invasive techniques such as dichotic listening studies or tachistoscopic examination of simultaneous visual presentations can be used to assess dominance. Detailed examination of the lips, tongue, and palate may require indirect laryngoscopy or bronchoscopy in order to see whether the vocal cords are moving normally and to be sure that there is no thickening, nodules, chronic inflammation, or subglotic tumors. A lateral x-ray of the neck can be very helpful. This will show the soft palate, tongue, and larynx and the size of the adenoidal pad. If this is combined with vocalization of sounds such as e and m, one can see the movement of the soft palate and also that it closes off the nasopharynx, i.e., a palatogram can be obtained (Hagerty et al., 1958). Nasal endoscopy using a small fiberoptic instrument will show the mobility of the soft palate and is used prior to consideration for pharyngoplasty. Tongue movements may be studied by painting the tongue with barium and performing cine or videofluoroscopy (Carden & Kemp, 1970; Powers,

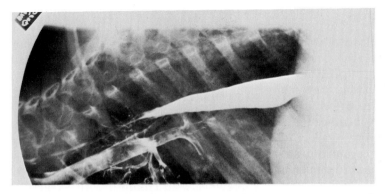

Fig. 5-15. X-ray to show bronchial overspill during a contrast swallow in a child with bulbar palsy.

1962). This latter technique has also helped enormously in viewing swallowing mechanisms, checking for overspill into the bronchial tree, looking for normal relaxation of cricopharyngeus muscle, and determining the presence or absence of reflux through the esophageogastric junction (Fig. 5-15). In selected cases (e.g., myoclonic movements of the palate), electromyography would be used. Electromyography of the larynx is beginning to be used more commonly in everyday practice. In individual cases physiologic measurements such as (1) measuring the intrabuccal pressure, (2) measuring the amount of drooling, and (3) using an isotope milk feed to measure overspill through the larynx may help in diagnosis and management.

MANAGEMENT OF THE CHILD WITH DYSARTHRIA

The speech pathology and speech therapy management of dysarthric children is considered in detail elsewhere in this volume, thus only some brief medical aspects will be considered here. The management is often dependent on the diagnosis, and the management of the child with normal intelligence who is locked in with a dyskinetic cerebral palsy is going to be different from that of a child with a progressive true bulbar palsy or a child with a brainstem tumor.

We have already discussed the importance of detailed assessment of all areas of function, i.e., gross motor, manipulative skills, self-help skills, visual and spatial development, social and emotional development, intelligence and education, complicating seizure disorder, and the disorder of communication. The resultant therapeutic profile involves many different professionals, and it is important that the role of each is understood prior to commencement of therapy (Johns, 1978).

Success in therapy will depend very much on the child's underlying intelligence, which is often the limiting factor in the use of various aids. One of the difficulties in management of the handicapped child is trying to keep realistic aims without becoming annihilistic. It is obviously pleasing that the child continues to make progress, and since brain development continues until 16–17 years of age one would expect a progressive increase in the child's abilities. In many cases the improvement is small and it becomes difficult to keep in perspective what the eventual outcome in terms of independence will be for the individual. Long-term studies in the acquisition of intelligible speech in children with dysarthria from cerebral palsy presents a rather gloomy picture from the point of view of any dramatic improvement, with 10–15 years of therapy aimed at exercises to the articulatory muscles (Ingram, 1960). This should be borne in mind when considering the use of an alternative communication system and should not be considered an either-or situation. The aim is to allow the child to communicate and it is vital that parents understand the aims and do not continuously correct the child's speech. Rather, they should attempt to understand the underlying idea, need, information, or emotion that he or she is trying to convey. The use of an alternative medium such as Blissymbolics does not lessen the amount of oral speech that the child uses but acts as a crutch, relieves anxiety, and may actually increase the amount of oral speech.

A further fundamental aim is to get the family to accept the handicap and not to wish that the child or the cirumstances were different. One should strive against a handicapped child being raised in a handicapped family, and this aim is not helped by wild claims of cures by one group or criticism by one professional that another professional's methods are of no use or that the child has come too late to that particular person, otherwise there would have been a miraculous cure. It is vital that the professional guards against using the family as a crutch for personal mental support and feeling that job satisfaction comes from the parents being totally dependent on him or her.

The aims, although often admirable, at times appear to be similiar to getting the blind to see, the deaf to hear, the lame to walk. Obviously one would like to get lip closure, improve the swallowing pattern, decrease the tongue thrust, and inhibit the primitive reflexes: one would like to cure the bulbar palsy but this is rarely possible. There is a place for formal articulation exercises such as getting the child to blow and suck at a straw, licking jam off his nose, and practicing tongue movements. Lack of use of the jaw will certainly result in stiffness and decreased movements at the temporomandibular joint. This may be very marked if one has to resort to tube feeding where secondary contractures may occur in the muscles in the same way that they would occur in an arm or a leg. Further risk is of dislocation of the temporomandibular joint, which is not uncommon in children with cerebral palsy, so that the tonic mouth opening may be maintained by secondary subluxation rather than continued muscle spasm.

Drooling is a common problem with all types of bulbar palsy and is rarely due to excessive production of saliva from excitation of the salivary nuclei but rather usually to failure of the tongue to move the saliva back as for a normal swallowing mechanism. The amount of drooling can be measured by using a form of dribble bibble in collecting the saliva, and this may amount to a liter or more in a 24-hour period. Drugs such as propanthaline will occasionally lessen the amount of saliva sufficient to prevent troublesome drooling, but in most cases this is unsatisfactory. Various types of feedback systems are available (Garber, 1971) so that as soon as the child starts to drool there is an auditory signal that indicates that he or she should voluntarily swallow. There are a series of tongue and bulbar exercises that might be helpful in individual cases. In severe persistent cases one may have to resort to recession of the ducts of the salivary glands back in the oropharynx so that the saliva tends to run downhill, i.e., backward rather than forward (Wilkie, 1970).

The use of drugs in bulbar problems is in clinical practice restricted to the use of anticholinergic drugs in myasthenia gravis. Surgery will certainly help in those cases of posterior fossa tumors, hydrocephalus, or conditions such as the Dandy–Walker syndrome with cystic dilatation of the fourth ventricle. Children with head injuries may need artificial ventilation over a long period of time and be severely dysarthric or anarthric, and it may be difficult to tell whether the child is anarthric or aphasic due to combined cortical or brainstem injury. The prognosis is, however, remarkably good. Most children recover speech and swallowing even after severe head injuries regardless of the system of therapy used.

Feeding difficulties are the first abnormality that require management and in the child with cerebral palsy may present at birth or in the first few weeks of life. Tube feeding is often necessary in the neonatal period; most infants will be weaned off the tube by 3–4 weeks after birth. Feeding may then be a traumatic experience for the mother as it may take over an hour with the child failing to thrive, looking thin, and being girny and irritable. It cannot be stressed enough that just as the aim of physical therapy is to achieve some form of mobility for the child, the aim of the speech therapist is to give the child the ability to communicate, and the aim of the occupational therapist is to give the child independent skills. The purpose of feeding, therefore, is to keep body and soul together as monitored by the child's growth. It is surprising how often children on feeding programs do not have a height and weight percentile or subcutaneous fat thickness monitored. The child's nutritional requirements should be calculated initially as those for the 25th centile for his or her age. This provides some measure as to the adequacy of the oral feeding regimen in terms of the daily shortcomings of the caloric needs of the child.

As the child gets older, immobility means that energy needs are less than that of a normal child, taking into consideration his or her growth parameters. The anxiety on the part of the mother to do everything for her child may result in obesity, which in a child, particularly with a lower motor neuron neuromuscular disorder, will further increase the handicap by increasing the load on weak muscles.

The seating of the child is vital so that the musculature is not thrown in to a tonic contraction as part of a mass extensor movement. The child must be seated without any strong contact to the paraspinal area in semiflexed position with the head forward. Avoidance of triggering re-flexogenic zones by the use of hard metal spoons, for example, has already been mentioned. It is essential to be aware of the total amount of food that is required in each feeding rather than just to accept that the child dipped the spoon in the food, got half of it to his or her mouth on three occasions, and is "clever" because he or she has actually managed to feed himself or herself.

Whether oral feeding is possible depends on the type of bulbar palsy. In the case of a true bulbar palsy where the protective reflexes have gone, oral feeding should not be attempted or a fatal aspiration may occur. In these children tube feeding or a gastrostomy are the only reasonable alternatives. The use of prolonged parenteral nutrition in young children is fraught with danger of infection. In small babies it may cause severe cholestasis or secondary malabsorption syndrome, and up to 75 percent will develop septicaemia. If neurologic examination plus cine or video recordings of the swallowing patterns show that the protective reflexes are present, then usually the child can be spoon fed. The primitive suck-ing and tongue rolling is not particularly effective in the child receiving milk from a bottle, which tends to pool in the mouth and splutter out at the side of the teat. Various types of plastic units for the administration of medication allow one to put food sufficiently far back on the tongue that it is swallowed rather than being pushed out. With correct position-ing, the use of the correct utensils, and a skilled operator, most children with a chronic pseudobulbar or extrapyramidal bulbar palsy can be fed orally and good nutrition is maintained. Some children with extrapyra-midal bulbar palsy in spite of very marked neurologic abnormality may develop sufficient bite and chew to eventually be able to manage a normal diet. The presence of free reflux into the nasopharynx must be remem-bered as recurrent otitis media and sinus infection may further add to the child's communication difficulties by causing chronic secretory otitis.

It has become obvious over recent years that many children who are immobile and spend their days unable to change position develop positional deformities. This includes asymmetry of the rib cage, scoliosis and windsweeping of the legs, and abnormalities of the position of hips and feet. Many of these children develop severe gastroesophageal reflux so that once food has entered the stomach it is freely refluxed into the esophagus, which can result in a true esophagitis and stricture. If feeding deteriorates in a child or attacks of screaming and food refusal occur, the possibility of peptic esophagitis should always be considered since treatment with alkali and cimetidine may result in a return to normal. Bleeding or stricture formation should be accepted as indications for surgery regardless of the severity of the child's handicaps, as it is indefensible to leave the child in pain or to starve to death. Free reflux means that there is also the possibility of recurrent aspiration. Repeated chest infections may be due to overspill during a period of tube feeding, or they may be due to recurrent reflux and the risk of acid aspiration. In the past, many hours were spent in articulation exercises, positioning, and attempting to inhibit the neurologic features of the various bulbar palsies, particularly in the case of extrapyramidal bulbar palsies in children suffering from cerebral palsy. Over recent years, a revolution has occurred partly with the introduction of new technology and new techniques but also with the realization that the child's comprehension and ability to communicate are of primary concern. The importance of checking for possible high-tone hearing loss and the correction of any loss from associated glue ears, together with the importance of a stimulating environment and if necessary the provision of structured language groups, has taken precedence over preoccupation with the child's pronunciation. Although many children with static bulbar palsies will eventually achieve comprehensible speech, one cannot wait 5 or more years for this development to occur and fail to allow the child to communicate. The advent of alternative communication systems, either manual such as Paget–Gorman or Makaton, or pictographic such as Blissymbolics, allows these children to communicate with their parents or with each other in a way that was not possible previously. The improvements in computer design so that a child with a generalized motor handicap can be interfaced with a computer and software that is applicable to the system such as Blissymbolics opened new horizons in that the handicap can now be circumvented rather than practiced.

The principles applied in the management of a child with mobility problems or learning disorders apply equally well to a child with a communication problem. One must first relieve the anxiety of chronic failure and circumvent the handicap, then develop areas in which the child has ability, and only finally practice the disability.

REFERENCES

Ardran, G. M., & Kemp, F. H. (1970). Some important factors in the assessment of oropharyngeal function. *Developmental Medicine, Child Neurology, 12,* 158–166.

Birrell, J. F. (1966). Palatal disproportion in children. *Journal of Laryngology and Otology, 80,* 706–717.

Blair, A., & Jones, A. (1983). Articulatory dyspraxia. *Developmental Medicine, Child Neurology.*

Bosma, J. F. (1973). *Oral sensation and perception, Development in the fetus and infant.* Bethesda, MD: US Department of Health, Education and Welfare. (NIH Publication No. 73-546). DHEW.

Brodal, A. (1981). *Neurological anatomy in relation to clinical medicine* (3rd ed.). New York: Oxford University Press.

Brown, J. K. (1969). Feeding reflexes in infancy. *Developmental Medicine, Child Neurology, 11,* 641.

Brown, J. K. (1976). Infants damaged during birth. In D. Hull (Ed.), *Recent advances in paediatrics.* London: Churchill Livingstone.

Brown, J. K. (1981). Learning disorders: A paediatric neurologists view. *Transactions of the College of Medicine of South Africa,* December, 49–104.

Brown, J. K. (1984). Disorders of speech. In J. O. Forfar & F. Arneil (Eds.), *Textbook of paediatrics.* London: Churchill Livingstone.

Chappell, G. E. (1973). Childhood verbal apraxia and its treatment. *Journal of Speech and Hearing Disorders, 38,* 362–368.

Crystal, D. (1980). *Introduction to language and pathology.* London: Edward Arnold.

Darley, F. L., Aronson, A. E., & Brown, J. R. (1975). *Motor speech disorders.* Philadelphia: Saunders. Denny-Brown, D. (1966). *The cerebral control of movement.* Liverpool, England: Liverpool University Press.

Drillen, C. M., & Ingram, T. T. S. (1966). *The causes and natural history of cleft lip and palate.* Edinburgh: E & S Livingstone.

Enderby, P. (1980). Frenchay dysarthria assessment. *The British Journal of Disorders of Communication, 15,* 165–173.

Farmer, A. & Lenicione, R. M. (1977). An extraneous vocal behavior in cerebral palsied speakers. *The British Journal of Disorders of Communication, 12,* 109–118.

Garber, N. B. (1971). Operant procedures to eliminate drooling behaviour in a cerebral palsied adolescent. *Developmental Medicine, Child Neurology, 13,* 641–644.

Geschwind, N. (1975). The apraxias: Neural mechanisms of disorders of learned movement. *American Scientist, 63,* 188–195.

Gilman, S., & Winans, S. S. (1982). *Mantar and Gatz's essentials of clinical neuroanatomy and neurophysiology* (6th ed.). Philadelphia: F. A. Davis.

Gomez, M. R., Clermont, V., & Bernstein, J. (1962). Progressive bulbar paralysis in childhood—Franzio-Londe's disease. *Archives of Neurology, 6,* 317.

Hagerty, R. F., Hill, M. J., Pettit, H. S., & Kane, J. J. (1958). Soft palate movement in normals. *Journal of Speech and Hearing Research, 1,* (4), 325–330.

Hagerty, R. F., Hill, M. S., Pettit, H. S., & Kane, J. J. (1958). Posterior pharyngeal wall movement in normals. *Journal of Speech and Hearing Research, 1,* (3), 203–330.

Hagerty, R. F., & Hill, M. J. (1960). Pharyngeal wall and palatal movement in postoperative cleft palates and normal palates. *Journal of Speech and Hearing Research, 3,* 59–66.

Ingram, T. T. S. (1959). Specific developmental disorders of speech in childhood. *Brain, 82,* 450–467.

Ingram, T. T. S. (1960). *Assessment of the results of speech and other therapies in cerebral palsy.* The Second National Spastics Society Study Group, Oxford.

Ingram, T. T. S. (1961). Speech defects and cerebral palsy. *Spastics Quarterly, 10,* 22–28.

Ingram, T. T. S. (1972). The assessment of a child in a speech clinic. The child with delayed speech. In R. Rutter & J. A. M. Martin (Eds.), *Clinics in developmental medicine no. 43* (pp. 68–82). London: Heinemann.

Johns, D. F. (1978). *Clinical management of neurogenic communicative disorders.* Boston: Little, Brown.

Martin, A. D. (1974). Some objections to the term "apraxia of speech". *Journal of Speech and Hearing Disorders, 39,* 53–64.

Martlew, M. (1981). The development of language. In K. J. Connolly & H. F. R. Prechtl (Eds.), Clinics in developmental medicine no. 77/78. London: Heinemann.

Meyerson, M. D., & Foushee, D. R. (1978). Speech language and hearing in moebius syndrome. *Developmental Medicine, Child Neurology, 20,* 357–365.

Mohr, J. P., Pessin, M. S., Finkelstein, S., et al. (1978). Broca's aphasia: Pathologic and clinical. *Neurology, 28,* 311–324.

Mutton, D. E., & Lea, J. (1980). Chromosome studies of children with specific speech and language delay. *Developmental Medicine, Child Neurology, 22,* 588–594.

Nylen, B. O. (1961). Cleft palate and speech. *Acta Radiologie* (Suppl. 203).

Powers, G. R. (1962). Cinefluorographic investigation of articulatory movements of selected individuals with cleft palates. *Journal of Speech and Hearing Research, 5,* 59–69.

Ratcliffe, S. G. (1982). Speech and learning disorders in children with sex chromosome abnormalities. *Developmental Medicine, Child Neurology, 24,* 80–84.

Renfrew, C. E. (1972). Speech therapy in the child with delayed speech. In R. M. Rutter & J. A. M. Martin (Eds.), *Clinics in developmental medicine no. 43,* (pp. 244–252). London: Heinemann.

Rosenbeck, J. C., & La Pointe, L. L. (1978). The dysarthrias. In D. F. Johns (Ed.), *Clinical management of neurogenic communication disorders.* Little Brown & Co., Boston: Little, Brown.

Rutter, M., & Martin, J. A. M. (1972). The child with delayed speech. In R. Rutter & J. A. M. Martin (Eds.), *Clinics in developmental medicine no. 43.* London: Heinemann.

Schiff, H. B., et al. (1983). Aphemia. *Archives of Neurology, 40,* 720–727.

Subtelny, J. D., Koepp-Baker, H., & Subtelny, J. D. (1961). Patal function and cleft palate speech. *Journal of Speech and Hearing Disorders, 26,* 213–224.

Wilkie, T. F. (1970). The surgical treatment of drooling. *Plastic and Reconstructive Surgery, 45,* 549–554.

Worster-Drought, C. (1968). Speech disorders in children. *Developmental Medicine, Child Neurology, 10,* 427–440.

Yoss, K. A., & Darley, F. L. (1974). Developmental apraxia of speech in children with defective articulation. *Journal of Speech and Hearing Research, 17,* 399–416.

Rachel E. Stark

6
Dysarthria in Children

Dysarthria has been defined as a speech disorder resulting from impairment of the neural mechanisms that regulate the movements of speech (Netsell, 1984). The definition is designed to exclude disorders resulting from impairment of neural mechanisms involved in the selection and sequencing of movements of the articulators in relation to the spatial–temporal goals of speech, i.e., those disorders referred to as dyspraxia or apraxia. These latter disorders, however, are subsumed in some classification systems under the term *central dysarthria*. In practice, it may be very difficult to distinguish dysarthria from dyspraxia in adults. In children, in whom these mechanisms are under development, it may be impossible.

Dysarthria in children may range in severity from complete anarthria, or lack of speech, to a disorder so mild that it may readily be confused with a resolving developmental articulation disorder. Developmental forms of dysarthria in children may show amelioration with age at least up to adolescence, or in the case of children with closed head trauma, over a period of at least 2 years postinsult. In the case of degenerative disorders, it may increase in severity with age.

The incidence of dysarthria among children is estimated to be 1–2/1000 (*ASHA*, 1980). The incidence is higher for males than females, the ratio being estimated at from 1.75:1 to 2:1 depending on the population studied (Cruikshank, 1976).

Speech and Language Evaluation in Neurology:
Childhood Disorders
ISBN 0-8089-1719-6

CLASSIFICATION

Dysarthrias in children have been classified according to (1) presumed etiology, (2) symptomatology, (3) presumed site of lesion. These three approaches to classification are not mutually exclusive.

Presumed etiologies include those associated with cerebral palsy (e.g., anoxia in the perinatal period, birth injury, hyperbilirubinema and others), closed head injury in later childhood, genetic anomalies, and the diseases and disorders of childhood referred to in Brown (chap. 5). It is frequently difficult, however, to ascribe dysarthrias in children to a particular etiology or etiologic pattern. Those that appear to have a genetic basis, for example, may be progressive in nature with gradual onset after a period of relatively normal development. Psychiatric explanation may be advanced in such cases (Batshaw & Haslam, 1976). Dysarthria classed with tardive dyskinesias and thought to be associated with the use of neuroleptics may also be attributable in part to genetic effects, i.e., to differences in physiologic makeup (Gaultieri & Hawk, 1980). It can be stated, however, that dysarthrias associated with problems in the neonatal period and present throughout the first 2 years of life are likely to require different approaches in assessment and intervention than those that are acquired after a period of normal speech and language development.

Classifications based on symptomatology include terms such as spastic dysarthria, athetoid dysarthria, dysarthria associated with dystonia, ataxic speech, etc. These diagnostic terms are usually based on patterns of impairment in control of the limbs and trunk documented in neurologic examination. Speech motor control, however, may be affected to a different extent and in a different manner from that observed in the limbs and trunk in children diagnosed as spastic, ataxic, or dystonic. Children with mild cerebral palsy may have severe dysarthria and, similarly, speech may be relatively unaffected and generally intelligible even to strangers in children with severe spastic quadriplegia (Brown, 1984). In addition, as Abbs, Hunker, and Barlow (1983) have shown, there are a number of significant physiologic and neurophysiologic differences among the subsystems that control speech movements and between these subsystems and those that control movement of the limbs. Speech motor patterns thus are not likely to be predictable on the basis of patterns of impairment of limb movement in the dysarthric individuals.

Sites of lesion are described in the clinical literature as *bulbar, suprabulbar, extrapyramidal,* and *cerebellar* (Espir & Rose, 1970). Bulbar palsy implies lesion to the cranial nerves, whose motor nuclei are in the medulla or bulbar portion of the brainstem. The sensory and motor nuclei of the cranial nerves, and the cranial nerves themselves, may be involved. Alternatively, the muscles may be affected at the most peripheral level by disorders involving the motor endplate as, for example, in myasthenia gravis. Weakness and lack of muscle tone is observed and the tendon reflexes may be reduced or absent. Muscle wasting and spontaneous contractions or fasciculations are present in later stages of the disease or disorder. Dysphagia and dysphonia may be present in addition to dysarthria, depending on the extent of involvement of the cranial nerves.

Pseudobulbar palsy results from bilateral lesions to corticobulbar tracts, i.e., of the upper motor neurons extending from the motor cortex to the brainstem. Most of the motor nuclei of the cranial nerves receive input from bilateral cortical sites, i.e., by a majority of crossed corticobulbar tracts originating in the contralateral hemisphere and by a smaller number of uncrossed corticobulbar tracts originating in the ipsilateral hemisphere. Thus if an upper motor neuron lesion is unilateral, the muscles supplied by a particular cranial nerve will still receive input from the unaffected side and pseduobulbar palsy will not be present. An exception to this rule occurs when that portion of the motor nuclei of the fifth cranial nerve subserving the muscles of the lower part of the face is involved. This portion receives input from crossed corticobulbar tracts only. Unilateral lesion to the corticobulbar tract carrying efferent impulses to these nuclei will give rise to contralateral paresis of the musculature of the lower face. In these cases, the more obvious weakness is for movements associated with emotional expression rather than with voluntary movements.

Pseudobulbar palsy is associated with increases in tone and in tendon reflexes as well as with paresis. Thus the jaw jerk may be increased. Dysphagia may be present in a significant number of cases as well as dysarthria.

Disorders of the extrapyramidal system and of the cerebellum are also associated with dysarthria in children. Distinctive patterns of dysarthric speech have been described in adults in relation to Parkinson's disease and multiple sclerosis (Aronson, 1981). In children, however, such distinctive patterns have not been reported.

Disorders that are primarily sensory–perceptual in nature may involve central or peripheral sites. MacNeilage, Rootes, and Chase (1967) described a 17-year-old dysarthric female with congenital loss of somesthetic sensibility and of sensitivity to pain, light touch, and temperature. Position sense was normal. Sensory receptors and nerves in the skin and oral mucosa had a normal appearance on microscopic examination. Thus the somesthetic disorder was thought to be at a higher information-processing level. This young woman was able to walk, grasp objects, and write legibly, although very slowly. There were no abnormalities of movement suggesting extrapyramidal or cerebellar involvement, however, and none suggesting localized damage to the motor cortex, pyramidal tract, or peripheral motor nerves.

Her speech consisted mainly of vowels, diphthongs and glottal stops. Rate of speech was slow, but intonation patterns were relatively normal. The patient relied more on the prosodic rather than the phonologic features of her speech in her communicative attempts.

Absence or impairment of more peripheral tactile sensitivity may be associated with dysarthria in its congenital form. Loss of oral tactile sensitivity induced experimentally in adults by means of topical anasthesia appears to be associated with alterations in the timing of articulatory gestures but not with a loss of precision and accuracy (Ringel & Steer, 1963). Rappaport (1972) and Zlatin (1972), however, reported the case of a child with congential sensory neuropathy as manifested on histologic examination by the absence of sensory nerve endings in the skin and the buccal mucosa. This child showed markedly delayed motor development. He was found to have a weak suck in infancy. An open mouth posture and drooling persisted in the first 3–4 years of life. He was able to feed himself, but he tended to project utensils into the lip tissue or, if they entered the mouth, to project them too far into the oral cavity and to trigger a gag reflex. His tongue was heavily scarred from accidental biting during feeding. He was unaware of spillage of food and would also continue gross chewing movements after a bolus of food had actually been swallowed.

Lip closure was achieved with relative ease on request, but lip rounding and protrusion were not observed and lip retraction was asymmetrical, probably because of an accompanying but unrelated mild right hemiplegia. Zlatin reports:

M. displayed only gross sucking and masticatory movements while eating. During swallowing he seemed to exhibit an antagonistic motion in that the anterior portion of the tongue appeared to protrude while the posterior portion manifested a retraction or partial 'somatic' swallowing pattern. M. was able to voluntarily protrude his tongue on midline (genioglossus function), swallow and open and close his mouth. He was unable to elevate or lateralize his tongue to command. He exhibited somewhat more discrete function of the lingual musculature during involuntary movements characterized by moderately good contraction of the vertical fibers (thinning or flattening) and fair contraction of transverse fibers (narrowing and lengthening) and genioglossus, styloglossus and superior longitudinal muscles (cupping). Repeated observations failed to reveal elevation or lateralizing movements of the tongue during speech or feeding activities.

In addition, discrete tongue-tip activity was not observed during speech. Instead, this child tended to thrust the tongue forward during speech and to employ blade and midtongue contact with the alveolar ridge, teeth, and midpalatal area. Back consonants (/k/ and /g/) appeared earliest. Bilabial sounds, (/b/, /p/, and /m/), which appear early in normal infants, were acquired late by this child and produced atypically. Sounds requiring less precision of movement (vowels and semivowels) were produced with greatest accuracy. Fricative consonants and consonantal clusters were acquired later than normal, and bilabial fricatives (/f/ and /v/) were produced atypically and inconsistently.

THEORETICAL CONSIDERATIONS

Dysarthrias in children are less well studied than those found in adults. Recent findings with respect to motor control systems in normal adults and in normally developing infants and young children may be helpful in establishing a theoretical framework for the study of dysarthria in children.

Central Motor Control Systems

According to classical descriptions, there are three independent motor systems concerned with posture and movement patterns: (1) the pyramidal system, controlling skilled voluntary movements; (2) the extrapyramidal system, controlling the postural adjustments that form the background for voluntary movement; and (3) the cerebellum, coordinating voluntary movement patterns. The more modern view is that these three systems are interconnected at many levels and interact in controlling voluntary movements in much more complex ways than were envisaged earlier. Recent studies have suggested the nature of the contributions made by these three systems as a result of their interactions. This position is clearly stated in Kandel and Schwartz (1981).

First, there are direct monosynaptic connections from the motor cortex to the motor neurons at the periphery. In higher primates, including man, direct pyramidal tract connections make possible the fractionation of movement, i.e., the ability to control individual muscles independently of one another. This ability is exemplified in the movements of the speech articulators and of separate digits in the adult human. Pyramidal and associated rubrospinal tract neurons start firing 20–50 msec before muscle contraction takes place.

The programs that are transmitted by the pyramidal tract are selected and modified, however, in the preceding 800 msec. Deecke, Scheid, and Kornhuber (1969) have shown that changes in potentials may be recorded over the motor cortex at least 800 msec before the initiation of voluntary movement of the finger. It is believed that the central nervous system (CNS) sets up programs that may be modified depending on information from the periphery. This modification is implemented by means of neurons in the basal ganglia and the deep cerebellar nuclei. DeLong (1974) has recorded single-unit activity in different regions of the basal ganglia in awake monkeys that were known, by virtue of their somatotopic organization, to be associated with the subsequent voluntary movement of a specific body part. This single-unit activity preceded not only the pyramidal tract activity but also that of the motor cortex and the cerebellum. This finding has suggested that the basal ganglia may play a role in the initiation of voluntary movement of the limbs and the digits. In addition, thalamocortical reverberatory circuits are involved in control of voluntary movement.

The cerebellum may also participate in the initiation of movement as well as in its fine coordination. Specifically, the motor association areas may act in cooperation with the lateral portions of the cerebellar hemispheres and with the dentate nuclei in the early phases of planning of voluntary movement. These neocerebellar areas receive input from the frontal association areas of cortex. They send their output to the motor cortex via the thalamus. Intermediate and older parts of the cerebellum may be involved in movement-to-movement control of sequences, once initiated. Thach (1980) has found in studies of awake monkeys that interposed neurons in these older parts, as well as neurons in the dentate nucleus, fire in close temporal association with phases of movement in a complex task in which the monkeys were trained. Interestingly, patterns of activity in the dentate neurons appeared to reflect the direction of each succeeding (and intended) movement and not the prevailing (ongoing) patterns of muscle contraction.

The intermediate parts of the cerebellum are kept informed of cortical commands by collaterals of pyramidal tract fibers. They may shape evolving movement patterns by the inhibitory action of Purkinji neurons on nuclear cells. The nuclear cells, in turn, may act on the red nucleus and thus on the motor cortex (Ghez & Fahn, 1981).

It is also probable that the cerebellum may store information about motor programs and that it is capable of learning new motor programs under special circumstances (Eccles, Ito, & Szentagothai, 1967). Normally, however, the motor cortex and supplementary motor cortex are predominantly involved in new motor learning. In speech motor learning the lower portion of the left third frontal convolution (Broca's area) plays a prominent part. The relative size of the cortical areas devoted to control of the orofacial and laryngeal musculature attests to the importance of this region in the human (Penfield & Roberts, 1959).

Speech Motor Control Systems

At a more peripheral level there are major differences between speech motor control and control of other movement systems (Abbs, 1981). These differences involve biomechanical properties of the oral structures such as inertia (less for the lips than for the upper limbs or even for the tongue) and connective tissue restraints (as implied by the joints, tendons, and ligaments present in the jaw and the limbs but not in the lips and tongue). They also have to do with associated neurophysiologic mechanisms. Thus, although the jaw, tongue, and larynx all have muscle spindles, only the closing muscles of the jaw are provided with spindles (not opening muscles). In addition, the spindle afferents from the larynx and tongue are configured differently from those of the jaw and the limbs. The lips do not have muscle spindles at all. These differences may reflect the need for reflex postural adjustments in the limbs and possibly the jaw, but not in the oral musculature.

As Abbs and colleagues (1981, 1983) have further noted, patterns of motoneuron recruitment are likely to be quite different for the oral and limb motor control systems. In addition, the patterns of recurrent and reciprocal inhibition that are manifest in the upper limbs do not appear to be in effect in oral structures innervated by the cranial nerves. Instead, control of inhibitory patterns may be effected at more central sites. It will be recalled that in primates the motoneurons of the lips, tongue, and jaw muscles receive monosynaptic inputs from cortical motor areas and that inhibitory cerebellar inputs are integrated in the efferent stimulus patterns thus transmitted (Dubner, Sessle, & Storey, 1978).

Additional major issues in the study of speech motor control have to do with the extent to which motor output is preconditioned, modulated, and/or refined on the basis of incoming afferent information (Abbs & Cole, 1982). It is regarded as unlikely that speech motor patterns are played out from prestored detailed muscle contraction programs without the possibility of movement-to-movement modification. Several findings contribute to this view:

- The speech motor system has the ability to compensate for unanticipated changes in position, or outside forces acting upon the musculature.
- The tongue and lips are capable of making compensatory adjustments in speech to fixation of the jaw (e.g., when a pipe stem or bite-block is held between the teeth) (Netsell, 1981).
- Speech is disrupted by the interruption or disruption of sensory information.

It appears likely, then, that afferent mechanisms are involved in speech motor control. These mechanisms could be primarily local closed-loop feedback processes or they could be open-loop feedforward processes that permit one subsystem (e.g., the lip subsystem) to influence timing and direction of force in another subsystem during speech (e.g., the tongue subsystem). Recent studies suggest that while closed-loop systems operating at the brainstem level may be involved in feeding (preventing injury to the tongue by biting, for example, as in the case of congenital sensory neuropathy described by Zlatin [1972]) and in speech motor learning in the first year of life, they are unlikely to have a major role once speech has become highly automatic and "overlearned." Open-loop, feedforward afferent systems are more likely to be involved in speech motor control in older children and adults.

Acquisition of Speech Motor Control in Infancy

The newborn infant is capable only of reflexive sound production. Sound production is constrained by the differences in the shape of the newborn infant vocal tract, which resembles that of the adult nonhuman primate more closely than that of the adult human (Bosma, 1975). Neurophysiologic constraints, however, are probably just as important in the first months of life, and are increasingly so throughout infancy.

Reflexive sound production includes cry and other discomfort sounds (fussing) and production of sounds associated with vegetative activity of the vocal tract. It has been suggested that cry vocalization in infants contributes to the later development of speech production (Lieberman, 1967; Stark, 1980). Lieberman (1967) advanced the hypothesis that infant cry constituted an "innate referential breath group" (p. 42). In his view, cry provided "the universal acoustic properties of the normal breath group that is used to segment speech into sentences" (p. 42). More recently, Wilder and Baken (1974) and Langlois and Baken (1976) have shown that respiratory behavior during cry resembles that of mature speech more closely than does ventilation in a resting state. The tidal volume increases during cry, the rate of respiration decreases, and the relative duration of expiration and inspiration changes. Specifically, these authors have shown that during cry, as in mature speech, the inspiratory phase is brief and is characterized by a sharp intake of air and expiration is prolonged. The ratio of the duration of the inspiratory phase to the total duration of the respiratory cycle (the 1-fraction) is accordingly different from that of breathing at rest, where the inspiratory and expiratory phases are approximately equal in duration. As a result, the time that is available for vocal or speech output within a respiratory cycle is greatly increased during cry and mature speech.

During cry, the infant gives up the otherwise obligatory pattern of nasal breathing and as a result produces open or vowel-like sounds. These sounds are frequently harsh and nasalized, possibly because of the tension of oropharyngeal musculature and related stretching of the oropharyngeal mucosal surfaces and the presence of a hypopharyngeal side cavity (Bosma, 1965). In addition, inspiration is audible and is frequently voiced. Voiced inspiratory sounds may be characterized by extreme pitch glides that are probably related to the high rate of air flowing during inspiration. Cry sounds show a variety of simple rhythmic patterns and are frequently interrupted by explosive sounds referred to as "glottal plosives" (Wasz-Hockert et al., 1968) or "coughs" (Stark and Schultz, submitted for publication). Coughs are viewed by Bosma, Truby, and Lind (1965) as an important mechanism, in addition to cry, in facilitating the newborn's transition to air breathing. These coughs are incorporated in cry. Coughs and harsh nasalized vocalic sounds are not found in later speech development. Simple rhythmic patterns of vocalization resembling those of cry are found, however, in subsequent developmental periods.

It has been suggested that anomalous cry features may be predictive of various forms of developmental delay and of sudden infant death syndrome (SIDS). Specific spectrographic features have been investigated from this standpoint (Colton & Steinschneider, 1980; Heinz, Stark, Condino, & Hege, 1983).

Vegetative sounds (e.g., clicks and buzzes) in the newborn are associated with primitive reflex activity of the vocal tract as well as with its reduced dimensions in the oropharyngeal region particularly. Tongue–epiglottic (and tongue–pharyngeal wall) contact is constantly being made and broken as a result of reflex activity within a restricted area (Sazaki, Levine, Laitman, & Crelin, 1977). Few vegetative sounds are voiced and they are as likely to be produced during inspiration as during expiration (Stark, Rose & McLagen, 1976).

Production of reflexive sounds is mediated at the brainstem level. Respiration and phonation in cry are coordinated through nuclei in the dorsal midbrain–pons region, the periacqueductal gray area having special importance, and the nucleus ambiguus. Cry phonation is coordinated with suck and swallow at this level, as may be deduced from the finding that anencephalic infants are capable of both cry and vegetative activity of the vocal tract.

If nervous system mechanisms above the brainstem level are of primary importance for subsequent vocal learning, then one might expect to see discontinuity of vocal development as higher level structures within the system mature and begin to exert control over lower-level structures. Each new level of organization should possess unique properties of structure and behavior. It has been hypothesized that three major landmarks of vocal development (cooing, reduplicated babbling, and expressive jargon) follow the initial reflexive soundmaking period (Stark, 1980). These landmarks reflect discontinuities of vocal and neural development. They could be viewed as "hardware" developments (see Klahr, 1978). It has also been hypothesized, however, that periods of expansion of vocal skills intervene between the major landmarks of vocal development. These expansions may be accompanied by continuing maturation within the functioning components of the vocal motor system. However, they may also reflect vocal learning as a result of social conditioning and/or inventiveness on the part of the infant as he or she experiences self-vocalizations through the auditory modality. These expansions of vocal skill may be thought of as "software" developments.

At 6–8 weeks of age the infant begins to produce reactive sounds, i.e., sounds such as cooing and laughter that are thought to be expressive of comfort, pleasure, and other feelings such as delight and interest. These sounds may be elicited by the vocalizations and smiles of adults or by the sight of colorful designs or of complex patterns of movement of objects.

Reactive soundmaking is chiefly important from a speech motor control point of view because it represents the acquisition of ability to initiate phonation in a noncry mode. Before 3 months of age, reactive sounds tend to be produced with the mouth partly or entirely closed. As a result these sounds may be heard as nasalized grunts or poorly resonated sounds. The ability to produce open vowel-like sounds in noncry at approximately 3 months of age appears to be associated with the disappearance of obligate nasal breathing. The author's observation suggests that this phenomenon, in turn, may be associated with a reduction in the absolute number of sensory nerve endings in the mucosa of the oropharyngeal region, i.e., of nerve endings that mediate tongue palatal and tongue pharyngeal wall contact (Munger, 1972). The vowel-like sounds produced are without the harsh nasalized quality of cry. Brief vegetative noises such as clicks and friction noises may be superimposed upon them. In laughter, which emerges at 4 months of age, the temporal structure of cry is incorporated, along with the explosive cough-like phenomena and voiced inspiratory sounds. The vowel-like sounds in laughter, however, have the harmonic structure of comfort sounds and are not harsh or nasalized.

Ontogenetically, development of speech motor control proceeds outward from the brainstem, i.e, both cephalward and caudalward (Bosma, 1975). It is likely that the onset of the first vocal landmark, i.e., phonation in reactive sound making, coincides with maturation and beginning functioning in speech motor control of the limbic system, specifically of the anterior cingulate area (Ploog, 1979). The cingulate area has been associated with initiation of vocalization, and the limbic system in its entirety with emotional expression in nonhuman primates and in humans (Jurgens & VonCramon, 1982).

Reactive soundmaking is followed by a period of expansion during which control of closed or consonant-like noises begin to be acquired and consonantal and vowel-like sounds begin to be combined with one another in simple sequences. Control of voice pitch in phonation is also acquired. These developments take place as the reflexive vegetative activity of the vocal tract (e.g., tongue protrusion and retraction and spontaneously occurring lip movements) begins to decline in extent and frequency of occurrence. In some infants control of pitch variation within extreme pitch ranges is first observed, and the consonantal noises and primitive consonant–vowel combinations appear later. In other infants these developments take place in the reverse order. These phenomena suggest that the infant is improvising in response to the discovery and practice of different sound types.

During the reactive period, elaboration of lower motor neuron systems as well as of limbic structures may be taking place. It is not clear how this elaboration may relate to the individual variation and different orders of development of sound types in different infants during the expansion period, which appears to be one of improvisation. Primate vocalization does not appear to offer a parallel for improvisation in vocal learning. In the primate species studied thus far, sound types employed by the adult are already present early in infancy and may be innate. For example, the "isolation peep," comfort sounds, shrieks, and trills that are produced by squirrel monkey infants appear to be genetically determined. Some of these sound types, however, may be analogous or acoustically similar to those produced by infants. The isolation peep, for example, is considered to be analogous to infant cry (Newman, in press). Different structures within the limbic system appear to be involved in the control of production of different squirrel monkey calls. Observation of the development of vocalization in human infants suggests that there could be analogous structures in the human limbic system that develop at different rates or according to different schedules from one human infant to another. They may do so in response to the infant's "discovery" and practice of different sound types.

Discovery implies that the infant is paying attention to the auditory feedback from his or her own vocalizations. Pathways have been discovered extending from the cingulate cortex of the squirrel monkey to the auditory association area. Cell nuclei within the auditory association cortex have been found to respond differentially to self-produced calls and similar calls recorded from other individuals in this species (Muller-Preuss, 1978). Similar mechanisms may become effective within the human infant in the first expansion period of vocal development.

The second major landmark of human vocal development is that of reduplicated babbling, i.e., the repetition of consonant–vowel syllables. Usually each syllable is heard as having the same consonant and the same vowel (as in /dadada/). However, careful listening reveals that there is often a general imprecision of articulation such that the target place of articulation for the consonant seems to remain the same throughout a given babbled vocalization, but the degree to which the target is attained may vary. The vocalization /dəjæjæjədə/, for example, might be a typical one at this age.

In babbling, the infant is able for the first time to open and close the mouth in accompaniment to phonation. The jaw and tongue may move together in an undifferentiated manner during this activity, but the ability to coordinate such movements with voicing suggests that cortical feedforward mechanisms may be in effect for the first time. The onset of reduplicated babbling coincides with the maturation of one or more layers of the cortical mantle in the motor face and larynx areas and/or of the analogous areas of the supplementary motor cortex (Milner, 1976, p 58).

It is also possible, however, that babbling has a higher-level "recognitory" function with respect to objects toward which the infant's gaze is directed. In normal infants the alternating opening–closing movements of tongue and jaw in reduplicated babbling may be strongly associated with visual inspection and/or manipulation and mouthing of objects (Stark, 1980), activities with which infants in these vocal developmental periods are intensely preoccupied.

Between 9 and 12 months two developmental changes are observed. First, there is a second expansion period in which sound types already acquired are elaborated and produced within a variety of intonation contours. Patterns are repeated in their entirety or with minor variations. It is probable that striatal and cerebellar circuits are undergoing extensive maturation at this time and make such elaborations possible. The second development is that of production of prewords or protowords. These utterances do not correspond in meaning to the words spoken by adults in the child's environment but they have some degree of phonetic consistency (Dore, Fraklin, Miller, & Ramer, 1976). They are not used symbolically but rather only in a general way in relation to recurring experiences or strongly felt needs and desires.

Finally, between 15 and 18 months true referential words are acquired. These are words or attempts at words from the language spoken in the child's environment. They refer to specific objects or actions. Their acquisition depends in part on the ability to imitate sounds. Imitation of speech sounds requires that the infant be able to coordinate a variety of oral gestures with phonation and respiration and also that he or she be able to make use of auditory templates in doing so.

Maturation of primary auditory association areas occurs during this period, as does maturation of tracts linking primary and secondary cortical motor areas with auditory association areas. The best known of these auditory–motor tracts is the arcuate fasciculus. Maturation of these cortical areas and of the tracts linking them is essential to the incorporation of segmental features and intonation contours of the language the infant hears in his or her own utterances.

In summary, the major landmarks of vocal development, i.e., phonation, reduplicated babbling, and single-word production, appear to be related to discontinuities of neural development. Mountcastle (1978) and others have stated, however, that the development of central control systems may be subject to modification on the basis of learning and experience. If learning and experience are important for vocal development, there should be aspects of continuity as well as of discontinuity in vocal development. Continuity of development does appear to be manifested between the major landmarks, i.e., in the first and the second expansion periods described previously.

CHARACTERISTICS OF DYSARTHRIA IN CHILDREN

Feeding Problems

Abnormal feeding patterns are present in some children with severe dysarthria, suggesting cranial nerve and/or lower motor neuron involvement. They may take the form of persistence of primitive oral reflexes or of failure of development of mature feeding patterns. Primitive oral reflexes include rooting reflexes (turning of the head toward the source of tactile stimulation in the orofacial area), the suck–swallow reflex, the phasic bite reflex (a rhythmical bite-and-release pattern with vertical movement of the jaw), lip reflexes and also the palmomental reflex (Prechtl & Beintema, 1965). In addition, a tongue lateralization reflex (with movement toward the source of tactile or chemical stimulation) has been described by Weiffenbach & Thach (1973). Other oral reflexes that persist in the older normal child and normal adult are the gag reflex and the jaw jerk. These reflexes may be depressed or hyperactive in the dysarthric child.

Persistence of the primitive oral reflexes beyond the first months of life makes mature patterns of feeding difficult if not impossible to acquire. Their presence has suggested to some investigators that speech motor control will be difficult to acquire also (Mysak, 1963).

Schedules for the development of mature feeding patterns have been proposed by Morris (1979) and by Mueller (1972). Delay in the emergence of lip retraction on spoon feeding, of jaw stabilization in drinking, and of differentiation of tongue and jaw movement in chewing in the first years of life may suggest abnormalities, including weakness and delay in maturation of the oral motor system, and may be predictive of dysarthria. In addition, inability to close the lips during feeding or when at rest after 6 months of age may suggest weakness of the lip musculature and may predict difficulty in the production of bilabial stops and/or of labiodental fricatives.

Oral Motor Characteristics

It has been suggested that dysarthria in children and adults is accompanied by significant restriction of oral nonspeech movements such as voluntary lateralization of the tongue or protrusion and retraction of the lips. Froeschels (1943), for example, suggested that nonspeech movements of the lips, tongue, and jaw should be evaluated in terms of the rate of repetition of such movements. Westlake (1951) advocated that adequacy of functioning of the oral motor system be assessed in terms of voluntary movements of the oral structures as well as of vegetative (feeding) activities in assessing "physiological readiness for speech."

Others have questioned the assumed relationship of restriction of movement during nonspeech activities and speech defectiveness. Irwin (1955), for example, in a study of 226 cerebral palsied children found that the relationship between nonspeech movements and speech articulation scores was too weak to be used for predictive purposes. He found that some children with severe involvement of the speech musculature were relatively proficient in the articulation of speech sounds and, vice versa, that some who performed well on tests of nonspeech movements had significant difficulty with speech articulation. Thus, prediction from oral nonspeech movement capabilities to phonetic ability was subject to considerable error.

Hixon and Hardy (1964), in a study of 50 cerebral palsied children diagnosed as spastic quadraplegics or athetoid quadraplegics, measured both repetitive speech and nonspeech movements. The repetitive movements were those of production of the nonsense syllables /mə/, /də/, and /gə/ and of the nonsense syllable sequence /pətəkə/ over a 10-second interval. They found that repetitive speech movements could be produced by these children at approximately twice the rate of nonspeech movements. In addition, ratings of speech defectiveness were found to correlate significantly more highly with rate of syllable production than with rate of production of nonspeech movements.

The authors point out that nonsense syllable production is presumably a more complex activity than production of movements such as opening and closing of the lips because it requires coordination of articulation, phonation, and respiration. The superiority of rate of syllable production over that of nonspeech movements thus appears somewhat paradoxical. However, the CNS has the potential of integrating highly complex activities. It may well be that since all of Hixon and Hardy's subjects were capable of speech, feedforward afferent mechanisms (both somesthetic and auditory) had been established and had facilitated rate of movements in repetitive-syllable production. A similar result with respect to rates of movement might well have been obtained from a group of matched normal control subjects.

It is noteworthy that production of the sequence /pətəkə/ proved more difficult and was reduced in rate compared with that of production of a single-syllable sequence. In the /pətəkə/ sequence, phonation must be turned on or off several times during production, and place of articulation is systematically varied. As we have seen, repetitive-syllable sequences, i.e., reduplicated babbling, appears earlier in the developmental sequence than sequences in which voicing and place of articulation for consonants is varied.

Production of the simpler sequences was more highly predictive of speech defectiveness than production of the /pətəkə/ sequence. In children with a greater degree of speech proficiency overall, i.e., in those who are said to be mildly dyspraxic, production of the /pətəkə/ sequence might well be more predictive of speech proficiency.

Speech Motor Characteristics

The speech of dysarthric children has been characterized as delayed and impaired in a manner not found in children without CNS system lesion. In the 1950s a series of studies were carried out with the aim of characterizing the speech of children manifesting spastic and athetoid cerebral palsy (Byrne, 1959; Lencione, 1953). These cross-sectional studies suggested that speech development is significantly delayed in cerebral palsied children but that it follows a similar course in cerebral palsied and in normal children. In cerebral palsied children, proficiency in producing consonantal sounds was greatest, for example, for bilabial sounds such as /w/ and /b/, which appear early in the acquisition of speech by normal infants. More complex tongue-tip and back of tongue sounds, all later appearing in the normal infant, were more often produced by older than by younger cerebral palsied children. Children with a diagnosis of athetosis tended to be more severely delayed than those with a diagnosis of spasticity.

In the aforementioned studies, vowels were more frequently produced without error than were consonants. A similar result has been reported by Huntingdon, Harris, Shankweiler, and Sholes (1967) for adult dysarthrics. The degree of precision required for production of consonants is greater than that required for vowel production. However, certain vowels, e.g., those with a mid or low front tongue position, were more accurately produced by the dysarthric children in Byrne's study than those requiring a higher front tongue position, (/e/ and /i/), lip rounding, (/o/ and /ɔ/ or diphthongization. In this respect also, the normal developmental sequence appears to be reflected.

Abnormal speech patterns found in dysarthric children are associated with the persistence of primitive oral reflexes or with interference from overflow movements or dyskinesic movement patterns affecting the oral musculature. Primitive reflexive movements are likely to inhibit the production of speech. These include jaw extension (a normal response to an object or person approaching the mouth of the infant of less than 5 months) and tongue protrusion–retraction movements (Peiper, 1963). These latter movements form part of the suck–swallow response but are manifested by infants of less than 5 or 6 months at times when they are not feeding. Jaw extension may inhibit articulatory activity of the tongue and lips, and tongue protrusion and retraction movements may inhibit phonation and pre-empt the voluntary movements of the tongue associated with production of vowels and consonants.

Athetoid and/or dystonic movements of the limbs and reflexes involving the trunk and limbs such as the Moro reflex and the tonic labyrinthine reflex may affect the stability of the shoulder girdle. As a result the control of speech may be indirectly affected. In addition, it has been suggested that primitive oral reflexes may be triggered by the asymmetrical tonic neck reflex and by the Moro reflex.

Love, Hagerman, and Taimi (1980) investigated the relationship of dysphagia and oral reflexes with speech performance in a group of 60 severely handicapped cerebral palsied individuals ranging in age from 3 to 26 years. Feeding behavior was assessed in these subjects by having them (1) bite a piece of toast, (2) suck and swallow 2 ounces of liquid through a plastic straw, and (3) chew a soft marshmallow and a piece of uncooked carrot. Performance was measured in terms of time taken to achieve a satisfactory result in terms of swallow. Primitive oral reflexes assessed included those affecting oral and pharyngeal areas (rooting, lip, mouth-opening, phasic biting, and suckle) and others affecting related structures (Sheppard, 1964).

Results indicated that 60 percent of the subjects performed adequately in feeding. For the remainder of the subjects, sucking through a straw was the most difficult task. This difficulty was thought to be associated with velopharyngeal dysfunction and with lack of sustained lip closure. Drooling was observed in only 12 subjects, and in 9 of these subjects swallowing was thought to be adequate. Inadequate deglutition thus may not be the only factor giving rise to drooling.

Infantile oral reflex patterns were found consistently in only 15 subjects, with the biting reflex being elicited most frequently. (Reflex biting is quite different from voluntary biting.) These results are at variance with those reported in Sheppard's original study in which the most frequent reflex was that of mouth opening and 84 percent of the subjects overall displayed abnormal oral reflex patterns. Both studies agreed, however, in finding that the number of subjects presenting primitive oral reflexes decreased with age from 5 to 25 years.

Speech proficiency was measured in the Love et al. (1980) study by means of a rating scale and a speech articulation test designed for use with cerebral palsied children. When subjects were divided into two groups on the basis of feeding proficiency, it was found that these two groups differed significantly in speech performance as assessed by both the rating scale and the articulation test. No significant relationship was found, however, between speech proficiency and oral reflex behavior. Taken together, these findings would appear to support Ingram's (1962) study in which he asserted that spontaneous feeding behavior has greater diagnostic and prognostic importance for the development of speech than does persistence of infantile oral reflexes.

Love and co-workers (1980) cautioned that although dysphagic subjects in general tended to have lower speech proficiency scores, the assumption should not be made that severe involvement of the oral musculature is the basis for both dysphagia and dysarthria or anarthria. Lack of speech may be associated with cognitive as well as oral motor deficits. Also, the occurrence of dysphagic symptoms does not necessarily predict with certainty the presence of dysarthria. The results of their study rather indicated possible independence or partial independence of speech and feeding.

Voice and resonance characteristics may also be affected in dysarthric individuals. Netsell (1969) has observed that velopharyngeal dysfunction with associated hypernasality of speech has a high frequency of occurrence in major clinical types of cerebral palsy. It is also found in children recovering from closed head trauma. Voice problems in both the cerebral palsied and the head-injured child may include weak, breathy voice, hoarse voice, and difficulty in initiating and/or sustaining phonation. Associated problems are abnormalities of rhythm and intonation of speech.

Sensory Deficits

Dysarthria in children, as in adults, is a sensorimotor problem. In the 1960s a number of studies concerned with oral sensory deficits concurred in indicating that such deficits play a role in the speech performance of the cerebral palsied. Oral tactile and oral stereognostic abilities both appeared to be implicated. Dato (1976) reported that recovery of oral somesthetic abilities was associated with speech improvement in a dysarthric youth recovering from a gunshot wound. In contrast, children with developmental articulation disorders do not show oral tactile or oral stereognostic deficits. In practice it is very difficult, however, to separate the effects of motor and sensory components of dysarthria. In addition, as Bishop, Ringel & House (1973) have concluded from a study of profoundly hearing-impaired children, oral stereognostic deficits may in some cases result from the failure of normal speech acquisition rather than giving rise to this failure.

Case Study

R. C., the only child of older parents, was born by caesarean section and was cyanotic at birth. A blood transfusion was considered necessary because of an RH incompatibility of mother and infant. Her sucking was weak in the neonatal period. Early development was relatively normal, however. She sat at 6 months, walked at 18 months, and was toilet trained at 2 years. Speech and language were somewhat delayed, but she was producing short, intelligible sentences by 3 years of age. At $4\frac{1}{2}$ years she began to fall a great deal and to run awkwardly. Seizures were suspected but not confirmed. Speech articulation defects were observed (it is not clear whether these represented a deterioration in speech motor skills or persisted from an earlier developmental period and became unacceptable when she entered nursery school). She became dysphonic, stuttered for a time, and gradually withdrew from social contacts, even avoiding eye contact and speaking only with her parents. They, in turn, became oversolicitous and very protective of her.

Her hearing was normal. She was found to be mildly to moderately retarded but eventually learned to read and write at a third-grade level. At 5 years of age, as her speech and voice became more markedly defective, a diagnosis of emotional disorder was suggested. However, her gait became increasingly abnormal, characterized by flexion of the lower limbs and "prancing" steps. Her speech and voice deteriorated until at $8\frac{1}{2}$ years she was completely aphonic, speaking only in a hoarse breathy whisper.

At 20 years of age, when first seen by the author, she could no longer whisper or produce recognizable articulatory movements for single-word production without a voice or breath source. Attempts to produce single syllables silently were attended by grimacing, tension in the shoulders, and head extension. A diagnosis of dystonia was finally confirmed. Bilateral involvement of the pyramidal tract and extrapyramidal rigidity were suggested.

On oral examination, it was found that R. C. had somewhat restricted lateral movement of the tongue, especially to the right. Downward movement of the tongue and voluntary opening of the mouth resulted in deviation of the mandible to the left. Lip movement appeared to be weak and she had difficulty in closing the lips firmly or keeping them closed. In spite of good movement of the soft palate and a brisk gag reflex, nasal emission was noted when she attempted to build up air pressure in the mouth, e.g., for producion of /pa/ and /da/. Diadochokinetic rates for movement of the tongue and lips (without voice) were below normal. Oral stereognosis appeared to be within normal limits.

Involuntary opening of the mouth and difficulty in closing it was first observed in her early 20s; thus chewing became impossible and feeding difficult. Treatment was principally in the form of drug therapies, although biofeedback (in the form of electromyographic (EMG) information) was tried unsuccessfully to facilitate mouth closing. She was taught some sign language but eventually used typing with the aid of a portable communication device in communicating with family members and others.

Assessment of dysarthria in children has not, until recently, made use of instrumentation to the same extent as in the case of adults. Techniques such as EMG, fiberoptics, and cineradiography are still considered to be too hazardous or unjustifiably invasive. Instrumental procedures such as palatography, measures of respiration and bite-block speaking, however, should be considered for use with children. Ultrasound may provide a useful approach to assessment in the future.

ASSESSMENT OF DYSARTHRIA

The first task in assessment of dysarthria in children is to determine the extent and nature of the speech impairment. It is important to assess the intelligibility of the child's speech, both to persons who are familiar with the child and to those who are not. In addition, the patterns of speech produced by the child should be assessed from an acoustic and a phonetic point of view. Phonetic analysis may provide the input to an analysis of the phonologic rule system employed by the child. Such an analysis may help differentiate children with dyspraxia or delayed development of speech (dyslalia) from those with dysarthria. If the child is not yet capable of speech, an inventory of the sounds that he or she is capable of producing should be derived in relation to the situational contexts in which they are produced and also their phonatory contexts (reactive vocalization, babbling, single-syllable production, etc.). It may be helpful in the case of the nonspeaking child to estimate the level of prespeech development of vocalization.

Secondly, the articulatory movements that the child employs should be studied. Much may be inferred about articulatory movement patterns from phonatory and acoustic analyses on the basis of what is known about articulatory–acoustic conversion in speech. Studies of the movements of speech per se, however, may provide information not otherwise obtainable. Studies of speech should include evaluation of voice and resonance characteristics, the prosodic aspects of speech, and the articulation of individual consonant and vowel sounds.

Studies of feeding behavior, primitive oral reflexes, voluntary nonspeech movements, and oral sensory capabilities may also be of great value. The results of such studies, however, should be interpreted in relation to the information obtained about the child's patterns of speech in standardized testing and observation. For example, lack of lip closure in feeding and drooling needs to be interpreted in relation to the child's ability to produce vowels with lip rounding and bilabial consonants. These studies may help identify children with dysarthria and may also indicate to what extent and in what manner different speech subsystems are affected.

Intelligibility

Intelligibility of speech may be assessed by means of a simple rating scale applied to the child's spontaneous speech such as that employed by Sheppard (1964), by more complicated psychophysical methods, or by having a group of listeners transcribe the child's attempt to read aloud or to imitate a set of words, phrases, or sentences. The listeners may be family members or naive or trained listeners who do not know the child. It is likely that all listeners will have less difficulty in transcribing phrases or sentences produced by the mildly dysarthric child than in transcribing single words, which by definition lack linguistic context. Parents who are able to understand a great deal of the spontaneous speech produced by their dysarthric child are frequently surprised at the difficulty they experience in transcribing single-word attempts of these same children.

Speech Proficiency

The child's speech proficiency must also be assessed in terms of accuracy of production of consonants and vowels in word and in phrase contexts. A standardized articulation test may be employed for this purpose. If the child is unable to name many pictures, a nonstandard approach may be necessary, e.g., the use of imitation or rote sentence-completion tasks. Nonsense syllables in repeated series or in unconstrained syllable production tasks may be included as well as words and phrases. The dysarthric child, unlike the dyspraxic child, is likely to show consistent error patterns on these tests.

Phonologic analyses of the child's speech should be employed in order to determine the rules for production of consonants and vowels in different contexts that the child employs. The results of phonologic analyses must be interpreted, however, in relation to the constraints that are imposed by the child's defective motor control system and not necessarily as reflecting the dysarthric child's level of knowledge of the phonologic system of the language spoken in his or her environment, as would be the case for the child with developmental delay in speech acquisition (i.e., the dyslalic child).

Acoustic analyses may be helpful as an aid or supplement to listener judgments (Kent & Netsell, 1975) and may reveal the fact that the dysarthric child has mastered some but not all of the fine motor aspects of particular articulatory contrasts, e.g., vowel duration before final voiced and voiceless stops. In addition, acoustic analysis may yield objective measures of such aspects as duration of articulatory events, fundamental frequency, and vowel formants, which may complement listener judgments of such features or provide indices of particular deficits or of progress made over time that are not available from listener judgments alone. Acoustic measurements are useful in analyzing vocalizations at a prespeech level. For example, they will confirm the presence of immaturities of control of phonation such as pitch breaks or subharmonic breaks and will provide measures of these phenomena; they also enable the speech pathologist to determine whether the child is capable of such skills as controlling pitch and intensity independently of one another.

Measurement of Articulatory Gestures

Articulatory movements may be studied by unaided direct observation or observation of cinephotographic data, and by more sophisticated techniques such as EMG, cineradiography, videofluorscopy, palatography, and ultrasound. With these techniques, which are not yet widely used, gestures not visible to the observer may be recorded and subjected to study. By means of videofluoroscopy, for example, velopharyngeal functioning during speech may be observed and the presence, extent, and dimensions of aperture at the velopharyngeal port during production of nonnasal sounds may be determined. Such measures may be helpful in planning for the use of a palatal prosthesis. EMG measurements may enable the speech pathologist to examine in greater detail the timing of gestures of lip, jaw, and/or tongue in the production of specified syllables in relation to one another. The use of the sophisticated National Microbeam X-Ray Facility at the University of Wisconsin, in all probability, will not be employed with children for some time. Techniques involving ultrasound, however, appear promising for the study of speech articulation and are likely to pose fewer hazards than conventional radiologic procedures. Other measures of movements associated with speech may be obtained by means of strain gauges placed on the chest wall or the mandible, plethysmography, and devices for measuring airflow and pressure. A summary of the aspects of vocalization or speech production that should be evaluated in the nonspeaking child and in the child with defective speech is provided in Table 6-1.

Table 6-1

Guidelines for Evaluation of Speech Motor Abilities in Children by Means of Standard Observation Procedures

Speech motor/vocal abilities: nonspeaking child
  Phonation
    Crying
    Laughing
    Quasiresonant nuclei (grunts, sighs)
    Vocant (vowel-like sounds) production
    Latency to onset of voluntary phonation
    Voice quality
  Consonantal sound production
    Primitive closants (consonant-like sounds)
    Sustained closants
    Ability to superimpose sustained closants on phonation
    Opening and closing
      Smooth transitions open to closed sounds with phonation
      Stop production
      Fricative production
    Ability to vary closant production
  Vocalic sound production
    Presence of mid and low front vocants
    Glides
    Production of high front and low back vocants
    Lip-rounding
    Diphthongs
  Pitch and intensity
    Variation in vocal effort
    High pitch
    Pitch breaks, extreme pitch glides
    Smooth pitch contours, high pitch
    Smooth pitch contours, normal pitch
    Smooth contours superimposed upon syllable production
    Independent variation of pitch and intensity
Speech motor abilities: speaking child
  Phonatory mechanism
    Valving efficiency
    Counting sustained phoneme production (S/Z)
      Number of seconds on 1 breath
  Vocal intensity
    Soft or loud
    Aphonic breaks
  Habitual pitch
    High or low
    Pitch breaks

(continued)

Table 6-1 (*continued*)

Prosody
  Increased or decreased rate
  Poor phrasing or inappropriate pauses
  Reduced intonation contours
  Reduced or inappropriate stress
Vocal quality
  Hoarse
  Harsh
  Strained
  Breathy noise (diplophonia glottal fry)
Resonance
  Hypernasal/hyponasal
  Nasal emission
  Short
    Minimal contrast word pairs
      bake/make
      mad/man
    Oral/nasal resonance phrases
      buy baby a bib
      make more money
Consonant production (rapid alternating speech movements)
  Diadochokinetic rates (per 5 sec; see Fletcher, 1972)
    Sequential ordering
    Phoneme selection accuracy
    Relative impairments of articulator movement
    Uneven loudness, pitch, or rate

	Trials	Mean	Observations
/pə/*	1 2 3		
/tə/*			
/kə/*			
/hə/			
/pətə/			
/təkə/			
/pətəkə/			

  Word repetitions
    Sequential ordering
    Phoneme selection accuracy
    Relative impairments of articulator movement; uneven loudness, pitch
    buddy
    Debbie
    doggy
    getting
    taco

(continued)

Table 6-1 (*continued*)

tiger
Becky
kitty

butterfly
buttercup
puppydog
umbrella

peanut butter
television
dictionary

refrigerator
Unconstrained syllable production (child produces model sequences, if
  possible, with use of visual feedback device)
Rate
Prosody
Diversity of syllables

* Greater than age 6: 4 sec; less than age 6: 3 sec.

Assessment of Oral Motor Abilities

The assessment of the oral motor abilities involved in feeding and in
producing voluntary nonspeech movements should be carried out with
the purpose of obtaining as much information about the motor subsystems involved in speaking as possible. For example, the motor subsystems involved in tongue movement may be assessed by asking the child
to raise the tip of the tongue to the upper lip several times in succession,
to produce a series of tongue clicks, or to lick an ice cream cone.

Assessment of feeding may be made by direct observation, with the
aid of cinephotography, and/or by videofluoroscopy or other imaging techniques. The approach to assessment should be as standard as possible and
repeated measurements should be obtained in order to estimate their
reliability. Clinically, the approach proposed by Love and colleagues
(1980) appears useful. For the prespeech infant, the rating scales proposed by Morris (1980) may prove instructive. Nutritive and nonnutritive
sucking should both be examined. For both infant or preschool child and
the older child, it is important to examine lip closure, lateral as well as
anterior posterior tongue movements, and the degree to which movements of tongue and jaw occur independently of one another.

In the assessment of primitive oral reflexes, the manner of elicitation should be as standard as possible (see Sheppard, 1964), and replications should be carried out at intervals long enough to ensure that short-term desensitization will not affect the results (Love et al., 1980). In addition, the child should be observed in naturally occurring feeding situations and during spontaneous speech. If jaw extension (mouth opening) or tongue protrusion–retraction is observed during speech, the circumstances under which they occur should be carefully noted.

In the study of voluntary nonspeech movements, the two sides of the face should be compared. Unilateral paresis of the face or of the tongue is not likely to impair speech production unless it is combined with other lesions. Its presence in a dysarthric child may suggest a mixed lesion affecting one or more subsystems.

Strength of movement of lips, tongue, and jaw may also be estimated bilaterally by opposing direction of movement. Different voluntary nonspeech movements may be sequenced as in the tests developed by Yoss and Darley (1974). Such tests may be influenced by comprehension of spoken instructions or, if the movements are produced in imitation of the examiner, by visual attention or visual memory. Ojemann (1983) has developed a procedure for use with adults in which the movement sequences to be carried out are presented in the form of a series of pictures, each picture representing a required gesture from the sequence. Stark (in preparation) has developed a test for children based on a similar approach. Each picture in a series represents a nonspeech sound or gesture that the child must produce. In addition, the pictures in the series are linked by a story line (e.g., in a three-picture sequence the same child is pictured drinking soda from a glass, making an appreciative sound, then smiling).

Cognitive and Linguistic Assessment

Cognitive and linguistic assessment should not be aimed primarily at obtaining an intelligence quotient (IQ) or age-related language score. Instead, the objective should be to determine the child's strengths and weaknesses in the auditory and visual modalities. As far as is possible, these two modalities should be assessed independently of one another. An information processing approach may be adopted and abilities assessed within an hypothesized hierarchy ranging from simple association of stimuli with one another, to discrimination of simple stimuli, to integration of stimuli into complex wholes and the ability to recognize parts and wholes, and finally to the ability to derive concepts from perceptual input and to integrate concepts with one another. Attention and memory must also be assessed.

It has sometimes been concluded that because the severely motorically disabled child is unable to explore the environment, he or she cannot be in a position to form concepts about events and objects in the environment. On the contrary, these children may develop higher-level cognitive and linguistic abilities in spite of their motor handicap. These abilities may be as important for speech acquisition as speech motor abilities per se.

Because of their severe motor handicaps, however, it is not possible for many dysarthric children to respond in a standard manner on cognitive or linguistic tests. It is therefore important to develop reliable and valid approaches to assessment in these areas that are nonstandard. Parents' reports should be considered carefully in deciding the response(s) to be elicited. Time limits may have to be extended, repetition of items employed, the child's attention specifically directed, and nonstandard test formats developed. Hypotheses should be developed and tested carefully in relation to the child's abilities. Unusual but isolated skills (the so-called splinter skills), such as pattern matching or word recognition, that have not been integrated into the child's conceptual framework should be identified, and overoptimistic assessments of the child's abilities based on observation of such splinter skills should be corrected.

Case Study

B. T., an 11-year-old boy, presented with mild obesity and a severe developmental speech motor problem. His speech was largely unintelligible to persons outside the immediate family. His hearing was normal and his full-scale IQ as measured by the WISC-R (1974) was 73 (verbal IQ, 72; performance IQ, 79). His reading and mathematical abilities were at a first-grade level; his drawing and handwriting were considered to be very poor.

Birth and neonatal histories were normal. Gross motor milestones were mildly delayed and fine motor skills were impaired. B. T. showed a mild delay in acquiring chewing in infancy. He was first able to dress himself at 5–6 years of age and did not begin to tie his shoe laces until he was 9 years of age. He presented as pleasant and easygoing but was subject to severe temper tantrums and destructive behavior at home. These outbursts occurred when he was teased about his speech by his family. His mother was best able to understand him, although his siblings (two brothers and one sister) were reported as able to follow much of what he said also. He was protected by his mother who spent much of her time reading to him, interpreting for him, and providing him with support. His dependence on his mother and his poor speech yielded the impression of infantilization.

On neurodevelopmental examination, cranial nerves were found to be intact. Motor strength and tone were normal. Mild choreiform movements were observed when arm extension had to be maintained. Sequencing of finger movements in a finger opposition task was poor and was accompanied by mirror movements on the opposite side. Finger opposition was poorest on the left, and dysdiadochokinesis was observed on the left. Overflow (mirroring) movements were present on the nontest side on both of these tasks. Performance on a finger identification task was poor bilaterally.

B. T.'s receptive age-related language scores ranged from a 5- to 8-year level. His auditory memory for digits was at a 3-year level only. Expressive language capabilities were estimated to be at a 3-year level.

Oral structures were within normal limits. Vegetative (feeding) movements of tongue and lips were within normal limits also. Sequenced oral volitional movements were performed with difficulty. Performance on this task was more accurate after verbal instruction than in response to demonstration by the examiner. Involuntary movements of the tongue were observed when the tongue was maintained in a protruded position, but these were gross choreiform movements, not those of fasciculation. Oral stereognosis was poor.

Intensive speech training over an extended period resulted in little improvement. B. T., therefore, was accepted into an experimental training program in which models of speech production and feedback of his attempts to match them were provided in the form of real-time visual spectrographic displays. He enjoyed this training and learned to produce a small set of words and phrases correctly with the aid of the visual displays. Once learned, these materials could be reproduced accurately without the aid of the displays. The articulatory skills acquired in specific contexts did not generalize to the production of other words or phrases. It was observed, however, that he could imitate new materials more accurately after training than before. With further specialized training, it might have been possible to improve his speech to a greater extent. However, since he came from a distant rural area, an extended period of training could not be arranged in his community. Instead, the decision was made to teach him sign language as a supplement to speech communication. Resources were available in his community for this purpose.

TREATMENT OF DYSARTHRIA IN CHILDREN

Over the past 40 years different approaches to the treatment of dysarthria in children have enjoyed popularity. In the 1940s and 1950s traditional approaches to speech therapy were employed. These included "exercises" to strengthen the muscles of speech, relaxation to reduce excessive tone where present, passive movement of the articulators and attempts to facilitate auditory–vocal learning. Little awareness of the need to address different subsystems of the speech motor system with different therapeutic techniques was evident. In the 1960s and 1970s, the neurodevelopmental approach came to be widely accepted. This approach stressed the importance of reflex inhibiting postures and of inculcation of normal feeding patterns as a basis for speech development. As we have seen, however, speech movements make use of neural circuits not employed in oral feeding patterns. Insufficient attention was paid to the identification of developmental sequences in prespeech soundmaking or to the facilitation of these sequences. Therefore such an approach may have only limited success in facilitating speech.

More recently, the use of augmentative communication systems has been stressed (see Blackstone, chapter 7). These systems (e.g., communication boards, sign language and synthetic speech) tend often to supplant rather than to augment speech that has low intelligibility, at least in certain communicative situations. Insufficient attention is frequently paid to speech improvement or facilitation when a communication system is recommended.

Each of these approaches to intervention has a contribution to make to the management of dysarthric children. In addition, however, attention should be paid to the normal sequence of development of speech and of prespeech soundmaking, and to its facilitation. Additional strategies should also be considered, including (1) the use of visual feedback, generated either in the form of displays of the acoustic features of speech or, at least in older children, of electromyographic data, (2) the use of palatal and other prostheses, and (3) the use of delayed auditory feedback or of simultaneous presentation through headphones of an auditory model and the child's own attempts to reproduce that model. If the child has an acquired dysarthria and is in a period of recovery, different strategies may have to be considered in different stages of recovery. In these, as in all cases, treatment should be based upon a careful, ongoing assessment of speech.

SUMMARY

Dysarthria in children needs to be differentiated from dyspraxia and from a developmental delay in the acquisition of speech articulation skills or dyslalia. It is traditionally believed that children with dysarthria will show difficulty in producing both vegetative or involuntary movements, such as those involved in feeding, as well as voluntary movements, particularly speech movements. The central motor control circuits in the nervous system for voluntary movements are quite different from those for reflexive movements. Peripheral closed-loop systems may be more important for feeding than for speech, even though some portions of a final common pathway are shared.

Dyspraxic children, on the other hand, are believed to have difficulty in sequencing voluntary oral movements, especially those of speech, but to have unimpaired oral vegetative movements. It is important, therefore, to assess the ability to sequence volitional oral movements in children with speech motor disorders, and to compare performance on such a task with that demonstrated on feeding skills (licking, biting, chewing, sucking, etc.) and in other vegetative activity.

Identification of dysarthria in children also requires that a careful assessment of speech proficiency and intelligibility be carried out. Differences in speech patterns are likely to be found in dysarthric, dyslalic, and dyspraxic children. Consistency of error patterns, for example, will often be greater for dysarthric than for dyspraxic children. Vowels will be more often correct than consonants in dysarthric children. Error patterns will less frequently be attributable to a lack of knowledge of the phonological rule system of the language.

In assessment of the dysarthric child, each of the subsystems involved in control of speech (i.e., those controlling movements of the lips, tongue and palate) should be examined separately. Cinematography and acoustic analysis of the speech signal may provide useful information with respect to these movements, but other techniques (e.g., use of bite blocks, ultrasound, and even electromyography) should be considered, at least with older children. Attempts should also be made to determine to what extent oral sensation may be reduced or abnormal in the affected children.

The approach to treatment should be based upon the results of careful assessment. A variety of approaches should be considered, including the use of an augmentative system for children whose speech is unintelligible to the naive listener. Even for those children whose repertoire is limited, the use of vocalization for the purposes of communication should be encouraged.

REFERENCES

Abbs, J. H. (1981). Neuromotor mechanisms of speech production. In J. K. Darby, Jr. (Ed.), *Speech evaluation in medicine.* New York: Grune & Stratton.

Abbs, J. H., & Cole, K. (1982). Consideration of bulbar and suprabulbar afferent influences upon speech motor control coordination and programming. In S. Grillner, B. Lindblom, J. Lubker, & A. Persson (Eds.), *Speech motor control.* New York: Pergamon Press.

Abbs, J. H., Hunker, C. J., & Barlow, S. M. (1983). Differential speech motor subsystem impairments with suprabulbar lesions: Neurophysiological framework and supporting data. In W. Berry (Ed.), *Clinical Dysarthria.* San Diego: College-Hill Press.

Aronson, A. E. (1981). Motor speech signs of neurologic disease. In J. K. Darby, Jr. (Ed.), *Speech evaluation in medicine.* New York: Grune & Stratton.

ASHA. (1980). Nonspeech communication: A Position paper. Ad Hoc Committee on Communication Processes and Nonspeaking Persons. *ASHA, 22,* 267–272.

Batshaw, M. L., & Haslam, R. H. A. (1976). Multidisciplinary management of dystonia misdiagnosed as hysteria. In R. Eldridge & S. Fahn (Eds.), *Advances in neurology Vol. 14.* New York: Raven Press.

Bishop, M. E., Ringel, R. E., & House, A. S. (1973). *Journal of Speech and Hearing Research, 16,* 257–266.

Bosma, J. F. (1975). Anatomic and physiologic development of the speech apparatus. In D. B. Tower (Ed.), *The nervous system. Vol. 3: Human communication and its disorders.* New York: Raven Press.

Bosma, J. F., Truby, H. M., & Lind, J. (1965). Studies of neonatal transition: Correlated cineradiographic and visual-acoustic observations. In J. Lind (Ed.), *Newborn infant cry.* Uppsala, Sweden: Almquist & Wiksells.

Brown, J. K. (1984). Disorders of speech. In J. O. Forfar (Ed.), *Textbook of paediatrics.* London: Churchill Livingstone.

Byrne, M. C. (1959). Speech and language development of athetoid and spastic children. *Journal of Speech and Hearing Disorders, 24,* 231–240.

Colton, R. H., & Steinschneider, A. (1980). Acoustic relationships of infant cries to the Sudden Infant Death Syndrome. In T. Murry and J. Murry (Eds.), *Infant Communication: Cry and Early Speech.* San Diego: College-Hill Press.

Cruikshank, W. M. (Ed.). (1976). *Cerebral palsy: A developmental disability* (3rd revised ed.). Syracuse, NY: Syracuse University Press.

Dato, D. P. (1976). Distinctive feature analysis of the speech of a head-injured, dysarthric child. Unpublished masters thesis, Georgetown University School of Languages and Linguistics, Washington, DC.

Deecke, L., Scheid, P., & Kornhuber, H. H. (1969). Distribution of readiness potential, pre-motion positivity, and motor potential of the human cerebral cortex preceding voluntary finger movements. *Experimental Brain Research, 7,* 158–168.

Delong, M. R. (1974). Motor functions of the basal ganglia: Single-unit activity during movement. In F. O. Schmitt & F. G. Worden (Eds.), *The neurosciences; Third study program.* Cambridge, MA: MIT Press.

Dore, J., Franklin, M. B., Miller, R. T., & Ramer, A. L. H. (1976). Transitional phenomena in early language acquisition. *Journal of Child Language, 3,* 13–28.

Dubner, R., Sessle, B., & Storey, A. (1978). *The neural basis of oral and facial functions.* New York: Plenum Press.

Eccles, J. C., Ito, M., & Szentagothai, J. (1967). *The cerebellum as a neuronal machine.* New York: Springer.

Espir, M. L. E., & Rose, F. C. (1970). *The basic neurology of speech.* Philadelphia: F. A. Davis.

Froeschels, E. (1943). A contribution to the pathology and therapy of dysarthria due to certain cerebral lesions. *Journal of Speech Disorders, 8,* 301–321.

Fletcher, S. G. (1972). Time-by-count measurement of diadochokinetic syllable rate. *Journal of Speech and Hearing Research, 15,* 763–770.

Ghez, C., & Fahn, S. (1981). The cerebellum. In E. R. Kandel & J. H. Schwartz (Eds.), *Principles of neuroscience*. New York: Elsevier/North-Holland.

Gualtieri, C. T., & Hawk, B. (1980). Tardiue dyskinesia and other drug-induced movement disorders among handicapped children and youth. *Applied Research in Mental Retardation, 1,* 55–69.

Heinz, J. M., Stark, R. E., Condino, R., & Hege, M. Acoustic analysis of cry of SIDS infants. *Journal of the Acoustical Society of America, 74,* S102–103.

Hixon, T., & Hardy, J. (1964). Restricted motility of the speech articulators in cerebral palsy. *Journal of Speech and Hearing Disorders, 29,* 293–306.

Huntingdon, D. A., Harris, K. S., Shankweiler, D., & Sholes, G. N. (1967). Some observations on monosyllable production by deaf and dysarthric speakers. *Status Report on Speech Research, 10,* 6.1–6.23.

Ingram, T. T. S. (1962). Clinical significance of the infantile feeding reflexes. *Developmental Medicine and Child Neurology, 4,* 159–169.

Irwin, O. C. (1955). Phonetic speech development in cerebral palsied children. *American Journal of Physical Medicine, 34,* 325–334.

Jurgens, V., & Von Cramon, D. (1982). On the role of the anterior cingulate cortex in phonation. A case report. *Brain and Language, 15,* 234–248.

Kandel, E. R., & Schwartz, J. H. (1981). *Principles of neural science.* New York: Elsevier/North-Holland.

Kant, R., & Netsell, R. (1975). A case study of an ataxic dysarthric: Cinefluoroscopic and spectrographic observations. *Journal of Speech and Hearing Disorders, 40,* 52–71.

Klahr, D. (1978). Open peer commentary on C. J. Brainerd's "The stage question in cognitive-developmental theory." *Behavioral Brain Sciences, 1,* 191–192.

Langlois, A., & Baken, R. J. (1976). Development of respiratory time factors in infant cry. *Developmental Medicine and Child Neurology, 18,* 732–737.

Lencione, R. M. (1953). A study of the speech sound ability and intelligibility status of a group of educable cerebral palsied children. Unpublished dissertation, Northwestern University, Chicago.

Lieberman, P. (1967). *Intonation, perception and language.* Cambridge, MA: MIT Press.

Love, R. J., Hagerman, E. L., & Taimi, E. G. (1980). Speech performance, dysphagia and oral reflexes in cerebral palsy. *Journal of Speech and Hearing Disorders, 45,* 59–75.

MacNeilage, P., Rootes, T., & Chase, R. A. (1967). Speech production and perception in a patient with severe impairment of somesthetic perception and motor control. *Journal of Speech and Hearing Research, 10,* 449–467.

Milner, E. (1976). CNS maturation and language acquisition. In H. Whitaker & H. A. Whitaker (Eds.), *Studies in neurolinguistics Vol. 1.* New York: Academic Press.

Morris, S. E. (1982). The normal acquisition of oral feeding skills: Implications for assessment and treatment. In M. M. Palmer (Ed.), New York: Therapeutic Media, Inc.

Mountcastle, V. B. (1978). An organizing principle for cerebral function: The unit module and the distributed system. In G. Edelman & V. B. Mountcastle (Eds.), *The mindful brain.* Cambridge, MA: MIT Press.

Mueller, H. A. (1972). Facilitating feeding and pre-speech. In P. H. Pearson & C.

E. Williams (Eds.), *Physical therapy services in the developmental disabilities.* Springfield, IL: Charles C. Thomas.

Muller-Preuss, P. (1978). Single unit responses of the auditory cortex in the squirrel monkey to self-produced and loudspeaker transmitted vocalizations. *Neuroscience Letters,* (Suppl. 1), S7.

Munger, B. L. (1973). The cytology and ultrastructure of sensory receptors in the adult and newborn primate tongue. In J. F. Bosma (Ed.), *Fourth symposium on oral sensation and perception.* Bethesda, MD: US Department of Health, Education, and Welfare.

Mysak, E. (1963). Dysarthria and oropharyngeal reflexology: A review. *Journal of Speech and Hearing Disorders, 28,* 252–260.

Netsell, R., Kent, R., & Abbs, J. (1978). *Adjustments of the tongue and lips to fixed jaw positions during speech: A preliminary report.* Paper presented to the Conference on Speech Motor Control, University of Wisconsin, Madison.

Netsell, R. (1981). The acquisition of speech motor control: A perspective with directions for research. In R. E. Stark (Ed.), *Language behavior in infancy and early childhood.* New York: Elsevier/North-Holland.

Newman, J. D. (in press). The infant cry of primates: An evolutionary perspective. In B. M. Lester & C. F. Z. Boukydis (Eds.), *Infant crying: Theoretical and research perspectives.* New York: Plenum Press.

Ojemann, G. (1983). Interrelationships in the brain organization of language-related behaviors: Evidence from electrical stimulation mapping. In U. Kirk (Ed.), *Neuropsychology of language reading and spelling.* New York: Academic Press.

Peiper, A. (1963). *Cerebral function in infancy and childhood.* New York: Consultants Bureau.

Penfield, W., & Roberts, L. (1959). *Speech and brain management.* Princeton, NJ: Princeton University Press.

Ploog, D. (1979). Phonation, emotion, cognition, with reference to the brain mechanisms involved. *Ciba Foundation Symposium 69.*

Precthl, H., & Beintema, D. (1965). *The neurological examination of the full-term newborn infant.* London: Heinemann.

Rappaport, J. L. (1972). Normal psychological development in the absence of oral and body surface sensation: A case report. In J. F. Bosma (Ed.), *Third symposium on oral sensation and perception: The mouth of the infant.* Springfield, IL: Charles C. Thomas.

Ringel, R. L., & Steer, M. D. (1963). Some effects of tactile and auditory alterations on speech output. *Journal of Speech and Hearing Research, 6,* 369–378.

Sazaki, C. T., Levine, P. A., Laitman, J. T., & Crelin, E. S. (1977). Postnatal descent of the epiglottis in man. *Archives of Otolaryngology, 103,* 169–171.

Sheppard, J. J. (1964). Cranio-oropharyngeal motor patterns associated with cerebral palsy. *Journal of Speech and Hearing Research, 7,* 373–380.

Stark, R. E. (1980a). Prespeech segmental feature development. In. P. Fletcher & M. Garman (Eds.), *Studies in language acquisition.* Cambridge, MA: Cambridge University Press.

Stark, R. E. (1980b). Stages of speech development in the first year of life. In G. H. Yenikomshian, J. F. Kavanagh, & C. A. Ferguson (Eds.), *Child phonology Vol. 1: Production.* New York: Academic Press.

Stark, R. E., Rose, S. N., & McLagen, M. (1976). Features of infant sound: The first eight weeks of life. *Journal of Child Language, 2,* 205–221.

Stark, R. E., & Schultz, N. (submitted for publication). Temporal pattern of cry in infants.

Thach, W. T., Jr. (1980). The cerebellum. In V. B. Mountcastle (Ed.), *Medical physiology Vol. 1* (14th ed.). St. Louis: C.V. Mosby.

Wasz-Hockert, O., Lind, J., Vuorenkoski, V., Partanen, T. J., & Valane, E. (1968). *The Infant Cry. Clinics in Developmental Medicine 29.* New York: Heine-mann.

Weiffenbach, J., & Thach, B. (1973). Elicited tongue movements: Touch and tests in the newborn human. In J. F. Bosma (Ed.), *Fourth symposium on oral sensation and perception: Development in the fetus and infant* (Report DHEW 73-S46). Superintendent of Documents. Washington, DC.

Westlake, H. (1951). Muscle training for cerebral palsied speech cases. *Journal of Speech and Hearing Disorders, 16,* 105–109.

Wilder, G. N., & Baken, R. J. (1974). Respiratory patterns in infant cry. *Human Communication, 3,* 18–34.

Zlatin, M. A. (1972). Development of speech, language, auditory and oral functions in the presence of congenital sensory neuropathy. In J. F. Bosma (Ed.), *The third symposium on oral sensation and perception: Development in the fetus and infant.* Springfield, IL: Charles C. Thomas.

Sarah W. Blackstone
Michael J. Painter

7
Speech Problems in Multihandicapped Children

The prevalence of speech impairment in the United States is estimated at 3.5 percent of those under 25 years (Fein, 1983). Although speech problems may occur in isolation, they are often secondary to other handicapping conditions: cerebral palsy, mental retardation, craniofacial anomalies, Down's syndrome, pervasive developmental disability/autism, hearing impairment, dysphasia/language disorders, traumatic brain injuries, or a combination of such problems. Other less common conditions associated with speech impairment include genetic, chromosomal, and metabolic disorders, e.g., cri du chat, dystonia musculorum deformans, spina bifida, Treacher Collin's syndrome, Hurler's syndrome, and osteogenesis imperfecta (Batshaw, 1981). This chapter will focus on the management of the speech-impaired child who is multihandicapped.

'Multi-handicapped' means concomitant impairments (such as mentally retarded–blind, mentally retarded–orthopedically impaired, etc.), the combination of which causes such severe educational problems that these children cannot be accommodated in special education programs solely for one of the impairments [Section 121a.5(b) of the Handicapped Act of 1975].

The authors are sincerely grateful to Ann Harris and Rachel E. Stark for their skilled editorial assistance during the preparation of this manuscript.

The prevalence of speech problems in the "multihandicapped" population is difficult to ascertain because so many diagnostic categories are included (see Brown, chap. 5); but according to a government survey (Governmental Affairs Review, 1981), nearly half (47.5 percent) of the children seen by speech–language pathologists in the United States have other primary handicapping conditions. The breakdown is as follows:

Mental retardation	19%
Specific learning disability	17.5%
Hearing impairment	2.8%
Emotional disturbance	2.5%
Orthopedic handicap	2%
Other health impairment	1%
Visual handicap	0.5%
Deaf-blind	0.2%

The epidemiology of multihandicaps in children is twofold: (1) Those with developmentally disabling conditions are children defined with abnormalities "beginning in fetal life or early childhood which precludes or significantly impedes normal physical and/or mental development" (Scheiner & McNabb, 1980). (2) Acquired conditions in children may be secondary to a degenerative process, traumatic injury, stroke, or other problem not present at birth. An acquired disability "originates before age 18, is expected to continue and constitutes a substantial handicap" (Scheiner & McNabb, 1980).

The expertise of one professional is inadequate to address the problems of the speech-impaired child with multiple handicaps (Holm, 1978). A position paper from the American Academy of Pediatrics (1978) agrees, stating that "teamwork is absolutely necessary to look at the whole child in a comprehensive manner." A clinical service delivery system should provide identification, assessment, plans for intervention, and therapeutic management of the child and family (Scheiner & McNabb, 1980). The system should also provide coordination of these services and evaluate their effectiveness over time. A primary role in this process should be assumed by those specifically trained in communication disorders, i.e., audiologists and speech–language pathologists. But successful management of the multihandicapped child with a concomitant speech impairment is an interdisciplinary task requiring the efforts of pediatricians, neurologists, psychologists, psychiatrists, occupational and physical therapists, educators, social workers, nurses, nutritionists, and others, as needed.

The remainder of this chapter will discuss some of the handicapping conditions commonly associated with speech disorders and will present clinical approaches used to identify, assess, and treat the communication problems of multihandicapped children.

DESCRIPTION OF THE PROBLEM

Speech production is a complicated process calling for the integration of respiratory, subglottic, glottic, pharyngeal, and oral movements effected by both smooth and skeletal muscles with complex innervation. In light of this, it is not surprising that the majority of neurologic disorders affect speech (Rood, 1983). The interaction of all movements necessary for speech production demands the functional integrity of the cerebral cortex, basal ganglia, cerebellum, and brainstem. Unfortunately, we are limited in our knowledge of the neuropathophysiology of speech problems in children.

We do know that the primary diagnoses of multihandicapped children are likely to be mental retardation, cerebral palsy, cleft palate, traumatic brain injury, Down's syndrome, and other congenital and acquired disabilities. Speech impairments constitute a diagnosis that is secondary to and often confounded by these primary handicapping conditions. The etiologic factors, then, that limit the child's ability to communicate and to develop expressive language and speech are both complex and numerous. They are as follows:

- Motor problems, e.g., paresis and/or discoordination of muscles involved in articulation, respiration, and phonation
- Sensory deficits, e.g., most commonly hearing impairment; however, increased or decreased oral sensitivity is also observed
- Language problems, e.g., difficulty with symbol acquisition and/or the grammatical and phonemic components of language
- Cognitive, neurologic, and behavioral factors, e.g., attentional and memory deficits, mental retardation, seizures, etc.

As the severity of CNS involvement increases, so does the extent of the handicapping conditions. Simply stated, the greater the damage to the CNS, the greater will be the functional impairment of the child. The pathophysiology of speech impairment in otherwise normal children has not been well described. The problem of description is clearly more complex in the multihandicapped child. The speech pattern will probably be severe and will probably be confounded by other disabilities (e.g., mental retardation). Ongoing collaborative research and clinical studies are required before we can understand the manner in which multiple etiologic factors interact in disrupting speech development. As disorders are classified and the neurophysiology better understood, our assessment and

treatment protocols should improve. A brief review of some multihandi-
capping conditions associated with speech impairment follows.

MENTAL RETARDATION

The largest subgroup of multihandicapped individuals is the mentally retarded subgroup. Mental retardation is defined as subaverage
intellectual functioning with deficits in adaptive behavior and with onset
during the developmental period (Grossman, 1973). The prevalence of
mental retardation in the United States is approximately 3 percent
(Scheiner & McNabb, 1980). The child who is mentally retarded is more
likely than the normal child to have developmental problems that prevent the acquisition of intelligible speech. Many studies have demonstrated that speech impairments are prevalent in mentally retarded children (Everhart, 1953; Healy et al., 1981; Siegel, 1963). Severity of mental
retardation is directly related to the occurrence of speech impairment.
Schlanger (1953) reported that 60 percent of children with intelligence
quotients (IQ) in the mild to borderline range of intelligence had speech
defects, while Sirkin and Lyons (1941) reported 75 percent with speech
defects in the moderate to severe range of intelligence. If one were to
randomly select three children with a diagnosis of severe mental retardation, all would probably have reduced speech intelligibility due to disorders of articulation, fluency, resonance, voice, or prosody. The disordered
processes of speech and language, however, would vary from child to
child, depending more on the child's other handicapping conditions (i.e.,
cerebral palsy, sensory impairment) than on his or her mental retardation.

AUTISM

Childhood autism is a male-dominated developmental disability
with an incidence reported at 4–5/10,000 births (Ritvo & Freeman, 1978).
It is a relatively rare disorder but does occur as often as profound deafness and more often than total blindness (Hinerman, 1983). In a report
submitted by Ritvo and Freeman to the National Society for Autistic
Children and to the American Psychiatric Association, the following
characteristics were described: (1) onset prior to age 30 months; (2) impaired social relationships; (3) failure to develop communication skills;

and (4) abnormal responses to the environment (Fay & Shuler, 1980; Hinerman, 1983).

No single cause for this syndrome has as yet been identified although neurophysiologic factors have been implicated. Most likely, there are several subtypes of the disorder, each with its own etiology (Hinerman, 1983). Ludlow (1983) reported that families of autistic children have an increased incidence of language and speech disorders. She suggests that autism may represent one mode of expression of a larger set of disorders with genetic influence. In addition to genetic factors, viral infections, metabolic disorders, and structural brain damage at or before birth, including brainstem lesions, are all being investigated as causal agents. The most valuable predictors of outcome for autistic individuals are intellectual functioning and speech and language abilities (Eisenberg, 1956; Harper & Williams, 1975; Rutter, 1978). Currently, the prognosis for this population is not favorable.

Autism generally occurs in conjunction with mental retardation with approximately 60 percent of these children classified in the severely retarded range (Ritvo & Freeman, 1978). In fact, the differential diagnosis of autism versus severe to profound mental retardation frequently results in professional controversy. The confusion probably originates from the autistic child's variable profile of development. The ability to learn and manipulate symbols is a relatively weak area among autistic children whereas visual or auditory matching skills may be relatively good. More specifically, we see autistic children in the clinic who can read printed words aloud (i.e., associate visual stimuli and auditory–motor functions) but who have no notion as to what the words mean (i.e., they cannot manipulate symbols in a meaningful way.) Findings support the theory of a central language disorder underlying the syndrome of autism (Prizant, 1983; Prutting, 1979; Wetherby & Gaines, 1982). Autism may be one form of a group of linguistic–cognitive impairments. An attempt is being made to clarify those domains of language functioning that tend to be the most severely impaired and those deficits that are most specific to autism.

It is estimated that nearly 50 percent of autistic children are at least semimute (Fay & Schuler, 1980.) Among autistic people who are verbal, approximately 75 percent are echolalic (Prizant, 1983; Schuler, 1975). Echolalia is defined as the "inappropriate repetition of words, phrases, or sentences previously spoken by others" (Hinerman, 1983). The speech of autistic individuals has been characterized as wooden, empty, parrotlike, and monotonous. The vocal quality of speakers may be hoarse, harsh, or hypernasal. Average pitch may be abnormally high. Poor volume control and guttural noises are common. Because these children rarely are motor impaired, articulation is generally intact (Boucher, 1976).

HEARING IMPAIRMENT

The prevalence of hearing impairment in children from birth to 16 years is estimated at 6.6/1000 for those with a significant bilateral hearing loss and 1.4/1000 for those with a severe to profound sensorineural hearing loss (Schein & Delk, 1974). Recently we have learned that as many as 15 percent of infants with hypoxic–ischemic CNS involvement have significant neurosensory hearing loss, i.e., hearing loss of sufficient severity to give rise to abnormalities of speech acquisition (Bergman, personal communication, 1984). In the cerebral palsied population of children aged birth to 15 years, the incidence of hearing impairment is disproportionately high, i.e., 20 times that found in the "normal population" (Morris, 1973).

Essentially all children with severe to profound hearing impairments will be speech impaired as well. Children with mild to moderate hearing impairment may have speech disorders too, but this depends on the configuration of the hearing loss, management of the problem, and presence of other handicapping conditions. The effects of recurrent bouts of otitis media on hearing and speech development are not yet well documented (Allen & Robinson, 1984). But it is worth noting that many children with neurologic disorders involving the tensor veli–palatini muscles can be expected to have eustachian tube dysfunction that results in chronic infections of the middle ear. Middle ear dysfunction is also observed in essentially all children with cleft palates. The kinds of speech impairments noted in the hearing impaired will depend on the configuration of the audiogram; however, articulation, resonance, and prosodic disorders are common. The child who has a speech problem and a hearing loss will require a habilitation program quite different from that provided to the neurologically impaired child who has a speech problem and normal hearing (Jaffe & Luterman, 1980).

CEREBRAL PALSY

Cerebral palsy is another diagnosis commonly associated with speech problems. The generally accepted definition of cerebral palsy is a "non-progressive disturbance of nervous system function characterized by abnormality of motor function and posture with an often associated aberrant movement disorder" (Eiben & Crocker, 1983). Although the term conveys little in the way of meaningful pathophysiology, the most important concept is that cerebral palsy is a nonprogressive process acquired early in life.

Speech disorders associated with cerebral palsy are primarily those

of pyramidal and extrapyramidal origin. Cerebral palsy usually originates in the perinatal period, most often due to asphyxia or hemorrhage
(Painter, 1984). Asphyxia still occurs in as many as 1 percent of deliv-
eries in modern obstetric units (Mulligan, Painter, & O'Donohue, 1980).
Prolonged partial asphyxia primarily affects the cerebral hemispheres,
but as the lesion progresses, involvement of the basal ganglia also occurs.
Acute total asphyxia results primarily in brainstem pathology (Meyers,
1975). Subependymal hemorrhage with interventricular extension
results in lesions that will extend to the descending corticobulbar pathways as well as the basal ganglia (Painter, 1984). As the subependymal
germinal matrix is the source of neurons and glia essential for neuronal
interconnection, impairment of both speech and language might be expected with this disorder.

The prevalence of cerebral palsy is approximately 2/1000 births
(Paneth & Kiely, 1984). As with the retarded population, children with
cerebral palsy are more likely to be multihandicapped and to have additional problems along with speech disorders. Tablan, as cited by Jones
(1975), reported that 88 percent of patients with cerebral palsy have
three or more disabilities. Among them are cognitive dysfunction, hearing loss, speech and language disorders, and seizures. Deafness is reported in 6–16 percent of those with cerebral palsy, and motor speech
disorders are described in as many as 68 percent of this group (Shapiro,
Palmer, Wachtel, & Capute, 1983).

According to a 1951 study of over 1000 patients in New Jersey
(Hopkins, Bice, and Colton, 1954), the most common "speech problem"
associated with cerebral palsy is dysarthria. Dysarthria was noted in 88.7
percent of the athetoid group (extrapyramidal cerebral palsy) and in 51.9
percent of the spastic group (pyramidal cerebral palsy). Yost and McMillan (1983) report a lower incidence of spastic children with dysarthria (44
percent).

Characteristics of dysarthric speech in cerebral palsy are described
in Chapter 6. Articulation, resonance, vocal quality, and prosody of
speech are affected secondary to primary motor impairment of musculature in the tongue, lips, velopharynx, larynx, rib cage, and diaphragm.

OROFACIAL AND CRANIOFACIAL ANOMALIES

One of every 750 white people in the United States is born with
craniofacial anomalies (McWilliams, Morris, & Shelton, 1984). The highest incidence is among the Japanese at 2.13/1000 (Nell, 1958). Craniofacial anomalies are associated with 154 genetic syndromes that include
clefting of facial structures as one of their features (McWilliams et al.,
1984). Statistics suggest sex differences in this diagnostic category. The

occurrence of cleft lip in males is nearly twice that noted in females (Oka, 1979); however, females compose more than 50 percent of those having isolated cleft palate.

The most common types of speech disorder observed in the cleft palate population are those of nasal resonance and distortions in production of oral consonants due to structural abnormalities and lack of velopharyngeal closure (Wells, 1971). In addition to abnormalities in the size of the velopharyngeal aperture, increased pharyngeal depth and insufficient velar length may affect the ability to achieve closure. Impairment in motor control of the musculature involved in velopharyngeal closure may give rise to speech problems (McWilliams et al., 1984). Articulation problems may occur as a result of structural defects of the lip and palate. Conductive and sensorineural hearing impairment, language problems, and mental retardation are all likely to coexist with oral structural anomalies.

CLINICAL MANAGEMENT OF THE MULTIHANDICAPPED CHILD

Team Approach

Handicapping conditions in children affect the entire family. The social aspects of developmental and acquired disabilities have particular importance for the communicatively impaired because functional independence depends so much on an individual's ability to communicate effectively. Clinical management of the multihandicapped includes the family and involves many professionals as well as local, state, and federal health care agencies and educational systems. Ideally, service delivery is integrated, utilizing available community resources and developing additional services as needed. Professionals who see the multihandicapped must work as a team (Holm, 1978). The role of the team is to identify goals, develop treatment priorities and strategies, and implement treatment procedures and evaluate their effects (Valletutti & Christoplos, 1977). Too many of our graduate programs in health services encourage a narrow discipline-specific focus. Today's professionals need additional training in leadership, case management, and how to function as a member of a team. For most, training is acquired "on the job," although continuing education courses are sometimes available (Jaffe, 1984).

Three major models of service delivery have been developed for implementation with the multihandicapped child: (1) the multidisciplinary team model, (2) the transdisciplinary team model, and (3) the interdisciplinary team model.

The *multidisciplinary team* is composed of professionals with interests and expertise in their particular disciplines and with respect to specific age-groups and diagnostic categories (Hart, 1977). Each has a clearly defined sector of discipline-specific responsibility agreed upon by the team as a whole. Since conflicting professional opinions and recommendations can arise that are difficult for families to handle, case coordination is a critical component of this model.

In the *transdisciplinary team* approach discipline borders are not observed. Skills developed in other health care fields are incorporated into the practice of each professional on the team. As a rule, the transdisciplinary team functions with one team member assuming most of the direct patient contact but obtaining consultation from other disciplines (McCormick & Goldman, 1979). The disadvantage of this model, as it applies to multihandicapped children, is that the specific expertise needed to treat multiple disorders adequately may not be available on a regular basis or may be at an unsophisticated level and therefore ineffective.

An *interdisciplinary team* defines professional roles case by case. Some members assume direct responsibility while others serve consultative roles, depending on the nature of the child's problems and needs at a particular time (Valletutti & Christoplos, 1977). The interdisciplinary team is mandated by P.L. 94-142 and elaborated through regulatory guidelines. Professionals on an interdisciplinary team must be knowledgeable in their own field and must know their discipline's limitations. The interaction of team members from a variety of disciplines is the basis of the interdisciplinary team approach. Some stability should be maintained over time, and this is often provided by the child's pediatrician. The local educational system and/or agencies with expertise in management of multihandicapped children may also offer a continuum of care. In principle, the interdisciplinary model is the most appropriate to the management of multihandicapped, speech-impaired children.

Changing Role of Team

The configuration of the management team will change over a child's life. As children develop, their needs and those of their families change. For example, during the first year or two a child with cerebral palsy may frequently visit the neurologist, pediatrician, and physical and occupational therapists. The focus is likely to be on home management issues such as feeding problems and positioning. Social service professionals may offer support to families after the diagnosis is provided. They may be able to clarify the nature of the child's problems for the family or direct them to available community resources, pertinent legislation, and emotional support groups. In the preschool and school-age years, intervention usually shifts to concerns about mobility, peer relations, communication, and education. The speech–language pathologist and special educator are likely to assume a more primary role. In adolescence, the focus of intervention changes once more. Issues of increased functional independence, prevocational training, adult living arrangements, and activities may again tap the expertise of special educators and speech–language pathologists, but occupational therapists, physical therapists, and vocational rehabilitation counselors become critical to the team as well.

IDENTIFICATION OF SPEECH PROBLEMS IN MULTIHANDICAPPED CHILDREN

Interdisciplinary Assessment

Delayed speech is a common first symptom of mental retardation, language disorders, and hearing impairment. Parents may become concerned about development during their child's first year of life, but physicians often wait to refer a child until after speech has failed to develop. In fact, prognostic statements regarding the potential for speech are difficult to make when the child is young, except in very severe or in very mild handicapping conditions.

Case Study

A 2-year-old child was referred to our clinic by his pediatrician because of delayed speech development. His parents reported that he was reluctant to imitate sounds and often "refused" to comply with their requests, yet they did not question his hearing. Occasionally, he produced a word that was intelligible but more typically he used gestures to communicate. He was reported as unusually "quiet" and as "not babbling much" as an infant. He had no history of eating or drinking problems, but he could not bite an apple, and did not chew meat. His parents and pediatrician wanted to know "why he wasn't talking." Was he retarded? Was he hearing impaired? Was he language delayed? Did he have oral/speech motor dysfunction? Were there contributing environmental factors?

To provide answers to these questions, professionals who are familiar with the problems of multihandicapped children must evaluate the child and discuss their findings. This patient was found to be a child with normal intelligence and hearing sensitivity. He had deficits in production and in understanding of connected language. He demonstrated motor speech discoordination. In addition, he had significant behavioral problems that responded well to behavior modification techniques and to a course of Ritalin.

Prompt establishment of a primary diagnosis in the multihandicapped child is crucial to the management of his or her developmental deficits. High-risk registries, neighborhood clinics, and legislation requiring identification of developmentally disabled children help alert professionals to children at risk for impaired speech development in the first year of life. Early identification of hearing impairment, cerebral palsy, and mental retardation as well as congenital abnormalities such as cleft lip and palate and Down's syndrome is now common. Many centers and agencies specialize in the management of developmentally compromised children. These include United Cerebral Palsy, Easter Seals, and Head Start programs, state-funded educational teams, crippled children's services, university-affiliated programs, and others. A description of evaluation procedures common in the practice of neurology, pediatrics, occupational and physical therapy, psychology, and social work is beyond the scope of this chapter. However, we will review approaches to the speech and language evaluation in relation to the data obtained by these other disciplines.

ASSESSMENT OF SPEECH PROBLEMS IN MULTIHANDICAPPED CHILDREN

The purpose of assessment is to establish a differential diagnosis, define problems, develop treatment goals, and predict the future communication outcomes and needs of the child. In this process it is critical to define accurately and carefully the factors interfering with a child's ability to speak and to communicate. Neurophysiologic factors must be given special consideration in the speech evaluation of multihandicapped children. The presence of bilateral corticospinal tract involvement, for example, must be documented in cases of pseudobulbar palsy. The effects of cranial nerve lesions must be discriminated from those deriving from use of seizure medications. Use of such medications may tend to disrupt cerebellar and extrapyramidal functions and may result in symptom complexes resembling those associated with cranial nerve lesions.

Most severely involved, multihandicapped children are identified as such within the first year of life. Appropriate intervention for these children can begin early. Identification of the problem occurs later for children with mild to moderate delays in communication development. Unfortunately, many parents of speech-delayed children are still told that their child will "outgrow the problem." In our clinical experience, parents who refer their child for a speech and language evaluation usually have legitimate concerns. As a rule, if a child is 2 years old, otherwise normal, and does not speak in short phrases that are intelligible to his parents, a complete audiologic and speech–language evaluation should be scheduled immediately.

Ideally the young child should be evaluated by professionals who have clinical expertise with developmentally young, "difficult to test" children, including those children with severe motor handicaps. The trend is for speech–language pathologists and audiologists to become specialized in their management of this population. Thus, in addition to the traditional clinical training in procedures for evaluation of hearing sensitivity and of speech and language development, professionals need training in the neuropathophysiology of speech problems and in assessment procedures appropriate for the developmentally young as well as the multihandicapped population. These professionals must also be trained in behavioral management and must become familiar with the spectrum of acquired as well as developmental disabilities.

Speech–language pathologists on an interdisciplinary team assess receptive and expressive language (vocabulary, verbal reasoning, grammatical components, connected language, etc.), articulation, oral and speech motor function, vocal parameters, nonspeech modes of communication, communicative functions expressed, and pragmatic and discourse skills. In order to interpret data obtained from a speech and language evaluation, information about the hearing status and cognitive abilities of the child must also be available. When assessing the multihandicapped child, information about medical factors, motor handicaps, seizures, and drug protocols is also critical.

Few norm-referenced measures are currently available to evaluate parameters of language and speech behaviors in multihandicapped individuals. Standardized testing procedures are often difficult to adhere to when a multihandicapped child has motor and/or cognitive handicaps. Test materials and procedures must often be adapted and additional measures obtained. Specific language tests will not be reviewed here, but adaptations of tests for the motor-impaired child can be accomplished in several ways. Spatially rearranging test materials to allow for nonverbal response modes such as eye gaze is one method. Using measures that require yes–no and/or multiple-choice responses is another.

For the purposes of this chapter we will concentrate only on the evaluation of speech behaviors in a clinical setting. Typically, the speech evaluation consists of structured observation procedures designed to elicit behaviors that provide information about a child's oral structures, phonemic repertoire, production of phonemic sequences, vocal quality, vocal resonance, speech intelligibility, and prosodic features of speech.

In young children the clinical assessment of speech behaviors is often difficult. In fact, to obtain a representative sample of expressive communication and speech motor behaviors in a clinic setting is sometimes impossible. Preschool children are simply less likely to "talk" or vocalize in unfamiliar surroundings. Nevertheless, professionals who work with the multihandicapped cannot afford to wait until these children become cooperative and "properly socialized" before making programmatic decisions.

Nor can most speech–language pathologists go to the child's home and make daily or weekly recordings of the child's vocalizations to ensure an adequate sample of the behaviors. Speech–language pathologists often rely heavily on parental report. Parental report is an effective way of screening the child's range of vocal and communicative behaviors. The most popular infant scales also rely on interview techniques. These scales, which incorporate questions about sound production, include the Receptive–Expressive Emergent Language Scale (Bzoch & League, 1971) and the Sequenced Inventory of Communication Development (Hendrick, 1975).

Another approach is to try to elicit vocalizations from the child. Since children are generally willing to eat and to play, provision of snacks and the use of familiar play routines may offer a particularly useful approach to the observation of behaviors. The clinician may set up a situation with the help of the parent that the child is likely to enjoy. Often the parent or sibling may participate while the clinician records the child's sound production. We find such direct elicitation procedures frequently increase vocalizations. Sytematic use of developmentally appropriate reinforcement is generally effective also. For example, the examiner may make a funny face every time the child vocalizes. Another technique is for the examiner to stop talking or ignore the child and talk to the parent. Then, when the child vocalizes, the examiner quickly reinforces any sound.

Another approach to assessment of early speech development has been developed by Morris. Her Pre-speech Assessment Scale (Morris, 1982b) rates prespeech behaviors from birth to 2 years. Feeding, respiration–phonation, and sound play are examined. Observation of overall postural tone and movement, head and trunk control, response to sensory stimulation, and response to specific treatment techniques are included. Considerable attention has been focused on assessment of eating and drinking skills. Despite their dependence, however, on the integrity of the same oral structures, and a final common neural pathway, no direct relationship can be shown to exist between feeding and speech behaviors.

A complete speech assessment includes an oral sensorimotor evaluation. This evaluation is dependent on the full cooperation of the child. Often we can complete a cursory examination of oral structures and their function during eating and drinking activities. With the developmentally older child, a more complete motor speech evaluation may be carried out. Several procedures are available, although few were actually developed for use with children. Many available scales focus on the differential diagnosis of verbal/oral dyspraxia versus dysarthria and the investigation of other etiologic factors. Yet, a clear diagnostic category of developmental dyspraxia has not emerged (Williams, Ingham, & Rosenthal, 1981). Please refer to chapters 5 and 6 for a complete discussion of this difficult area.

As the child becomes older, standardized articulation tests may be used to elicit speech-production responses. It is important, however, to evaluate speech sounds in a variety of real-speech contexts. A typical articulation test requires the child to imitate or name pictures and objects. English phonemes are tested in various positions in words. Some approaches are also designed to analyze phonologically the speech samples obtained. Finally, a speech intelligibility measure should be obtained as a means of ascertaining the extent to which the child's speech problem actually interferes with his or her ability to communicate.

Because multihandicapped children have often experienced years of failure and have undergone multiple evaluations, we often find them reluctant to participate in any speech-related activities. It is therefore essential to assess them in as naturalistic and supportive an environment as possible.

Interpretation of Assessment Data

Evaluation is the key to intervention. Data obtained from the interdisciplinary team evaluation should be used to identify, describe, and prioritize the problems that require intervention. The complaint that a child has delayed speech does not necessarily mean that intervention should be provided. The child with speech abilities that are delayed secondary to mental retardation but that are commensurate with the child's cognitive and language abilities and communication skills will not require speech intervention. However, if a child's "speech" or communicative use of vocalizations is significantly delayed in comparison with his or her cognitive and language abilities, and if his or her speech is ineffective for the purposes of communication, then therapy should be provided.

Because the description of the clinical course of speech disorders in the major diagnostic groups has not been undertaken, prognostic statements cannot be made with confidence except in the case of very severe or very mild handicapping conditions. For example, J. P. is a severely retarded 3-year-old boy with cerebral palsy who has significant oral motor dysfunction and a persistence of abnormal oral reflexes. Because of these problems, he is unable to accept food orally and is fed through a gastrostomy tube. He is unlikely to develop functional speech. D. K., on the other hand, presents a much less severe problem. He is a 3-year-old of normal intelligence with delayed speech thought to be secondary to motor speech discoordination. The speech and language evaluation also revealed deficits in some areas of language acquisition. He is likely to develop functional speech but may have residual expressive language deficits for many years, and he is at risk for a language-based learning disability.

In general, factors that indicate a good prognosis are as follows: (1) normal or superior intelligence; (2) relatively mild sensory and/or motor impairment; (3) family involvement and advocacy; and (4) early intervention.

While maturational and intellectual factors cannot be manipulated, environmental factors may be (Moser, 1983). Environmental factors are critical to prognosis. The family's needs and resources thus should be evaluated in relation to the child's. The ideal family has the energy and resources necessary to optimize the child's experiences and advocate for the child over the years of programming and intervention by numerous professionals. Realistically, all families experience problems and stress in dealing with the day-to-day care of their multihandicapped children. These problems are compounded by the number of treatment visits and professional appointments that must be made and the financial strains experienced. Some families manage to cope with these stresses and develop new skills and strengths that enable them to support their child's development. Others, however, find it extremely difficult, if not impossible, to care for their handicapped child. These families are in particular need of support and understanding.

TREATMENT

Following the interdisciplinary evaluation treatment decisions are made. This section will introduce some general considerations with respect to the clinical management of speech problems of multihandicapped children and will describe some approaches to treatment. The medical management of the speech-impaired child will not be addressed. Although not discussed in this chapter, medical management by the otolaryngologist, neurologist, radiologist, and surgeon may be indicated and appropriate evaluation by such specialists must be provided. In some cases treatment may be provided by the speech–language pathologist and medical specialist as a team. For example, surgery to correct craniofacial anomalies may precede speech and language intervention. The speech–language pathologist will establish short and long term goals that reflect the conclusions of the interdisciplinary team as a whole. As a result the expectations of the professionals, family, and ultimately the child are likely to be realistic.

The ability to communicate is the right of each individual and is a behavior that is taken for granted. Communication occurs in a variety of modes, including speaking, gesturing, head nods, facial expression, writing, signing, pointing, etc. When a child's communicative needs outweigh his or her ability to communicate using speech, he or she will experience communicative dissonance, i.e., there will be a dissociation between his or her desire to make requests, comment, tease, ask, and answer questions, etc., and his or her ability to express these needs and thoughts using speech. This situation can occur at a surprisingly early age and is likely to be present in children by the time they reach a developmental level of 18–21 months. A child who experiences communicative disso- nance encounters increasing frustration, isolation, and dependence; therefore, intervention should be provided promptly. For children who are considered at risk for the development of speech (e.g., those with severe oral and speech motor dysfunction or moderate to severe hearing impairment), preventive steps should be taken to prevent or minimize the development of communication problems for the child and his or her communication partners.

Intervention procedures should have two primary goals: (1) the re- duction of the discrepancy between the child's communicative needs and abilities, i.e., enhancement of communication in all situations; and (2) facilitation of the child's speech or vocal production skills. Objectives are to remediate deficits interfering with speech production, to teach the child how to use his or her existing speech or vocal abilities more effec- tively in communication, and/or to provide compensatory techniques that will permit the child to communicate in spite of speech production defi- cits. A number of treatment strategies are discussed in the following sections. Unfortunately research is still limited on the efficacy of these approaches.

Articulation Therapy

Articulation therapy uses learning theory techniques to increase a child's speech intelligibility through specific training in production of phonemes, phonemic sequences, words, phrases, and sentences. In tradi- tional articulation therapy the speech–language pathologist selects an error sound (e.g., /k/) and teaches the child to produce the sound cor- rectly. The child then practices the sound in various phonemic contexts. Picture cards or word lists are frequently used as stimulus materials for older children. For the developmentally younger child, learning theory paradigms can be employed within naturalistic settings. For example, objects selected for the child to play with might contain the target pho- neme (e.g., /d/) so that the child will have ample opportunity to practice the sound repeatedly during the session.

Articulation therapy has only limited success when used with chil- dren whose speech disorders are neurologically based or caused by orofa- cial anomalies that directly affect speech sound production (McWilliams et al., 1984). Limited success is reported with children who are diagnosed with developmental dyspraxia. The approach is only minimally effective with severely retarded children. Children with impaired hearing may improve when articulation therapy is combined with auditory training procedures. The approach is most likely to be successful with children of normal intelligence whose hearing sensitivity in the speech ranges (250–4000 Hz) is not poorer than 80 db and when good educational and family support are present.

Neurodevelopmental Treatment

Berta Bobath, a physical therapist, and Karel Bobath, a neurologist, developed the neurodevelopmental treatment (NDT) approach in England (Bobath & Bobath, 1972). The approach has been used extensively in the United States and Europe, particularly by physical and occupational therapists. However, the 8-week NDT course is offered to speech–language pathologists also. The approach requires that the motor-impaired child experience normal movement patterns. Handling techniques are employed that provide optimal positioning, inhibit primitive reflex patterns, and facilitate normal movement patterns, including the normal oral movement patterns underlying speech. The emphasis may be on positioning and moving the limbs and trunk rather than mouth parts. The child's ability to speak is affected not only by the oral musculature but also by other muscle groups, particularly those of the chest, neck, and head. Most speech–language pathologists who work with the multihandicapped child are influenced by the NDT approach although relatively few have completed NDT training. Davis (1978) and others advocate early intervention with neurologically impaired infants, the goals being to establish normal muscle tone and neuromuscular patterns.

Oral and Speech Motor Facilitation

The goal of this approach is to improve the range, speed, and accuracy of movements of the lips, tongue, and jaw through oral and speech motor exercises. Much of the current sensorimotor programming for the neurologically speech-impaired child is based on the work of Mueller (1975). The speech–language pathologist trained in oral and speech motor facilitation provides a discrete sensory input to the articulators (i.e., firm touch, vibration, brushing, icing) with the intent of eliciting a specific motor response (i.e., lip rounding, tongue protrusion, cough, swallow). The techniques progress from simple to more complex movement patterns. Many speech–language pathologists use modified techniques as part of or preceding direct speech/articulation training. Mysak (1980) considers stimulation of listening, speech postures, hand movements, and basic speech movements as fundamental to neurospeech therapy. His approach reflects an emphasis on relaxation, normalization of tone, posture, and movement, and facilitation of integration of movement patterns and elimination of reflexes. He recommends isometric exercises and resistance techniques to increase muscle strength and tone and to improve motor function in neurologically impaired children.

Feeding Therapy

Feeding therapy attempts to use the elements of oral–speech movements that occur during eating and drinking to elicit sound production or speech prerequisites. The basic approach was described by Mueller (1975) and has undergone minimal changes since. Love and Associates (1980) reported a trend, although not systematic, for children with adequate eating and drinking skills to have better speech. However, although the same structures are utilized, the neurophysiologic patterns are different. No evidence currently exists that relates the practice of oral feeding movements to improved speech development. Nevertheless, feeding time is still considered a good context for intervention. Mealtimes are likely to be periods during which a young child will vocalize, practice sounds, exercise movements of tongue and lips, and interact with a communication partner. Morris (1982a) used the activities of eating and drinking with some success as an integral part of her assessment tool and treatment strategies.

Augmentative Communication

A common sequela of severe cognitive and/or physical impairment is an inability to produce intelligible speech. Although most multihandicapped children with severe motor, sensory, and/or cognitive impairments develop communicative use of their voice, it may be limited to calling for attention, requesting, laughing, crying, and protesting. For these children functional speech may not be obtained for many years or may be an unrealistic goal at any future time. The American Speech–Language–Hearing Association has estimated that approximately one million nonspeaking individuals currently reside in the United States. Non-speaking persons are defined as a group of individuals for whom speech is temporarily or permanently inadequate to meet all of his or her communication needs, and whose inability to speak is not due primarily to a hearing impairment (ASHA, 1981). Of these, 900,000 are developmentally disabled, 500,000 have an acquired disability such as head trauma, and 140,000 have a progressive neuromuscular pathology. Historically, nonspeaking persons were either enrolled in a protracted course of speech therapy, often unsuccessful, or were denied treatment because of the severity of the problem and resulting poor prognosis for developing intelligible speech. Many different approaches have been tried increasingly over the past decade to help such children communicate and thus have the means to learn more about what is happening around them. Efforts have been made to teach them sign language, to have them communicate through picture boards, and more recently to operate electronic devices and microcomputers.

Augmentative communication approaches should be considered when a child experiences or is likely to encounter communicative dissonance. Augmentative approaches, which include the use of gestures, manual sign systems, mechanical and electronic communication aids, speech aids, and computers, are used to supplement an individual's vocal skills, enhance an individual's communication abilities, and/or facilitate certain communication skills. These approaches may improve a child's ability to respond, construct messages, engage in conversation, write, or have access to computers. An *unaided* augmentative approach does not require a physical device and refers to gestures, manual sign systems, and facial expressions. An *aided* approach is one that uses a physical object or device such as a language board, a mechanical or electrical aid, or a microcomputer. A dedicated communication aid is a device that is used solely for communication. Commercially available home and hand-held computers are now being used to enhance the communication skills of handicapped individuals. Some off-the-shelf computers permit the child to carry out educational and leisure activities as well as to engage in conversation and to write and prepare messages. Hardware, firmware, and software exist that permit even the most severely motor-impaired individual access to communication aids and computers (Vanderheiden, 1982). The communication processes are different, however, when augmentative communication aids are used. Technology does not yet offer a true communication prosthesis to the user. During conversational exchanges, the rate of message transmission is very slow, the content of messages is telegraphic, and the conversational pattern is not normal (Blackstone & Cassatt, 1983; Calculator & Dolloghan, 1982; Harris, 1982). Future studies will help determine how to facilitate the use of augmentative approaches with children to make communication more efficient and rewarding.

The speech–language pathologist works in conjunction with the family, teachers, occupational and physical therapists, rehabilitation engineers, computer programmers, and others to evaluate and prescribe appropriate augmentative approaches. Generally, multihandicapped children will benefit from more than one approach at any one time and throughout their lives. Many decisions must be made regarding the child's present and future communication needs, and the cognitive, environmental, language, motor, and behavioral factors that affect the child must be considered. If a communication aid is recommended, questions must be raised as to how the child will operate the device (e.g., point directly, use a special code, use a switch interface), the output options that are included with the device (e.g., synthesized speech, printer, LED display, LCD display, digitized speech), and the symbol system that is most appropriate (e.g., pictures, Blissymbolics, orthographs). It is essential that the child and family receive training in all augmentative approaches introduced. As technology becomes increasingly available and affordable, new means of talking and communicating are possible. Communication augmentation options have greatly improved the social, education, and vocational potential for multihandicapped children.

SUMMARY

The multihandicapped child with communication problems secondary to a speech impairment presents a challenge to professionals from a variety of disciplines. Service delivery to these children and their families is generally provided within the framework of three models. The most effective model may often be the interdisciplinary model. In the past many of these children were denied services. Now, the needs of even the most severely impaired are being addressed.

Five of the more common primary handicapping conditions associated with speech impairment in children are mental retardation, hearing impairment, cerebral palsy, autism, and craniofacial anomalies. The speech-language pathologist necessarily plays a primary role on any team concerned with children who have communication disorders. Current clinical management practices used by speech–language pathologists must include identification, evaluation, and treatment of speech disorders in multihandicapped children. The reader is cautioned that the scope of this chapter is necessarily broad in order to present an overview. The reader should not conclude that the content is in any way an inclusive review of current clinical practices with multihandicapped, speech-impaired children.

REFERENCES

Allen, D. V., & Robinson, D. O. (1984). Middle ear status and language development in preschool children. *ASHA*, 26, 33–37.

American Academy of Pediatrics. (1978). Committee on Children with Handicaps: Position paper.

ASHA, Ad Hoc Committee on Communication Processes and Non-speaking persons (1981). Position statement on nonspeech communication. *ASHA*, 28, 577–81.

Batshaw, M. L., & Perrett, Y. M. (1981). *Children with handicaps: A medical primer* (pp. 191–351). Baltimore: Paul H. Brookes.

Beadle, K. R. (1981). Speech and language disturbances in childhood development. In J. K. Darby (Ed.), *Speech evaluation in medicine* (pp. 279–294). New York: Grune & Stratton.

Blackstone, S. W., & Cassatt, E. L. (1984). *Communicative competence in communication aid users and their partners.* Presented at Third International Conference on Augmentative and Alternative Communication, M.I.T., Boston.

Bobath, K., & Bobath, B. (1972). Cerebral palsy. Part 1. Diagnosis and assessment of cerebral palsy. Part 2. The neurodevelopmental approach to treatment. In P. H. Pearson & C. E. Williams (Eds.), *Physical therapy services in the developmental disabilities.* Springfield, IL: Charles C. Thomas.

Boucher, J. (1976). Articulation in early childhood autism. *Journal of Autism and Childhood Schizophrenia, 6,* 297–302.

Bzoch, K. R., & League, R. (1971). *Assessing language skills in infancy.* Gainesville, FL: Tree Life Press.

Calculator, S., & Dolloghan, C. (1982). The use of communication boards in a residential setting: An evaluation. *Journal of Speech and Hearing Disorders, 47,* 281–287.

Davis, L. (1978). Pre-speech. In F. P. Connor, G. G. Williamson, & J. M. Siepp (Eds.), *Program guide for infants and toddlers with neuromotor and other developmental disabilities.* New York: Teachers College Press, Columbia University.

Eiben, R. M., & Crocker, A. C. (1983). Cerebral palsy within the spectrum of developmental disabilities. In G. H. Thompson, I. L. Rubin, & R. M. Bilenker (Eds.), *Comprehensive management of cerebral palsy* (pp. 19–25). New York: Grune & Stratton.

Eisenberg, L. (1956). The autistic child in adolescence. *American Medical Association Archives of Neurology and Psychiatry, 112,* 607–612.

Everhart, R. W. (1953). The relationship between articulation and other developmental factors in childrren. *Journal of Speech and Hearing Disorders, 18,* 332–338.

Fay, W. H., & Schuler, A. L. (1980). *Emerging language in autistic children* (pp. 1–50). Baltimore: University Park Press.

Fein, D. J. (1983). The prevalence of speech and language impairments. *ASHA, 25,* 2–37.

Flower, R. M. (1981). Neurodevelopmental disorders in childhood. In J. K. Darby (Ed.), *Speech evaluation in medicine* (pp. 309–340). New York: Grune & Stratton.

Governmental Affairs Review. (1981). *2:2,* p. 12.

Grossman, A. J. (1973). *Manual on terminology and classification of mental retardation and association of mental deficits.* Baltimore: Garanmond-Predemark Press.

Harper, J., & Williams, S. (1975). Age and type of onset as critical variables in early infantile autism. *Journal of Autism and Childhood Schizophrenia, 5,* 25–36.

Harris, D. (1982). Communication interaction processes involving nonvocal physically handicapped children. *Topics in Language Disorders, 2,* 21–37.

Hart, V. (1977). The use of many disciplines with the severely and profoundly handicapped. In E. Sontag (Ed.), *Educational programming for the severely and profoundly handicapped* (pp. 391–396). Reston, VA: Council for Exceptional Children. Division on Mental Retardation.

Healey, W. C., Ackerman, B. L., Chappe II, C. R., Perrin, K. L. & Stormer, J. (1981). The prevalence of communicative disorders: A review of the literature. Final Report. Rockville, MD: American Speech - Language - Hearing Association.

Healey, W. C., & Karp-Nortman, D. C. (1975). The hearing-impaired mentally retarded: Recommendations for action. Rockville, MD: American Speech - Language - Hearing Association.

Hendrick, D. L., Prather, E. M., & Tobin, A. R. (1975). *The sequenced inventory of communication development.* Seattle, University of Washington Press.

Hinerman, P. S. (1983). *Teaching autistic children to communicate* (pp. 1–37). Rockville, MD: Aspen Systems Corp.

Holm, V. A. (1978). Team issues. In K. E. Allen, V. A. Holm, & R. L. Schiefelbusch (Eds.), *Early intervention: A team approach* (pp. 99–115). Baltimore: University Park Press.

Hopkins, T., Bice, H. V., & Colton, K. (1954). *Evaluation and education of the cerebral palsied child.* Washington, DC: International Council for Exceptional Children.

Jacobson, J. W., & Janicki, M. P. (1983). Observed prevalence of multiple developmental disabilities. *Mental Retardation, 21,* 3, 87–94.

Jaffe, B. F., & Luterman, D. M. (1980). The child with a hearing loss. In A. P. Sheiner & I. F. Abroms (Eds.), *The practical management of the developmentally disabled child* (pp. 250–268). St. Louis: C. V. Mosby.

Jaffe, M. B. (1984). Neurological impairment of speech production: Assessment and treatment. In A. Holland (Ed.), *Speech disorders in children* (pp. 157–185). San Diego: College-Hill Press.

Jones, M. (1975). Differential diagnosis and natural history of the cerebral palsied child. In R. Samilson (Ed.), *Orthopedic aspects of cerebral palsy.* Philadelphia: Lippincott.

Love, R. J., Hagerman, E. L., & Taimi, E. G. (1980). Speech performance, dysphagia and oral reflexes in cerebral palsy. *Journal of Speech and Hearing Disorders, 45,* 59–75.

Ludlow, C. L., & Cooper, J. A. (1983). *Genetic aspects of speech and language disorders* (pp. 1–20). New York: Academic Press.

McCormick, L., & Goldman, R. (1979). The transdisciplinary model: Implications for service delivery and personnel preparation for the severely and profoundly handicapped. *American Association for the Education of the Severely and Profoundly Handicapped Review, 4,* 152–161.

McWilliams, B. J., Morris, H. L., & Shelton, R. L. (1984). *Cleft palate speech.* Ontario: B. C. Decker.

Meyers, R. E. (1975). Perinatal asphyxia: The neurologist's viewpoint. In K. Adamsons & H. A. Fox (Eds.), *Preventability of perinatal injury.* New York: Liss.

Morris, S. E. (1982a). *The normal acquisition of oral feeding skills: Implications for assessment and treatment.* Boston: Therapeutic Media.

Morris, S. E. (1982b). *The pre-speech assessment scale.* Clifton, NJ: J. A. Preston.

Morris, T. (1973). Hearing impaired cerebral palsied children and their education. *Public Health, 88,* 27.

Moser, H. W. (1983). Prevention of psychosocial mental retardation. In G. H. Thompson et al. (Eds.), *Comprehensive management of cerebral palsy* (pp. 75–83). New York: Grune & Stratton.

Mueller, H. A. (1975). Feeding, speech. In N. R. Finnie (Ed.), *Handling the young cerebral palsied child at home* (2nd ed.). New York: Dutton.

Mulligan, J. C., Painter, M. J., & O'Donohue, P. D. (1980). Neonatal asphyxia II. Neonatal mortality and long term sequealae. *Journal of Pediatrics, 96,* 903.

Mysak, E. D. (1980). *Neurospeech therapy for the cerebral palsied* (3rd ed.). New York: Teachers College Press, Columbia University.

Nell, J. V. (1958). A study of major congenital defects in Japanese infants. *American Journal of Human Genetics, 10,* 398.

Oka, S. W. (1979). Epidemiology and genetics of clefting: With implications for etiology. In H. K. Cooper, R. L. Harding, W. M. Krogman, M. Maxaheri, & R. T. Millard (Eds.), *Cleft palate and cleft lip: A team approach to clinical management and rehabilitation of the patient.* Philadelphia: W. B. Saunders.

Painter, M. J. (1984). Neurological sequealae of birth. In J. J. Sciarra (Ed.), *Practice of obstetrics and gynecology.* Hagerstown, MD: Harper & Row.

Palmer, M. (1947). Studies in clinical techniques. II. Normalization of chewing, sucking and swallowing reflexes in cerebral palsy: A home program. *Journal of Speech Disorders, 12,* 415.

Paneth, N., & Kiely, J. (1984). Clinics in developmental medicine and child neurology, 87: The epidemiology of the cerebral palsies. In F. Stanley & E. Alberman (Eds.), *The Spastics International Medical Publication.* Oxford: Blackwell Scientific Publications Limited.

Prizant, B. M. (1983). Language acquisition and communicative behavior in autism: Toward an understanding of the "whole" of it. *Journal of Speech and Hearing Disorders, 48,* 296–307.

Prutting, C. (1979). Process: The action of moving forward progressively from one point to another on the way to completion. *Journal of Speech and Hearing Disorders, 44,* 3–30.

Ritvo, E. R., & Freeman, B. J. (1978). NSAC definition of syndrome of autism. *Journal of Autism and Childhood Schizophrenia, 8,* 162–167.

Rood, S. (1983). Anatomy and physiology of speech. In C. E. Bluestone & S. Stool (Eds.), *Pediatric otolaryngology.* Philadelphia: W. B. Saunders.

Rutter, M. (1978). Diagnosis and definition. In M. Rutter & E. Schopler (Eds.), *Autism: A reappraisal of concepts and treatment.* New York: Plenum Press.

Schein, J., & Delk, C. (1974). The deaf population of the United States. Silver Springs, MD: National Association of the Deaf.

Scheiner, A. P., & McNabb, N. A. (1980). The child with mental retardation. In A. P. Scheiner & I. F. Abroms (Eds.), *The practical management of the developmentally disabled child* (pp. 184–221). St. Louis: C. V. Mosby.

Schlanger, B. B. (1953). Speech examination of a group of institutionalized mentally handicapped children. *Journal of Speech and Hearing Disorders, 18,* 339–349.

Schuler, A. L. (1975). Echolalia: Issues and clinical applications. *Journal of Speech and Hearing Disorders, 44,* 411–434.

Shapiro, B. K., Palmer, F. B., Wachtel, R. C., & Capute, A. J. (1983). Associated dysfunctions. In G. H. Thompson, I. L. Rubin, & R. M. Bilenker. *Comprehensive management of cerebral palsy* (pp. 87–97). New York: Grune & Stratton.

Siegel, G. M. (1963). Verbal behavior of retarded children assembled with pre-instituted adults. In R. Schiefelbusch (Ed.), Language studies of mentally retarded children. *Journal of Speech and Hearing Monograph Supplement, No. 10.*

Thompson, G. H., Rubin, I. L., & Bilenker, R. M. (1983). *Comprehensive management of cerebral palsy.* New York: Grune & Stratton.

Valletutti, P. J. & Christoplos, F. (1977). *Interdisciplinary approaches to human services* (pp. 1–11). Baltimore: University Park Press.

Vanderheiden, G. (1982). Computers can play a dual role for disabled individuals. *Byte, 7* (7), 1–8.

Wells, C. G. (1971). *Cleft palate and its associated speech disorders.* New York: McGraw-Hill.

Wetherby, A. M., & Gaines, B. H. (1982). Cognition and language development in autism. *Journal of Speech and Hearing Disorders, 47,* 63–70.

Williams, R., Ingham, R. J., & Rosenthal, J. (1981). A further analysis of developmental apraxia of speech in children with defective articulation. *Journal of Speech and Hearing Research, 24,* 496–505.

Yost, J. G., & McMillan, P. M. (1983). Communication disorder. In H. Thompson et al. *Comprehensive management of cerebral palsy* (pp. 157–171). New York: Grune & Stratton.

III. GENETICS IN SPEECH AND LANGUAGE DISORDERS

Judith A. Cooper
Christy L. Ludlow

8

The Genetics of Developmental Speech and Language Disorders

Many childhood communication disorders are secondary to trauma or infections occurring prenatally, at birth, or during early childhood (Dennis & Whitaker, 1976; Hecaen, 1976). Further, mental retardation, reduced hearing sensitivity, infantile autism, and other psychiatric disorders are all associated with impaired speech and language development. Despite the frequent occurrence of childhood speech and language impairments secondary to other disorders, the bases for most deficits remain unknown. Children with developmental misarticulations, language disorders, or stuttering generally have negative histories regarding medical, neurologic, psychiatric, and environmental factors that might be etiologic. Such disorders may be the result of particular genotypes, or combinations of genes. A genetic basis for developmental speech and language problems has been implicated or suspected for many years since often family members of children with such problems have similar communicative impairments (Arnold, 1961; Luchsinger, 1970). With recent developments in the field of behavioral genetics, the tools for identifying genetic aspects of speech and language disorders may be within our reach.

A brief review of certain basic concepts in genetics seems relevant at this point. Normally, an individual has 23 pairs of chromosomes, or nu-

---

Speech and Language Evaluation in Neurology:
Childhood Disorders
ISBN 0-8089-1719-6

cleoprotein bodies, which carry the genes. Twenty-two of these pairs are labeled *autosomal*. The remaining pair are termed *sex chromosomes,* and are two X chromosomes in females and an X and Y in males. Pairs of genes occupy particular locations on each chromosome pair. If these pairs, or alleles, are identical, an individual is described as *homozygous* at that location, and *heterozygous* if not identical.

Various genetic abnormalities have been documented, including single gene defects, chromosomal aberrations, and multifactorial traits. The concepts of a dominant trait (expression of a trait when the gene is only one chromosome of a pair) and recessive trait (expression of a trait requires the gene be present on both chromosomes of a pair) are important in interpreting and predicting single gene defects (Pashayan, 1975). If the mutant gene is on an autosomal chromosome, it is termed *autosomal,* while if it is on a sex chromosome, it is *sex-linked.* Examples of single gene defects include Tay-Sachs (autosomal) and hemophilia (sex-linked). Genes, however, are not always expressed phenotypically, that is, the result of the interaction of genotypic and environmental factors may not necessarily be visible. *Reduced penetrance* describes traits that may not be expressed by individuals carrying the principal gene or genes conditioning them. Expression of an abnormal genotype, therefore, may vary across members of a family or society, resulting in differing characteristics and severity. Chromosomal aberrations may be the result of translocations (abnormal arrangements of genetic material) or alterations in the number or structure of chromosomes (Pashayan, 1975). Down's syndrome and cri du chat syndrome are the result of chromosomal aberrations. Multifactorial traits reflect a type of genetic transmission in which numerous genes, with varying loci, are related to the manifestation of a trait. Usual patterns of inheritance cannot explain these traits, which would include certain developmental and psychiatric disorders.

Behavioral genetics involves the investigation of the contributions of both heredity and environment to individual behavioral differences (Plomin, DeFries, & McClearn, 1980). Examination of the influence of environment and genotype is possible by comparing individuals who differ only in their genotype but were reared in similar environments, such as adopted children reared together. Conversely, to examine the effects of genotype, individuals are compared who have the same genotype but were reared in different environments, such as monozygotic (or identical) twins adopted into different homes and reared apart. The recent emergence of the discipline of behavioral genetics has altered the investigation of the hereditary bases of many behavioral traits, including specific cognitive abilities, psychopathology, and intelligence.

The purpose of this chapter is to discuss (1) the current state of knowledge regarding genetic aspects of developmental speech and language disorders, (2) procedures for identification of a familial disorder with a possible genetic basis, and (3) issues related to genetic counseling.

CURRENT STATUS: REVIEW OF THE LITERATURE

Developmental Speech and Language Disorders

Primary developmental speech and/or language disorders are those not secondary to hearing loss, mental retardation, documented brain damage, or autism. Most studies suggesting a genetic basis for primary developmental language disorders have been descriptive case studies (e.g., Arnold, 1961; Luchsinger, 1970). Methodologic problems often accompany such studies, affecting the validity of findings. For example, subject selection criteria are unclear, and definitions of the communicative disorders are not specified or confirmed by formalized testing. Use of parental report to establish a positive family history has accompanying difficulties. Family reports of developmental language disorders can be altered by (1) the passage of time affecting the accuracy of recollections, (2) a family's willingness to acknowledge problems in other family members, and (3) the reporter's perceptions of what constituted a disorder or problem.

A few studies of speech- and language-delayed children have examined karyotypes, or the characteristics of an individual's chromosomes, including number, size, and shape. Garvey and Mutton (1973) studied 9 children with impaired expressive abilities and found sex chromosome abnormalities in 3 cases. In a similar study, Mutton and Lea (1980) found four of 88 individuals with severe speech and language disorders had chromosomal anomalies, a greater incidence than would be expected in the normal population. It is unlikely, however, that chromosomal deviations are present in a large portion of speech- and language-impaired children since other investigations have found no major or minor chromosomal abnormalities in this population (Tuncbilek, Kurultay, & Belgin, 1978; Hier, Atkins, & Perlo, 1980). Subject selection criteria (particularly intelligence) may have affected the results of Garvey and Mutton and of Mutton and Lea since chromosomal abnormalities are more frequent in the mentally retarded than in the normal population (Adler, 1976; Siegel-Sadewitz & Shprintzen, 1982).

Although relatively few children with developmental language disorders have sex chromosome anomalies, when children with such anomalies are studied, many are found to have communication impairments (Bender, Fry, Pennington, Puck, Salbenblatt, & Robinson, 1983). Males with Klinefelter's syndrome (two or more X chromosomes in addition to the Y chromosome), 47 XYY syndrome, or females with trisomy X frequently exhibit delays in language and articulatory development (Nielsen, Sorenson, & Sorenson, 1981; Pennington, Puck, & Robinson, 1980). The delayed speech associated with the 47 XYY subjects may be similar to verbal dyspraxia (Ratcliffe, 1982), although not all studies have supported this view (e.g., Bender et al., 1983). In addition to communicative impairments, individuals with sex chromosome abnormalities frequently encounter academic difficulties (Annell, Gustavson, & Tenstam, 1970; Haka-Ikse, Steward, & Cripps, 1978). An exception is the sex chromosome aberration, Turner's syndrome, which is often associated with impaired nonverbal performance and normal verbal skills (Hier et al., 1980; Nielsen & Sillesen, 1976).

Few studies have focused on the genetic bases of developmental speech misarticulations. Some individuals with these disorders have been included in studies of genetic aspects of delayed or impaired language development (Arnold, 1961; Mutton & Lea, 1980). Few investigations, however, have studied phonologic or articulatory disorders independently. McLaughlin and Kriegsman (1980) documented a family with Renpenning's syndrome, or nonspecific X-linked mental retardation, with developmental verbal dyspraxia as a predominant feature. They reported pedigree information suggestive of an X-linked pattern of transmission for the dyspraxia.

Developmental speech and language problems are often associated with subsequent academic problems, particularly reading disorders. A genetic basis for dyslexia has been considered since the early 1900s (see Hallgren, 1950, for a review). The few chromosomal analyses that have been done thus far with these individuals, however, have failed to reveal obvious abnormalities (Hier et al., 1980). An increased occurrence among males (Zahalkova, Vrzal, & Kloboukova, 1972), a strong family history of dyslexia (Silver, 1971), and similarities between the disabilities of family members and those of the child with the disorder (Childs & Finnuci, 1979; Omenn & Weber, 1978) are all suggestive of a genetic component to dyslexia. However, although investigators have frequently documented the generation-to-generation transmission of this disorder, no one pattern or mode of transmission appears capable of explaining the variety of pedigrees reported. A recent development was the suggestion of a linkage between a gene influencing dyslexia and chromosome 15p heteromorphism (Smith, Pennington, Kimberling, & Lubs, 1983). More investigation is needed, however, to determine if this pertains to only one specific type of dyslexia.

Stuttering

Of the developmental communication disorders, stuttering has received the most attention from behavioral geneticists. Accumulated evidence suggests the following:

- Relatives of a stutterer have an increased risk of stuttering. This is further increased if one parent is a stutterer (Andrews & Harris, 1964; Pauls & Kidd, 1982).
- Monozygotic twins have a significantly greater incidence of concordance for stuttering than dizygotic (or fraternal) twins (Howie, 1981b).
- A strong sex effect is prominent: males are affected between three and four times more frequently than females (Ehrman & Parson, 1976; Porfert & Rosenfield, 1978). The risk of stuttering among relatives of female stutterers seems greater than the risk among relatives of male stutterers (Andrews & Harris, 1964).
- There is lack of support for a learning or environmental theory. For example, many parents who stuttered recovered prior to the birth of the case under investigation (Kidd, Riech, & Kessler, 1973). There are reports of adopted children who stutter with no stuttering history in the adopted family (Bloodstein, 1961). Finally, most siblings of stutterers are nonaffected (Chakravartti, Roy, Rao, & Chakravartti, 1979).

Despite strong evidence of a nonenvironmental basis for stuttering, a genetic explanation is not readily apparent. Kidd, Riech, and Kessler (1973) have suggested that stuttering may involve a dominant gene with a single locus and two alleles (variants of a gene with the same locus on a particular chromosome). If an individual is homozygous for the normal allele, stuttering would not occur. If an individual is homozygous for the stuttering allele, stuttering would almost always occur. Heterozygosity would be associated with stuttering 25 percent of the time in males but only 4 percent of the time in females, and environmental factors would affect only those individuals with heterozygosity. In contrast, other investigators claim stuttering may be wholly polygenic or multifactorial. For example, Andrews and Harris (1964) suggested that stuttering may be transmitted similarly to stature and intelligence, and that no one gene is essential. Rather, a number of genes may act together creating an underlying predisposition. Most investigators agree that the exact method of transmission has yet to be determined (Chakravartti et al., 1979; Howie, 1981a, 1981b; Kidd, Heimbuch, & Records, 1981). It is probably that further headway cannot be made in this area until the pathophysiologic bases of stuttering is determined. Without an understanding of the processes underlying the development of stuttering, it is difficult to know what factor should be identified for association with a genetic mutation.

Genetic Disorders Associated With Speech and Language Deficits

Many genetic abnormalities, in addition to those involving the sex chromosomes, are associated with impaired communicative skills. Such abnormalities may give rise to communication disorders by interfering with brain development and/or functioning, resulting in impaired cognitive and/or speech production abilities (Adler, 1976).

Siegel-Sadewitz and Shprintzen (1982) present a listing of 105 genetic syndromes, with descriptions of the communication pathology encountered in each. For example, Beckwith-Wiedemann syndrome is frequently associated with macroglossia affecting speech articulation, while Mobius syndrome includes bilateral facial paralysis and frequent hypoglossal motor nuclei anomalies. Thus by knowing a particular medical syndrome, it is often possible to predict the type of communicative deficits. However, although particular anomalies are associated with each syndrome, the effects of such anomalies on the development of communicative skills will vary. For example, children with Down's syndrome differ significantly in their pattern and severity of communicative skills. Thus considerable care must be taken in the assessment and diagnosis of communicative deficits in clients presenting genetic syndromes because of variability in phenotypic expression and the potential effects of the syndrome on the development of communicative skills.

Two other childhood disorders which have associated communication impairments and may be affected by genetic factors are autism and Gilles de la Tourette syndrome. Autism is characterized by the following:

- Onset before 30 months of age
- Pervasive lack of responsiveness to other people
- Gross language deficit
- If speech is present, peculiar speech patterns (e.g., immediate/ delayed echolalia, metaphorical language, pronominal reversals)
- Bizarre responses to various aspects of the environment (e.g., resistance to change, peculiar interest in objects) (American Psychiatric Association, 1980).

Research on infantile autism has recently begun to focus on a possible genetic bases for the disorder. However, chromosomal analyses of autistic children have failed to reveal abnormalities (Spence, 1976). There are, nonetheless, other findings suggestive of a genetic component. These include the altered sex ratio among affected individuals, i.e., a higher incidence among males (Spence, 1976), and an increased incidence, albeit small (2 percent), of autism in siblings of autistic individuals. Although this percent appears low, it is 50 times that of the general population (Folstein & Rutter, 1977; Ross & Pelham, 1981). In addition, significant familial clusterings of cognitive disabilities in the siblings of autistic children have been reported (August, Stewart, & Tsai, 1981). Determining what might be the mode of inheritance has been difficult because of the low incidence of marriage or parenthood among autistics. Infantile autism may represent a combination of brain development anomalies and cognitive abnormalities (Folstein & Rutter, 1977).

Gilles de la Tourette syndrome is characterized by the following (Shapiro, Bruun, Shapiro, & Sweet, 1978):

- Age of onset between 2 and 15 years of age
- Multiple involuntary muscular and verbal tics
- Symptoms that wax and wane
- Slow change in symptoms, usually over a 3-month period
- Chronic lifelong illness

In addition to the verbal and nonverbal tics, language and speech abnormalities occur in over 50 percent of cases, including a poverty of speech and poor elaboration skills (Ludlow, Polinsky, Caine, Bassich, & Ebert, 1982). Although the mode of transmission of Tourette's syndrome has not been determined, some evidence indicates a possible genetic component to the disorder (Kidd & Pauls, 1982). An increased ratio in males over females, in Ashkenazi Jews, and the increased incidence of tics in family members suggests the possibility of complicated genetic transmission (Shapiro et al., 1978).

IDENTIFICATION OF A GENETIC COMPONENT

One criticism of behavioral genetics is that the final proof of inheritance must lie in the location of the genetic mutation or allele responsible for the disorder. Thus far, few if any complex traits addressed in behavioral genetics have been so defined. For many disorders, therefore, such techniques only contribute information on the degree of statistical association between behavioral traits and similar or dissimilar genotypes, and do not identify the biologic cause or specific genetic mechanisms. Behavioral genetics, however, can provide the first step in determining whether there is a genetic component to a disorder (Fuller & Thompson, 1978).

Several observable factors might lead one to suspect a genetic contribution to a disorder (Pauls & Kidd, 1981):

- A higher concordance among monozygotic twins than among dizygotic twins
- Significant occurrence of a trait within families
- Genetic linkage of a trait with an identifiable allele at a marker locus
- A higher incidence of a trait among biologic offspring of affected individuals than among the biological offspring of unaffected individuals, including those raised in adoptive homes

Whereas some behavioral traits may more closely reflect genetic differences, such as mental retardation in some genetic syndromes, most are reflective of the interaction of both genotype and environment. There are traits or behaviors that occur frequently within families but that are not genetic. Kaplan (1976) noted that sociocultural and psychogenic influences may facilitate transmission of a behavioral trait as consistently as genetic factors. Environmental factors that are not genetic include language type, dialect, diet, and religion. These factors may show a concentration in families or cultures, being transmitted from parent to child (Pauls & Kidd, 1981). Care must be taken in ascribing a genetic basis to a speech and language disorder simply because of an increased incidence within the family.

Twin studies provide good information on the relative contributions of genotype and environmental conditions in behaviors or disorders (Hrubec & Robinette, 1984). Since monozygotic twins have the same environment and genotype, differences in speech and language development between twins provide information on the degree of variation in a communicative disorder independent of both the genotype and the environment. Dizygotic twins, on the other hand, provide information on the degree of variation in speech and language when the environment is highly similar but there are differences in genotype. A comparison of the similarities and differences in speech and language development between monozygotic and dizygotic twin pairs is thus useful for examining differences when the environment is the same but the degree of similarity in genotype varies. Adoption studies are also useful for examining the relative contributions of genotype and environment on variations in speech and language development. Although rare, the instances of monozygotic twins being separated at birth and reared in different environments are most useful for examining the effects of environment on variations in behavioral development independent of genotype. Although the genotypes are more dissimilar in dyzygotic twins, examination of the differences in such twins when reared apart, in comparison to when they are reared together, can be useful for studying the effects of differences in environment. Finally, the degree of similarity between adopted siblings and natural siblings, where the environment is similar in both instances but there is a greater variation in genotype between adopted siblings, can be used to examine questions regarding the effects of genotypic variation. Since the occurrence of adopted siblings and natural siblings is relatively common, the degree of concordance in traits between siblings in each group is often an initial approach to determining whether the degree of variations in genotypes has an influence on the occurrence of a particular trait.

To document the occurrence in a family of a trait or disease over several generations, a pedigree should be developed. The proband (the affected individual from whom the family was identified) is usually indicated on the pedigree by an arrow. Male and female family members are indicated by squares and circles, and individuals demonstrating the trait are indicated by solid symbols. To develop a pedigree, information must be collected regarding the occurrence of the disorder in family members other than the proband. Pedigrees have been reported that illustrate positive family histories of stuttering (Kidd & Records, 1979), dyslexia (Kimberling & Brookhouser, 1981; Smith, Pennington, Kimberling, & Lubs, 1983), learning disabilities (Silver, 1971), developmental dyspraxia (McLaughlin & Kriegsmann, 1980) and developmental language disorders (Arnold, 1961). Routine formulation of pedigrees by service providers of children with developmental speech and language disorders would be an initial step in ascertaining the frequency of positive family histories and variations in patterns of inheritance. Certain pedigrees suggest possible modes of inheritance. When a child presents a trait and has an affected parent, the disorder may be autosomal dominant. When the child's disorder is not present in the parents, however, the disorder must be autosomal recessive. Sex-linked recessive inheritance may pertain when male children present a disorder and their mothers do not, but may carry the mutant gene. The aforementioned patterns may not be applicable or explanatory for most developmental speech and language disorders. For example, a mutant gene does not always give rise to the aberrant disorder, or when it does, the degree of severity may vary widely (Pashayan, 1975).

Familial studies are most useful for determining a possible mode of inheritance. The identification of a genetic basis, however, also requires the determination of the location of a specific gene, allele, or mutation responsible for a particular trait. Gene mapping is the determination of the location of specific genes on chromosomes. At the present time, approximate locations on chromosomes are known for less than 1 percent of human genes (Kimberling, 1983). Large families with a high frequency of occurrence of a specific trait are used in genetic-linkage studies. The trait characteristics should be uniform across individuals exhibiting it to provide assurance that the same gene or genetic mutation is responsible for the trait in all individuals exhibiting the disorder. Within the kindred, the degree of association of a marker gene for which the location is known is examined for association with the occurrence of the trait being studied.

When the trait being studied is found to be highly associated with a marker gene, then the two may lie in the same chromosome in close proximity. Genetic-linkage studies are extremely time consuming and success if dependent on having an adequate number of marker genes and a large enough number of multigenerational families with the same trait to heighten the chance of finding linkage with a marker gene. For these reasons, few successful studies have been completed in communicative disorders, but this should change.

GENETIC COUNSELING

An individual or family might seek genetic counseling for a variety of reasons. An affected child may have been born, and the family wishes to know the risk to subsequent, yet unborn, children. An individual considering marriage may have questions about disorders known to occur in the future partner's family, or in his or her own race or ethnic group. According to Plomin, DeFries, and McClearn (1980), there are three important steps in genetic counseling: formulation of a precise diagnosis, obtainment of detailed pedigrees, and explanation of expected risks and burdens. The responsibility of counseling most often falls upon a medical specialist with graduate training in genetics. The counseling process generally avoids advising a family about what should be done but rather focuses on informing the family of the range of possible outcomes of a particular pregnancy and of possible alternatives or solutions. With amniocentesis, techniques are available for identifying genetic disorders prenatally. Chromosomal abnormalities such as occur in Down's syndrome can be identified. In addition, significant progress is being made in the number of single gene disorders that can be identified such as sickle cell anemia and Tay-Sachs disease (Plomin et al., 1980). The speech-language pathologist, as part of a multidisciplinary team, provides speech and language assessment of children with confirmed genetic disorders. Following such an assessment, information regarding the prognosis for acquisition of speech and language skills should be provided by the speech–language pathologist, with estimates of prognosis for future children best provided by a genetic counselor.

Is genetic counseling appropriate for families of children with developmental speech and language disorders? In the case of hereditary deafness, a family may want to seek counseling regarding the risk to future offspring. A genetic counselor can provide valuable input regarding the possible basis for the disorder. Other communicative disorders, such as stuttering, are much less predictable. As with autism and Gilles de la Tourette syndrome, however, the knowledge that such disorders can occur in higher concentrations in some families may alleviate parental guilt regarding environmental or behavioral causes. Further, when a high incidence of such communicative disorders appears in a family history, the counselor might be able to provide information on the expected risks of the disorder to future children.

REFERENCES

Adler, S. (1976). The influence of genetic syndromes upon oral communication skills. *Journal of Speech and Hearing Disorders, 41,* 136–138.

American Psychiatric Association. (1980). *Quick reference to the diagnostic criteria from diagnostic and statistical manual of mental disorders,* (3rd ed.). Washington, DC: Author.

Andrews, G., & Harris, M. (1964). *The syndrome of stuttering.* Lavenham, Suffolk: Lavenham Press.

Annell, A-L., Gustavson, K-H., & Tenstam, J. (1970). Symptomatology in schoolboys with positive sex chromatin (The Klinefelter Syndrome). *Acta Psychiatrica Scandinavica, 46,* 71–80.

Arnold, G. E. (1961). The genetic background of developmental language disorders. *Folia Phoniatrica, 13,* 246–254.

August, G. J., Stewart, M. A., & Tsai, L. (1981). The incidence of cognitive disabilities in the siblings of autistic children. *British Journal of Psychiatry, 138,* 416–422.

Bender, B., Fry, E., Pennington, B., Puck, M., Salbenblatt, J., & Robinson, T. (1983). Speech and language development in 41 children with sex chromosome anomalies. *Pediatrics, 71,* 262–267.

Bloodstein, O. (1961). Stuttering in families of adopted stutterers. *Journal of Speech and Hearing Disorders, 26,* 395–396.

Chakravartti, R., Roy, A. K., Rao, K. U. M., & Chakravartti, M. R. (1979). Hereditary factors in stammering. *Journal de Genetique Humaine, 27,* 319–328.

Childs, B., & Finucci, J. M. (1979). The genetics of learning disabilities. *Human Genetics: Possibilities and Realities, 66,* 359–376.

Dennis, M., & Whitaker, H. A. (1976). Language acquisition following hemidecortication. *Brain and Language, 3,* 404–433.

Ehrman, L., & Parsons, P. A. (1976). *The genetics of behavior.* Sunderland, MA: Sinauer Associates.

Folstein, S., & Rutter, M. (1977). Infantile autism: A genetic study of 21 twin pairs. *Journal of Child Psychology and Psychiatry and Allied Disciplines, 18,* 297–321.

Fuller, J. L., & Thompson, W. R. (1978). *Foundations of behavior genetics.* St. Louis: C. V. Mosby.

Garvey, M., & Mutton, D. E. (1973). Sex chromosome aberrations and speech development. *Archives of Disease in Childhood, 48,* 937–941.

Haka-Ikse, K., Stewart, D. A., & Cripps, M. H. (1978). Early development of children with sex chromosome aberrations. *Pediatrics, 62,* 761–766.

Hallgren, B. (1950). Specific dyslexia: A clinical and genetic study. *Acta Psychiatrica et Neurological,* (Suppl. 65), 1–287.

Hecaen, H. (1976). Acquired aphasia in children. *Brain and Language, 3*, 114–134.

Hier, D. B., Atkins, L., & Perlo, V. P. (1980). Learning disorders and sex chromosome aberrations. *Journal of Mental Deficiency Research, 24*, 17–26.

Howie, P. M. (1981a). Concordance for stuttering in monozygotic and dizygotic twin pairs. *Journal of Speech and Hearing Research, 24*, 317–321.

Howie, P. M. (1981b). Intrapair similarity in frequency of disfluency in monozygotic and dizygotic twin pairs containing stutterers. *Behavior Genetics, 11*, 227–238.

Hrubec, Z., & Robinette, C. D. (1984). The study of human twins in medical research. *New England Journal of Medicine, 310*, 435–441.

Kaplan, A. R. (1976). *Human behavior genetics.* Springfield, IL: Charles C. Thomas.

Kidd, K. K., Heimbuch, R. C., & Records, M. A. (1981). Vertical transmission of susceptibility to stuttering with sex modified expression. *Proceedings of the National Academy of Sciences, 78*, 1–658.

Kidd, K. K., & Pauls, D. L. (1982). Genetic hypotheses for Tourette syndrome. In A. J. Fredhoff & T. N. Chase (Eds.), *Gilles de la Tourette syndrome.* New York: Raven Press. 1982.

Kidd, K. K., & Records, M. A. (1979). Genetic methodologies for the study of speech. In X. O. Breakfield (Ed.), *Neurogenetics: Genetic approaches to the nervous system.* New York: Elsevier.

Kidd, K., Reich, T., & Kessler, S. (1973). A genetic analysis of stuttering suggesting single major focus. *Genetics, 72*, S137.

Kimberling, W. J. (1983). Linkage analysis of communication disorders. In C. L. Ludlow & J. A. Cooper (Eds.), *Genetic aspects of speech and language disorders.* New York: Academic Press.

Kimberling, W. J., & Brookhouser, P. E. (1981). Biochemical and cytogenetic techniques for the study of communication disorders. *Laryngoscope, 91*, 238–249.

Luchsinger, R. (1970). Inheritance of speech defects. *Folia Phoniatrica, 22*, 216–230.

Ludlow, C. L., Polinsky, R. J., Caine, E. D., Bassich, C. J., & Ebert, M. H. (1982). Language and speech abnormalities in Tourette syndrome. In A. J. Friedhoff & T. N. Chase (Eds.), *Gilles de la Tourette syndrome.* New York: Raven Press.

McLaughlin, J. F., & Kriegsman, E. (1980). Developmental dyspraxia in family with X-linked mental retardation (Renpenning syndrome). *Developmental Medicine and Child Neurology, 22*, 84–92.

Mutton, D. E., & Lea, J. (1980). Chromosome studies of children with specific speech and language delay. *Developmental Medicine and Child Neurology, 22*, 588–594.

Nielsen, J., & Sillesen, I. (1976). Follow-up till age 2–4 of unselected children with sex chromosome abnormalities. *Human Genetics, 33*, 241–257.

Neilsen, J., Sorensen, A. M., & Sorensen, K. (1981). Mental development of unselected children with sex chromosome abnormalities. *Human Genetics, 59*, 324–332.

Omenn, G. S. & Weber, B. A. (1978). Dyslexia: Search for phenotypic and genetic heterogeneity. *American Journal of Medical Genetics, 1*, 333–342.

Pashayan, H. M. (1975). The basic concepts of medical genetics. *Journal of Speech and Hearing Disorders, 40,* 147–163.

Pauls, D. L., & Kidd, K. K. (1981). Genetics of childhood behavior disorders. In B. B. Lahey & A. E. Kazden (Eds), *Advances in clinical child psychology, Vol. 4.* New York: Plenum Press.

Pauls, D. L., & Kidd, K. K. (1982). Genetic strategies for the analysis of childhood behavioral traits. *Schizophrenia Bulletin, 8,* 253–266.

Pennington, B., Puck, M., & Robinson, A. (1980). Language and cognitive development on 47 XXX females followed since birth. *Behavior Genetics, 10,* 31–41.

Plomin, R., DeFries, V. C., & McClearn, G. G. (1980). *Behavioral genetics: A primer.* San Francisco: Freeman.

Porfert, A. R., & Rosenfield, D. B. (1978). Prevalence of stuttering. *Journal of Neurology, Neurosurgery, and Psychiatry, 41,* 954–956.

Ratcliffe, S. G. (1982). Speech and learning disorders in children with sex chromosome abnormalities. *Developmental Medicine and Child Neurology, 24,* 80–84.

Ross, A. D., & Pelham, W. E. (1981). Child psychopathology. *Annual Review of Psychology, 32,* 243–278.

Shapiro, A. K., Bruun, R. D., Shapiro, E. S., & Sweet, R. D. (1978). *Gilles de la Tourette syndrome.* New York: Raven Press.

Siegel-Sadewitz, V., & Shprintzen, R. J. (1982). The relationship of communication disorders to syndrome identification. *Journal of Speech and Hearing Disorders, 47,* 338–354.

Silver, L. B. (1971). Familial patterns in children with neurologically based learning disabilities. *Journal of Learning Disabilities, 4,* 349–358.

Smith, S. D., Pennington, B. F., Kimberling, W. J., & Lubs, H. A. (1983). A genetic analysis of specific reading disability. In C. L. Ludlow & J. A. Cooper (Eds.), *Genetic aspects of speech and language disorders.* New York: Academic Press.

Spence, M. A. (1976). Genetic studies. In E. R. Ritvo (Ed.), *Autism: Diagnosis, current research and management.* New York: Spectrum.

Tuncbilek, E., Kurultay, N., & Belgin, E. (1978). Are sex chromosome abnormalities a factor in speech delay?. *Archives of Disease in Childhood, 53,* 831.

Zahalkova, M., Vrzal, V., & Kloboukova, E. (1972). Genetical investigations in dyslexia. *Journal of Medical Genetics, 9,* 48–52.

John K. Darby
Kenneth K. Kidd
Luigi Luca Cavalli-Sforza

9
Molecular Genetics in Speech and Language Disorders

The purpose of this chapter is to present information from behavioral genetics, molecular genetics, and DNA polymorphism research that is relevant to the genetic features of speech and language disorders. The chapter will briefly review (1) the molecular mechanisms of inherited disease, (2) linkage analysis, (3) the human genome mapping project, (4) DNA polymorphism methodology, (5) neurogenetic aspects, (6) dyslexia, and (7) stuttering.

The unique genetic makeup of each individual is in large part responsible for human diversity. Specific genes and gene combinations determine such individual features as eye, hair, and skin color, body structure, and vulnerability to environmental stress factors (including infectious disease) and genetic disorders. Behavioral traits such as temperament, certain psychiatric and communication disorders, and even specific components of intelligence may result from gene–environment interaction. Animal models illustrating the specificity of interactional trait responses provide amazing examples of genetically programmed stimulus–response patterns as can be seen in (1) imprinting of ducks, (2) bird-dog response to birds, (3) cocker spaniel response to nets or startle stimuli, and (4) squirrel monkey response to snakes.

About 3000 genetic disorders are currently catalogued (McKusick,

---

Speech and Language Evaluation in Neurology:
Childhood Disorders
ISBN 0-8089-1719-6

1983); this number is increasing. The recent advances in DNA technology have provided current understanding and methodologies that are suitable to the task of elucidating specific molecular mechanisms, diagnosis, and treatment of genetic diseases. Moreover, these techniques can be directly applied to neurogenetic disorders, thus ushering in a new era for genetics and neuroscience.

MECHANISMS OF INHERITANCE

The human genome or DNA complement is composed of about 3.2 billion nucleotide base pairs. The sequence of specific base pairs encodes the genetic information just as the sequence of letters on this page encodes the meaning. An exact replica of the DNA sequence is found in practically each individual cell of the body, but the specific base sequence code is unique for each person because of numerous minor variations. The arrangement of the DNA into chromosomes is, however, uniform for all humans in its sequential arrangement of genes, and approximately 100,000 to one million genes are encoded in the DNA sequence. These genes are differentially expressed in various tissues or cells throughout growth and development. The genes are expressed by transcription into messenger RNA (mRNA) copies that migrate from the cell nucleus to cytoplasmic ribosomes, which read and translate the mRNA code into sequences of amino acids, which form proteins. The proteins provide the building blocks for cell structure as well as regulate the metabolism and function of each cell. The function of proteins is dependent on their three-dimensional geometric structure, which is determined by their amino acid sequence, which is in turn determined by the DNA coding base pair sequence. A mutation in the DNA base pair sequence, therefore, can have disastrous consequences for protein structure and thus for some aspect of cell function.

The prototypic example of these concepts has been elucidated in sickle cell anemia where a point mutation in the 18th nucleotide (Chang & Kan, 1981) of the gene coding for β globin, a component of hemoglobin, has resulted in a substituted amino acid in the sixth position in the sequence of the protein which produces an alteration in the three-dimensional configuration of hemoglobin. This results in an abnormality of red blood cell structure that causes the abnormal clogging and clotting in arterioles, finally determining the thrombotic tissue destruction characteristic of sickle cell anemia. Knowledge of the specific molecular alteration characteristic of this disease now provides a variety of potential diagnostic and treatment approaches (such as repression of gene expression by azacytidine) that were previously inconceivable.

An important step in the solution to each of the 3000 known genetic

diseases thus lies with the discovery of the specific DNA and RNA alterations relevant to the disorder. Such information, even in gene–environment disorders, is now obtainable, but much work is required.

LINKAGE ANALYSIS

During reproduction, maternal and paternal DNAs (chromosomes)
in each parent recombine into a unique new sequence that is transmitted
to the child. Since the genome retains its gene sequence and chromosomal
sequence uniformity and integrity (despite individual base pair diversity), this allows for the tracking of the parental source of DNA through
family pedigrees providing that genes or DNA segments can somehow be
marked from their source. Considerable individual nucleotide variation
exists, which provides the opportunity for recognizing DNA segments by
acting as a source of "markers." These DNA polymorphisms are termed
restriction fragment length polymorphisms (RFLPs), and their usefulness in diagnosis of disease was first shown by Kan & Dozy (1978), and for
genetic linkage analysis by Botstein, White, Skolnick and Davis (1980),
and Wymam and White (1980).

If either a dominant or a recessive disease is evident from a family
pedigree, then any specific cloned gene can be tracked through the pedigree to see if it segregates jointly with the disease. When this happens we
speak of linkage. An example of the pedigree of a dominant disease (Huntington's chorea, A) and a recessive linked marker (a) is the following:

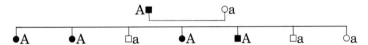

Here there are only two types of progeny, which are identical to one of the
two parents. Linkage is complete. If it is not complete, recombination
(expressed in percentage units called centimorgans) is the frequency with
which linked markers separate (e.g., in pedigrees like the above, the
relative frequency of individuals with the disease and "a" marker, or
without the disease and the "A" marker). A large kindred (50–200 family
members) or multiple smaller families showing the inherited disease
need to be tested to ascertain whether linkage is present beyond possible
doubts due to statistical fluctuation. The statistical analysis may be accomplished by mathematical computation of the odds for and against
linkage (Morton, 1955), as programmed by Ott (1974). For a more detailed review, see Conneally and Rivas (1980).

A successful application of this method in Huntington's chorea was
described by Gusella, Wexler, Conneally, Naylor, Anderson, et al. (1983).

HUMAN GENOME MAPPING PROJECT

The process of linkage analysis will be greatly facilitated by a complete linkage map of the human genome. This can be done in a preliminary, somewhat coarse way by dividing the genome into approximately 320 DNA segments of 10 centimorgans (recombination units) by use of spaced RFLPs as markers. However, since DNA clones cannot be obtained or characterized with such uniformity, practical constraints require that 400–600 such markers will be necessary for this initial map of the genome (Bishop & Skolnick, 1983).

A DNA clone can be assigned to its correct chromosomal region by somatic cell hybridization (Giles & Ruddle, 1981a) and/or hybridization in situ (Giles & Ruddle, 1981b). Each of these methods utilizes radioactive tagging of the DNA clone to isolate and identify the specific chromosome location of the DNA segment. If a polymorphism is known, the recombination distance (in centimorgans) to neighboring RFLPs can be determined by pedigree analysis.

Many labs throughout the world are currently collaborating to provide the necessary DNA clones to map the human genome at 10 centimorgan intervals. Currently, nearly 40 percent of the human genome can be studied for disease linkage, assuming a large data set and straightforward inheritance patterns (and phenotypic expression) using available markers (K. K. Kidd, personal communication, 1985).

DNA POLYMORPHISM METHODOLOGY

DNA is extracted from white blood cells obtained by a 30-ml venepuncture (Bell, Karam, & Rutter, 1981). The isolated DNA is then digested by any one of 80 or more different commercially available restriction enzymes that cut the DNA at a specified base code sequence. For example, the enzyme Eco RI will divide the DNA from one cell nucleus into 500,000 to one million separately sized pieces by cutting at its unique nucleotide recognition sequence (Maniatis, Fritsch, and Sambrook, 1982). Many cells will be treated together and supply identical copies of the fragments. These DNA fragments are then placed in an agarose gel and subjected to an electric field that forces the fragments to migrate various distances through the gel. The migration distance is inversely proportional to individual fragment lengths or molecular weights. The various DNA fragments are then transferred by ionic and osmotic gradients to a charged filter paper that exactly replicates their position on the gel by the Southern method (1975). This filter paper is then bathed in a salt solution containing the "hot" probe, that is a cloned

DNA segment or gene made radioactive (Rigby, Dieckman, Rhodes, & Berg, 1977), at a suitable temperature; the two complementary strands forming DNA dissociate and the probe associates specifically (hybridizes) with its complementary DNA strand (Watson & Crick, 1953) by hydrogen bonding. The filter paper is then removed, radioactive DNA that has not hybridized is washed away, and the paper is placed on x-ray film for a period of 3-10 days at $-70°C$. The image of the radioactive segment is recorded on the radiosensitive x-ray film, and a replica of the hybridized clone fragment on the filter paper is seen by the visual impression made on the film.

The sizes of the gene fragments present on the filter which have been revealed by their hybridization with the radioactive probe can then be compared among various individuals. The polymorphic variation in genes allows the proper tracking and differentiation of paternal and maternal gene segments, and linkage with disease can be studied. A linkage relationship may thus be detected or excluded by the analysis of an adequate number of families.

NEUROGENETIC ASPECTS

The human brain is the most complex of all the organs and its development and structure is largely determined by genetic information. The brain contains roughly 8 billion neurons, each with an average of 1000 interconnections, thus making it numerically more complex than the genetic DNA sequence. Brain communication (neurotransmission) and metabolism are largely regulated by ongoing DNA-RNA control mechanisms. Over twice as many genes are involved in brain function (100,000–200,000) as in other tissues (Hahn, Van Ness, & Chaudhari, 1982; Kaplan & Finch, 1982).

Some genes relevant to nervous system development and neurotransmission have already been cloned, e.g., pro-opiomelanocortin gene (Chang, Cochet, & Cohen, 1980), and nerve growth factor (Scott, Selby, Urdea, Quiroga, Bell, & Rutter, 1983; Ullrich, Gray, Berman, & Dull, 1983). Linkage studies with these clones are currently underway in neurologic and psychiatric disorders. Geneticists have also identified inherited differences for certain brain enzymes (e.g., see Weinshilboum, 1975), and it has been noted that some synthesize or metabolize neurotransmitters more rapidly than others.

Genetic variations in nerve, brain, and muscle function can clearly affect communication via intermediate mechanisms as seen, for example, in myasthenia gravis, muscular dystrophies, and Huntington's chorea. It has yet to be demonstrated, however, that speech and/or language function can be directly and specifically affected by genetic mechanisms. Dyslexia and stuttering offer two disorders where this could be the case.

DYSLEXIA

Dyslexia is a common disorder, perhaps involving 10 percent of the population (Critchley, 1964), that is more frequent in males and that is marked by clinical heterogeneity. It is a familial disorder and in some cases is possibly transmitted through an autosomal-dominant mode of inheritance (Zahalkova, Vrzal, & Klobovkova, 1972). Dyslexia has been subdivided into two major clinical subtypes by Finucci and Childs (1983) on the basis of severity, intelligence quotient (IQ), and dysphonetic spelling errors.

Neuropathologic Features

Galaburda (1983) has reported a case of dyslexia with the following significant left hemispheric neuropathologic findings:

- Micropolygyria in the posterior superior temporal gyrus
- Multiple areas of focal cortical dysplasia involving the entire left hemisphere but most densely in the posterior half
- Distortion of normal cortical layering and the presence of abnormally large pyramidal neurons in the deeper layers
- Increased width of subcortical white matter
- Abnormal size and placement of neurons bilaterally in the lateralis posterior (LP) and medial geniculate nuclei of the thalamus

Galaburda (1983) has suggested a model to explain these findings, which could be attributed to a single genetic defect in neuron migration of telencephalic cells into the LP–pulvinar anlage at 16–20 weeks of gestation, which could give rise to the bilateral thalamic lesions. The unilateral cortical defects could theoretically be secondary to these thalamic defects due to the differential in growth rates between the left and right cerebral hemispheres. Galaburda suggests that subsequent right hemisphere invasion could explain the presence of excessive white matter in the left hemisphere, thus resulting in the cerebral asymmetry observed in these cases.

Linkage Analysis

Smith, Pennington, Kimberling, and Lubs (1983) have reported preliminary evidence for the linkage of dyslexia to chromosome 15q by a chromosomal heteromorphism analysis. They reported a lod score of 3.24 at 24 map units. For disorders with such diagnostic uncertainties as dyslexia, this statistical support for loose linkage must be interpreted with great caution. It is suggestive, but does not constitute proof. It was also noted that dyslexia in their selected families appeared to be inherited as an autosomal-dominant trait and that the sex ratio between boys and girls (1.44:1) was not statistically significant, although males were more severely affected. Smith and associates selected 9 families where the dyslexia was present in each of three consecutive generations; a reading level 2 years below grade level with no intellectual or motor problems present was also necessary for diagnosis and inclusion in the study. It is impossible to make generalizations from this highly selective sample to all cases of dyslexia. It is most likely that the type of dyslexia seen in this study was only one of several different forms, each with a different cause.

Even though these interesting neuropathologic and linkage analysis studies must be considered as preliminary findings, and confirmatory studies are required, they provide strong impetus toward further research.

STUTTERING

Stuttering is a disruption in the timing and smooth flow of speech with onset prior to age 12 years. The lifetime incidence is nearly 3 percent (Andrews & Harris, 1964), and the ratio of affected males to affected females is somewhere between 5:1 and 2:1 (Van Riper, 1971). The associated features of stuttering include eye blinks, head jerks, and facial grimaces that are not part of the basic disorder and are believed to be secondary features acquired through behavioral reinforcement.

Differential Diagnosis

Stuttering must be distinguished from cluttering, a disorder characterized by speech so rapid that syllables and words are omitted, resulting in unintelligible utterances. Cluttering may be improved by conscious slowing of speech or in stressful circumstances, in contradistinction to stuttering. Cluttering may show autosomal-dominant inheritance (Op't Hof & Uys, 1974) whereas stuttering rarely shows such a simple pattern (Kidd, 1983).

Table 9-1
Distribution of Stuttering Among First-Degree
Relatives of Adult Stutterers

	Male Probands	Female Probands
Fathers	18%	20%
Mothers	4.4%	12%
Brothers	19%	23%
Sisters	4%	13%
Sons	24%	36%
Daughters	9%	18%

Spontaneous Recovery

The frequency of spontaneous recovery in stuttering is reported to
range from 36 percent (Cooper, 1972) to 80 percent (Sheehan & Martyn,
1966). Seider, Gladstien, and Kidd (1983) found recovery rates of 66 percent in females and 46 percent in males. When stuttering persisted into
adulthood, recovery was unlikely.

Cerebral Laterality

Tests of dichotic listening have shown that stutterers exhibit a left-
ear (right hemisphere) preference for words and sentences in dichotic
reception whereas nonstutterers show a right-ear (left hemisphere) preference for such materials (Curry & Gregory, 1969; Perrin, 1969). Sommers, Brady, and Moore (1975) found that the left-ear preferences decreased with age and suggested that hemispheric lateralization of speech
may continue to develop at slower rates in stutterers as compared with
normals.

Genetics

Stuttering is familial (Bloodstein, 1981; Kidd, Kidd, & Records,
1978; Van Riper, 1971) and family histories have been reported as positive in 24–80 percent of index cases with a median of 42 percent. Kidd
(1983) has reported the frequencies of stuttering among first-degree relatives (see Table 9-1). The data indicate (1) that the frequency is greater in
males than in females, and (2) that the frequencies within affected families are higher than found in the general population.

Twin studies have reported concordance for stuttering as ranging from 1.9 percent (Graf, 1955) to 20 percent (Nelson, Hunter, & Walter, 1945). Howie (1981) reported 58–63 percent concordance in monozygotic (MZ) twins and 13–19 percent in dizygotic (DZ) twins. Proband concordances were 75 percent for both male and female MZ twins but only 45 percent for male DZ twins and 0 percent for female DZ twins. Small sample sizes and uncertainty over possible ascertainment biases make these estimates of twin concorances difficult to interpret.

Genetic Transmission Hypothesis

These genetic data illustrate that stuttering exhibits vertical transmission and that sex-modified expression of the phenotype is present (Kidd, Heimbuch, & Records, 1981). Kidd (1983) has suggested a single major locus model with three genotypes, each with sex-specific probabilities of phenotypic expression. This is a sex-modified intermediate mode of inheritance with gene-environment interaction. In this model heterozygotes would stutter if they have a stressful environment while homozygotes might not stutter if they have a benign or ameliorating environment.

When this model is applied to the Yale study (2000 participants), the stutterer gene frequency is 4 percent (heterozygote frequency of 8 percent) and less than 2 in 1000 individuals are homozygous. Phenotypic expression is zero for normal male and female homozygotes and penetrance is nearly 100 percent for homozygotes for the stuttering allele. In the heterozygote, penetrance is 40 percent for males but only 11 percent for females. These parameters predict a lifetime incidence of 4 percent for males and 1 percent for females. While this model provides a working hypothesis, it is not sufficient to explain all aspects of the familial pattern of stuttering (Cox & Kidd, 1983). A more recent analysis of the data suggests that a major locus may not be present (Cox, Kramer, and Kidd, 1984).

The difficulties in analyzing the data on stuttering emphasize the need for an alternate methodology to elucidate the inheritance mode in stuttering. Genetic analyses with polymorphic DNA markers offer such an opportunity.

CONCLUSION

This chapter has attempted to provide a review and synthesis of information from behavioral and molecular genetics that may be used as a guide in understanding the potential clinical applications of the "new genetics" in neurogenetic, biobehavioral, and speech and language disorders. While much information is lacking at the level of molecular detail, the principal concepts, strategies, and scientific techniques of recombinant DNA methods offer optimism for the study of genetic disease. Suitable strategies of research can be devised to investigate the problems of diagnosis, etiology, molecular pathogenesis, management, treatment, and even cures for genetic diseases. The major obstacle to productive research at this juncture appears to be the amount of time, money, and manpower necessary to carry out the required strategies. While current techniques have been streamlined, there appear to be no major shortcuts available to the necessary large-scale clinical and laboratory teamwork efforts required to study a disease by these strategies. Conversely, the potential rewards are much greater than previously possible.

REFERENCES

Andrews, G., & Harris, M. M. (1964). *The syndrome of stuttering. Clinics in developmental medicine, no. 17.* London: Spastics Society Medical Education and Information in association with William Helinvemann.

Bell, G. I., Karam, J. H., & Rutter, W. J. (1981). Polymorphic DNA region adjacent to the 5' end of the human insulin gene. *Proceedings of the National Academy of Science, 78,* 5759–5763.

Bishop, D. T., & Skolnick, M. H. (1983). Genetic markers and linkage analysis. In C. T. Caskey & R. L. White (Eds.), *Banbury Report 14 Recombinant DNA applications to human disease.* (pp. 251–261). New York: Cold Spring Harbor Laboratory.

Bloodstein, O. (1981). *A handbook on stuttering.* Chicago: National Easter Seal Society for Crippled Children and Adults.

Botstein, D., White, R. L., Skolnick, M., & Davis, R. W. (1980). Construction of a genetic linkage map in man using restriction fragment length polymorphisms. *American Journal of Human Genetics, 32,* 314–331.

Chang, A. C. Y., Cochet, M., & Cohen, S. N. (1980). Structural organization of human genomic DNA encoding the pro-opiomelanocortin peptide. *Proceedings of the National Academy of Science, 77,* 4890–4894.

Chang, J. C., & Kan, Y. W. (1981). Antenatal diagnosis of sickle cell anemia by direct analysis of the sickle mutation. *Lancet,* November, 1127–1128.

Conneally, P. M., & Rivas, M. L. (1980). Linkage analysis in man. *Advances in Human Genetics, 10,* 209–266.

Cooper, E. B. (1972). Recovery from stuttering in a junior and senior high school population. *Journal of Speech and Hearing Research, 15,* 632–638.

Cox, N. J., & Kidd, K. K. (1983). Can recovery from stuttering be considered a genetically milder subtype of stuttering? *Behavior Genetics, 13,* 129–139.

Cox, N. J., Kramer, P. L. & Kidd, K. K. (1984). Segregation analysis of stuttering. *Genetic Epidemiology, 1,* 245–253.

Critchley, M. (1964). *Developmental dyslexia.* London: William Heinemann.

Curry, F. K. W., & Gregory, H. H. (1969). The performance of stutterers on dichotic listening tasks thought to reflect cerebral dominance. *Journal of Speech and Hearing Research, 12,* 73–82.

Finucci, J. M., & Childs, B. (1983). Dyslexia: Family studies. In C. L. Ludlow & J. A. Cooper (Eds.), *Genetic aspects of speech and language disorders* (pp. 157–168). New York: Academic Press.

Galaburda, A. M. (1983). Definition of the anatomical phenotype. In C. L. Ludlow & J. A. Cooper (Eds.), *Genetic aspects of speech and language disorders* (pp. 71–84). New York: Academic Press.

Giles, E. G., & Ruddle, F. H., (1981a). Gene localization using interspecific somatic cell hybrids. In L. M. Schwartz & M. M. Azar (Eds.), *Advanced cell biology* (pp. 1105–1113). New York: Van Nostrand Reinhold.

Giles, E. G., & Ruddle, F. H. (1981b). Gene localization using nucleic acid hybridization. In L. M. Schwartz & M. M. Azar (Eds.), *Advanced cell biology* (pp. 1114–1123). New York: Van Nostrand Reinhold. Graf, O. I. (1955). Incidence of stuttering among twins. In W. Johnson (Ed.), *Stuttering in children and adults*. Minneapolis: University of Minnesota Press.

Gusella, J. F., Wexler, N. S., Conneally, P. M., Naylor, S. L., Anderson, M. A., Tanzi, R. E., et al. (1983). A polymorphic DNA marker genetically linked to Huntington's disease. *Nature, 306,* 234–238.

Hahn, W. E., Van Ness, J., & Chaudhari, N. (1982). Overview of the molecular genetics of mouse brain. In F. O. Schmitt, S. J. Bird, & F. E. Bloom (Eds.), *Molecular genetic neuroscience* (pp. 323–334). New York: Raven Press.

Howie, P. M. (1981). A twin investigation of the etiology of stuttering. *Journal of Speech and Hearing Research, 24,* 317–321.

Kan, Y. W. & Dozy, A. M. (1978). Polymorphism of DNA sequence adjacent to the human β-globin structural gene: Relationship to sickle cell mutation. *Proceedings of the National Academy of Science, 75,* 5631–5635.

Kaplan, B. B., & Finch, C. E. (1982). The sequence complexity of brain ribonucleic acids. In I. R. Brown (Ed.), *Molecular approaches to neurobiology* (pp. 71–98). New York: Academic Press.

Kidd, K. K. (1983). Recent progress on the genetics of stuttering. In C. L. Ludlow & J. A. Cooper (Eds.), *Genetic aspects of speech and language disorders* (pp. 197–213). New York: Academic Press.

Kidd, K. K., Heimbuch, R. C., & Records, M. A. (1981). Vertical transmission of susceptibility to stuttering with sex-modified expression. *Proceedings of the National Academy of Sciences USA, 78,* 606–610.

Kidd, K. K., Kidd, J. R., & Records, M. A. (1978). The possible causes of the sex ratio in stuttering and its implication. *Journal of Fluency Disorders, 3,* 13–23.

Maniatis, T., Fritsch, E. F., & Sambrook, J. (1982). *Molecular Cloning* (pp. 98–99). New York: Cold Spring Harbor Laboratory.

McKusick, V. A. (1983). *Mendelian inheritance in man* (6th ed.). Baltimore: Johns Hopkins University Press.

Morton, N. E. (1955). Sequential tests for the detection of linkage. *American Journal of Human Genetics, 7,* 277.

Nelson, S. F., Hunter, N., & Walter, M. (1945). Stuttering in twin types. *Journal of Speech Disorders, 10,* 335–343.

Op't Hof, J., & Uys, I. C. (1974). A clinical delineation of tachyphemia (cluttering): A case of dominant inheritance. *South African Journal of Medical Sciences, 48,* 1624–1628.

Ott, J. (1974). Estimation of the recombination fraction in human pedigrees; efficient computation of the likelihood for human linkage studies. *American Journal of Human Genetics, 26,* 588–597.

Perrin, K. (1969). An examination of ear preference for speech and non-speech in a stuttering population. Unpublished doctoral dissertation, Stanford University, Stanford, CA.

Rigby, P. W. J., Dieckman, M., Rhodes, C., & Berg, P. (1977). Labeling deoxyribonucleic acid to high specific activity in vitro by nick translation with DNA polymerase I. *Journal of Molecular Biology, 113,* 237–251.

Scott, J., Selby, M., Urdea, M., Quiroga, M., Bell, G., & Rutter, W. J. (1983). Isolation and nucleotide sequence of a cDNA encoding the precursor of mouse nerve growth factor. *Nature, 302,* 538–540.

Seider, R. A., Gladstien, K. L., & Kidd, K. K. (1983). Recovery and persistence of stuttering among relatives of stuttering. *Journal of Speech and Hearing Disorders, 48,* 402–409.

Sheehan, J. G., & Martyn, M. M. (1966). Spontaneous recovery from stuttering. *Journal of Speech and Hearing Research, 9,* 121–135.

Smith, S. D., Pennington, B. F., Kimberling, W. J., & Lubs, H. A. (1983). A genetic analysis of specific reading disability. In C. L. Ludlow & J. A. Cooper (Eds.), *Genetic aspects of speech and language disorders* (pp. 169–178). New York: Academic Press.

Sommers, R. K., Brady, W. A., & Moore, W. H. (1975). Dichotic ear preferences of stuttering children and adults. *Perceptual and Motor Skills, 41,* 931–938.

Southern, E. M. (1975). Detection of specific sequences among DNA fragments separated by gel electrophoresis. *Journal of Molecular Biology, 98,* 503–517.

Ullrich, A., Gray, A., Berman, C., & Dull, T. J. (1983). Human β-nerve growth factor gene sequence highly homologous to that of mouse. *Nature, 303,* 821–825.

Van Riper, C. (1971). *The nature of stuttering.* Englewood Cliffs, NJ: Prentice-Hall.

Watson, J. D., & Crick, F. H. C. (1953). Molecular structure of nucleic acid. A structure for deoxyribose nucleic acid. *Nature, 171,* 737–738.

Weinshilboum, R. M., Schrott, H. G., Raymond, F. A., Weidman, W. H., & Elveback, L. R., (1975). Inheritance of very low serum dopamine beta hydroxylase activity. *American Journal of Human Genetics, 27,* 573–585.

Wyman, A. R. & White, R., (1980). A highly polymorphic locus in human DNA. *Proceedings of the National Academy of Science, 77,* 6754–6758.

Zahalkova, M., Vrzal, V., & Klobovkova, E. (1972). Genetical investigations in dyslexia. *Journal of Medical Genetics, 9,* 48–62.

Index